Using Narrative Writing to Enhance Healing During and After Global Health Crises

Jennifer Lynne Bird
Oxbridge Academy, USA

A volume in the Advances in Medical Diagnosis, Treatment, and Care (AMDTC) Book Series

Published in the United States of America by
IGI Global
Medical Information Science Reference (an imprint of IGI Global)
701 E. Chocolate Avenue
Hershey PA, USA 17033
Tel: 717-533-8845
Fax: 717-533-8661
E-mail: cust@igi-global.com
Web site: http://www.igi-global.com

Library of Congress Cataloging-in-Publication Data

Names: Bird, Jennifer Lynne, author.
Title: Using narrative writing to enhance healing during and after global health crises / Jennifer Lynne Bird.
Description: Hershey, PA : Information Science Reference, [2022] | Includes bibliographical references and index. | Summary: "This authored book explains how there is a growing body of evidence that suggests that patients who actively write about their health conditions are able to process worries, concerns, frustrations and fears and gradually convert negative thoughts into more positive thoughts and an overall more positive attitude toward their situation"-- Provided by publisher.
Identifiers: LCCN 2021030082 (print) | LCCN 2021030083 (ebook) | ISBN 9781799890515 (hardcover) | ISBN 9781799890522 (paperback) | ISBN 9781799890539 (ebook)
Subjects: LCSH: Health education. | Narration (Rhetoric) | Narrative medicine.
Classification: LCC RC489.W75 B57 2022 (print) | LCC RC489.W75 (ebook) | DDC 615.8/5163--dc23
LC record available at https://lccn.loc.gov/2021030082
LC ebook record available at https://lccn.loc.gov/2021030083

This book is published in the IGI Global book series Advances in Medical Diagnosis, Treatment, and Care (AMDTC) (ISSN: 2475-6628; eISSN: 2475-6636)

British Cataloguing in Publication Data
A Cataloguing in Publication record for this book is available from the British Library.

For electronic access to this publication, please contact: eresources@igi-global.com.

Advances in Medical Diagnosis, Treatment, and Care (AMDTC) Book Series

ISSN:2475-6628
EISSN:2475-6636

Mission

Advancements in medicine have prolonged the life expectancy of individuals all over the world. Once life-threatening conditions have become significantly easier to treat and even cure in many cases. Continued research in the medical field will further improve the quality of life, longevity, and wellbeing of individuals.

The **Advances in Medical Diagnosis, Treatment, and Care (AMDTC)** book series seeks to highlight publications on innovative treatment methodologies, diagnosis tools and techniques, and best practices for patient care. Comprised of comprehensive resources aimed to assist professionals in the medical field apply the latest innovations in the identification and management of medical conditions as well as patient care and interaction, the books within the AMDTC series are relevant to the research and practical needs of medical practitioners, researchers, students, and hospital administrators.

Coverage

- Patient-Centered Care
- Experimental Medicine
- Chronic Conditions
- Critical Care
- Cancer Treatment
- Medical Procedures
- Alternative Medicine
- Disease Prevention
- Medical Testing
- Emergency Medicine

IGI Global is currently accepting manuscripts for publication within this series. To submit a proposal for a volume in this series, please contact our Acquisition Editors at acquisitions@igi-global.com or visit: https://www.igi-global.com/publish/.

The Advances in Medical Diagnosis, Treatment, and Care (AMDTC) Book Series (ISSN 2475-6628) is published by IGI Global, 701 E. Chocolate Avenue, Hershey, PA 17033-1240, USA, www.igi-global.com. This series is composed of titles available for purchase individually; each title is edited to be contextually exclusive from any other title within the series. For pricing and ordering information please visit https://www.igi-global.com/book-series/advances-medical-diagnosis-treatment-care/129618. Postmaster: Send all address changes to above address.

Titles in this Series

For a list of additional titles in this series, please visit: www.igi-global.com/book-series/advances-medical-diagnosis-treatment-care/129618

Handbook of Research on Pathophysiology and Strategies for the Management of COVID-19
Omar El Hiba (Chouaib Doukkali University, Morocco) Jayakumar Radhakrishnan (Veterans Affairs Medical Center, USA) Tiziano Balzano (University Hospital HM Puerta del Sur, Spain) and Faical Isbaine (Emory University USA)
Medical Information Science Reference • © 2022 • 352pp • H/C (ISBN: 9781799882251) • US $425.00

Strategies to Overcome Superbug Invasions Emerging Research and Opportunities
Dimple Sethi Chopra (Punjabi University, India) and Ankur Kaul (Institute of Nuclear Medicine and Allied Sciences, India)
Medical Information Science Reference • © 2021 • 319pp • H/C (ISBN: 9781799803072) • US $225.00

Integrated Care and Fall Prevention in Active and Healthy Aging
Patrik Eklund (Umea University, Sweden)
Medical Information Science Reference • © 2021 • 348pp • H/C (ISBN: 9781799844112) • US $345.00

Cases on Applied and Therapeutic Humor
Michael K. Cundall Jr. (North Carolina A&T State University, USA) and Stephanie Kelly (North Carolina A&T State University, USA)
Medical Information Science Reference • © 2021 • 267pp • H/C (ISBN: 9781799845287) • US $255.00

Artificial Intelligence for Accurate Analysis and Detection of Autism Spectrum Disorder
Sandeep Kautish (Lord Buddha Education Foundation, Nepal & Asia Pacific University of Technology & Innovation, Malaysia) and Gaurav Dhiman (Government Bikram College of Commerce, India)
Medical Information Science Reference • © 2021 • 224pp • H/C (ISBN: 9781799874607) • US $295.00

Diagnostic and Treatment Methods for Ulcerative Colitis and Colitis-Associated Cancer
Ashok Kumar Pandurangan (B. S. Abdur Rahman Crescent Institute of Science and Technology, India)
Medical Information Science Reference • © 2021 • 309pp • H/C (ISBN: 9781799835806) • US $295.00

Enhancing the Therapeutic Efficacy of Herbal Formulations
Rajesh Kumar Kesharwani (Nehru Gram Bharati (Deemed), Prayagraj, India) Raj K. Keservani (Faculty of B. Pharmacy, CSM Group of Institutions, Prayagraj, India) and Anil K. Sharma (GD Goenka University, India)
Medical Information Science Reference • © 2021 • 367pp • H/C (ISBN: 9781799844532) • US $265.00

IGI Global
PUBLISHER of TIMELY KNOWLEDGE

701 East Chocolate Avenue, Hershey, PA 17033, USA
Tel: 717-533-8845 x100 • Fax: 717-533-8661
E-Mail: cust@igi-global.com • www.igi-global.com

Table of Contents

Foreword

Individuals who are experiencing illness are often riddled with negativity and anxiety. A growing body of evidence suggests that patients who actively write about their health conditions are able to process worries, concerns, frustrations and fears and gradually convert negative thoughts into more positive thoughts and an overall more positive attitude toward their situation. As a medical physiologist and professor of wellness, I am keenly aware of the importance of cultivating a positive attitude in all avenues of life, but perhaps especially during illness because negative stressors, if left unchecked, can wreak havoc on multiple biological and psychological systems. Through a cascade of events the result is unnecessary cellular and system damage, oxidative stress, and an impaired ability to repair damaged tissues. Furthermore, over-stimulation of the hypothalamic-pituitary-adrenal (HPA) axis in response to increased levels of psychological stress exacerbates the inflammatory process and can result in stress-mediated depression, which further has a negative effect on one's health. Not only does this cascade of negativity and stress impair healing, it actually leads to the development of disease conditions.

There is also a disturbing and inequitable distribution of stress in our society. Namely, people earning low income are likely to experience more stressors and concomitant stress-mediated depression owing to subjective experiences and emotions that result from income insecurity, lower social status, disempowerment and stigma. And as stated above, stress-mediated depression serves as a trigger for pathophysiological processes that influence both physical and mental well-being, and social and emotional stressors negatively impact cell-mediated immunity and health.

Unfortunately, stress is not the only risk factor that is over-represented for people earning low income. Every risk factor for developing non-communicable diseases –the largest source of preventable death--is inextricably linked to the social determinants of health and exacerbated for individuals of low socioeconomic status. Concomitantly, individuals living in poverty endure worse health outcomes compared to people in other social strata. What an empowering thought it is that writing holds healing powers, and writing is free. However, solutions to social inequities is never that easy and opportunities are not always united with the most deserving recipients.

This point is evidenced when one recaps promises to reduce these health disparities. The National Academy of Medicine report, *Unequal Treatment: Confronting Racial and Ethnic Disparities in Healthcare*,1 made front-page news when released in March 2002. That was 18 years ago. Even before the National Academy of Medicine report, in 2000 the Healthy People 2010 campaign2 highlighted and set targets for reduction of health disparities. That was 20 years ago. The American Medical Association was committed to disparities reductions by 2004 if not earlier. Most importantly, the Accreditation Council for Graduate Medical Education (ACGME) began requiring health disparities education for residents since at least 2004. Therefore, one would expect that after 2 decades of national focus on health disparities and 15 years of required curricula, nearly all internal medicine residency programs would include a disparities curriculum. However, this is not the case.

Books such as this one by Dr. Jennifer Bird shine a light on how simple solutions can offer so much healing. Dr. Bird's book teaches us that writing can be healing. It is my hope that Dr. Bird's book will reach an audience that may be moved to take action to connect therapeutic writing with the people who are at highest risk for poor health and who can benefit the most from simple solutions.

C. Jayne Brahler
University of Dayton, USA

Preface

Dear Reader,

I love my book *Using Narrative Writing to Enhance Healing* and didn't plan on revising it two years after the initial publication. I also didn't plan on surviving a pandemic either. This experience led to my desire for reflection and revision.

Someday I know people will gather in person again (such gatherings can begin to happen as I write this sentence in July 2021), but what alternatives exist for people who need a community of support in the meantime? Would my students still enjoy my innovative teaching methods in the era of online learning? Could my role as a health coach evolve once hospitals became immersed in caring for coronavirus patients? It became time for new narratives.

THIS BOOK'S PURPOSE

One of my goals as a writer remains to provide the most helpful information possible for my community of readers. I want to acknowledge strategies for coping with the pandemic while simultaneously providing optimism for new beginnings when the pandemic eventually ends.

This book about narratives, *Using Narrative Writing to Enhance Healing During and After Global Health Crises,* will introduce or reintroduce you to how narrative writing can help you. I have used narrative writing in my classroom, at my church, and in medical settings. I share research to show the effectiveness of writing in disciplines I have not personally experienced, and I share narratives from my own life to illustrate how writing has positively affected my healing from both physical and emotional pain. Doyle (2013) shares, "when you write your truth, it is a love offering to the world because it helps us feel braver and less alone" (p. 25). Finding the courage to write my truth takes vulnerability but becomes worth it when my students, colleagues, or readers tell me they felt comfortable sharing their stories because I shared mine. Even in a worldwide crisis such as the pandemic, I read and watched news stories of people showing grace and kindness to each other. It motivated me to find moments of joy in my life. I agree with Doyle, who writes "so that's why I write – to find the treasures in the suffering" (p. 228). Because of lockdowns and travel bans, the news served as my only connection to pandemic narratives in other countries around the world. How could I expect the narrative of my life in the United States to apply to anyone else? I don't want to make any assumptions about the pandemic struggles other people experienced. I can't know everyone's story in every part of the world, but I want to provide useful information. This book will give you resources to rebuild your life as the world emerges from the pandemic.

After a trauma such as the pandemic, however, it may become difficult to share our narratives with each other. Brown (2020) believes, "the greatest casualty of trauma – the thing that trauma often takes away from us – is the emotional, and sometimes even physical, safety that is necessary for us to be vulnerable" (p. xix). While everyone has a different narrative, we share the common experience of humanity and need to create safe spaces for each other. The world shares the collective experience of a pandemic, and each person who experienced the pandemic has a narrative. When we create space to share our narratives with each other, we open the door for compassion, empathy, and understanding.

DISCLAIMER

The strategies and treatments discussed in this book do not take the place of a visit with a medical professional such as a physician, physical therapist, psychiatrist, or other trained specialist. I do not advocate attempting any treatment plan on your own. I encourage you to feel inspired by the stories, but please consult a medical professional if you are experiencing physical or emotional pain.

RECURRING THEMES

As a teacher of literature, I love exploring themes, especially when themes recur in a text. Therefore, I deliberately placed themes to reappear during various places in this book. Some of the themes, such as narrative inquiry and multigenre writing, appear in multiple chapters. The theory of narrative inquiry and the practice of multigenre writing provide the foundation for presenting research in an innovative method, as well as honoring the first person voice during the sharing of narratives. Narrative writing gives writers the opportunity to share part of themselves with the reader. In the following sections, I introduce themes which reemerge throughout this narrative, like threads in an elaborate tapestry connecting to form a beautiful picture.

NARRATIVE INQUIRY

In all of the chapters of this book, I use the qualitative interpretive research theory of narrative inquiry, which embodies the sharing of stories. Clandinin and Connelly (2000) explain when describing narrative inquiry, "what may have appeared to be insignificant nothingness at the time they were composed as field texts may take on a pattern as they are interwoven with other field texts in the construction of research texts" (p. 104). Studying narratives helps researchers find patterns in stories to assemble pieces of the research puzzle, much like an academic game of connect the dots. I love narrative inquiry because I want to know how people find meaning in the themes of their stories.

Narrative inquiries remain ongoing. As I write these words, I witness athletes in the 2020 Olympics (postponed to 2021 because of the pandemic) focus conversations in the news on their mental health in addition to their physical athletic performances. I reference mental health throughout this book, but the emerging worldwide mental health narrative motivated me to highlight it here. Boyes (2015) believes, "building resiliency is one way you can prevent yourself from getting derailed by anxiety" (p. 46). I view this idea as resiliency coexisting with anxiety. The students and teachers (including myself) at my school demonstrated both resilience and anxiety during the pandemic. Resilience made my anxiety manageable, but it also became essential for me to acknowledge my feelings and talk or write about them. I lived with both anxiety and resilience: When anxiety knocked me down, resilience helped me get up again. If you are not okay, that is okay. Tell someone.

COLLABORATIVE NARRATIVES

I feel grateful that my research and writing journey meant my path crossed with team members who shared my interests. Heard (1995) explains, "the more honest I am with myself about my own needs, the better I can guide my readers into giving me the kind of help I truly need" (p. 131). Joining a research team requires honesty and authenticity. Sharing part of my life in narratives led to the honor of collaborating with an outstanding team of writers. Thanks to my cousin Robin Perry Newkirk and my friends Claudia Jayne Brahler, Susannah Brown, Valerie Bryan, Ann Musgrove, Jillian Powers, Ryan Urenda, and Eric Wanner for writing the original IGI publications with me which inspired ideas for this book. Thanks to my cousin Melissa Bird for creating medical artwork from an X-ray of my spine that appeared on the cover of the original publication and which the publisher chose again for the revision.

I feel honored that Dr. Claudia Jayne Brahler wrote the forward to this book. Jayne's enthusiasm for research inspires me to complete my best work. She challenges me to think about research from a different perspective. In the middle of a research study, Jayne reminded me that as an English teacher, I brought my unique skills to our research team. So how did I plan to use my gifts? With renewed motivation, I grabbed a different pen, curled up on a couch outside Jayne's office on the University of Dayton campus, and scored surveys from physical therapy patients. During another visit to Dayton, Jayne invited me to attend a school visit where she met with high school students in a drop out recovery program who succeeded in completing a college level medical math class that Jayne had developed and offered for dual high school and college credit. I observed Jayne interact with teachers and students at the school in a wonderful opportunity watching an expert in her fieldwork element. She developed an impressive hybrid model of both online instruction and face to face meetings years before other schools adopted this mode of instruction due to the pandemic. I look forward to working with her again in the future.

Physical therapist Dr. Eric Wanner and I analyze research differently, which results in us working well together. I like to focus on larger themes and finding connections with patient narratives, while Eric studies every detail of surveys patients complete to make sure we don't miss anything. Despite our different approaches, we still have inter-rater reliability scoring percentages over 90% when scoring patient surveys. He also challenges me to write better by finding the essential ideas in my wandering first drafts. I appreciate him giving me the opportunity to share his writing in this book, and I look forward to working with him again in the future too.

WRITING MEETS MEDICINE

As a high school English teacher and college professor of future teachers, I knew writing could help students feel better emotionally. Every year my students read *The Freedom Writers Diary* and watch the corresponding movie *Freedom Writers.* Just like the Freedom Writers, my students write in journals and in conferences with me report how the writing helps them process their emotions. I relate to the words of Gruwell and the Freedom Writers (1999) who write, "maybe the end of our journey is really just the beginning" (p. 277). I feel the same way about this research journey. Discovering that writing held physical healing benefits in addition to emotional healing benefits, I added a new chapter to my research. Psychologist Pennebaker (1997) describes his research study where college students who wrote about thoughts and feelings related to a trauma had fewer visits to the health center and reports, "I'll never forget the initial thrill of finding that writing about traumas affected physical health" (p. 35). Jayne, Eric, and I found a trend showing patients who used more positive language on the short answer questions of a survey we designed showed higher healing gains on objective physical therapy measurements.

In her medical research about outlook and aging, Tindle (2013) discusses, "our outlook is the lens through which we view the world" (p. 5). She discovered a connection between positive outlook and health and elaborates, "a positive outlook is good medicine" (p. 6). Tindle determined that positive outlook influences the one percent of patients who achieve ideal cardiac health, but wanted to know more about the script inside the patients' heads. When I read that, I felt like jumping up and down while screaming like a teenager at a concert, because I saw the connection. English teachers have used writing for years to know the script in students' heads, usually in the form of prompts that require students to write responses in journals. Cameron (1998) explains, "when a writer writes from the heart of what matters to him personally, the writing is often both personal and powerful" (p. 218). Writing from the heart reveals the writer's thoughts and emotions. Since English teachers and doctors typically don't work in the same circles, connecting the fields of writing and medicine promotes the sharing of knowledge and conversations that lead to new discoveries.

PRACTICING SELF-COMPASSION

I can be my own worst critic. The self-critical voice in my head sometimes says things I would never say to another person. Especially now, after the world experienced the pandemic, people need to show compassion to themselves and others. Neff (2021) explains, "tender self-compassion harnesses the energy of nurturing to alleviate suffering, while fierce self-compassion harnesses the energy of action to alleviate suffering – when these are fully integrated, they manifest as caring force" (p. 5). Together as a community, we can work to alleviate suffering either through nurturing or action and become a caring force for positive change. Some people may want to return to activities they experienced before the pandemic sooner than other people do, and both choices are okay. Neff discusses a research study which shows the benefits of self-compassion and describes, "researchers recruited participants on Facebook and asked them to write a compassionate letter to themselves once a day for seven days" (p. 126). She continues, "they then tracked the well-being of participants over time, and found that compared to the control group, those who wrote with self-compassion were less depressed for three months afterward. Even more remarkable, they reported feeling happier for six months" (p. 127). The research illustrated another way writing helps people, demonstrating that writing leads to improved health whether people write about a trauma or about compassion.

Everyone experienced some kind of stress during the pandemic. Gilbert (2016) provides the definition, "the word stress comes from the Latin word for compression, and that compression is what prematurely ages us – compacting us, physically and emotionally, into a feeling of frailty and brokenness" (p. xvi). Stress has a negative impact on health, and stress management strategies such as self-compassion and journal writing help put the broken pieces of a life back together. David (2016) studied Pennebaker's writing experiments and elaborates, "in each study, Pennebaker found that the people who wrote about emotionally charged episodes experienced a marked increase in their physical and mental well-being. They were happier, less depressed, and less anxious. In the months after the writing sessions, they had lower blood pressure, better immune function, and fewer doctor visits" (p. 90). David investigated why using words to express emotions helped the research participants and concluded, "the writers in these experiments who thrived the most began to develop insight" (p. 92) and "by dissolving the entanglement that had built up between their impulses and their actions so they could see their experience in context, and form a broader perspective, they flourished despite it all" (p. 92). Writing about experiences doesn't change the past, but makes people more aware of the present in order to move from surviving to thriving in the future.

TEACHING, HEALTH COACHING, AND STEPHEN MINISTRY

I wear three hats in my professional life, but they integrate beautifully into my wardrobe. I view my narratives through the lenses of my experiences. I explain why strategies relate to both the field of education and the field of medicine. Kanold (2017) describes how a colleague "highlighted the mission and principles of the Mayo Clinic as a model for educators to follow" (p. 232). The audience of educators followed the advice to read the Mayo Clinic's mission and principles and "replace the word patient with student" (p. 232). Medical professionals focus on the needs of patients, while education professionals focus on the needs of students.

As a high school English teacher, I experienced an unusual school year during the pandemic. Nevertheless, my students and I demonstrated resilience. Goff (2018) shares, "it's given me a lot of comfort knowing we're all rough drafts of the people we're still becoming" (p. ix). Just like a rough draft of an essay evolves over time, people evolve over time. Even though I didn't feel the same resilience on the first day of the school year as I did on the last, I needed to set an optimistic tone for my classroom so students would feel safe.

As a Stephen Minister at my church, I offered prayers to people who needed comfort. Talking to someone on the phone or on a video call provides a different dynamic than holding someone's hand during a prayer, but in the absence of physical presence, the words need to resonate. Goff (2017) believes, "it's not often that we have the chance to lean over our own lives and try to make sense of them" (p. 2). During the pandemic, parts of life didn't make sense. In those moments, it becomes essential to focus on what I could control and give the rest up to a higher power.

As a National Board Certified Health and Wellness Coach, I shared with my school's health and wellness committee the strategies I learned working with patients. Health coaching focuses on using vision and values to set goals. Neff (2021) explains, "in short, goals are something we do, values are something we live" (p. 185). One of my favorite questions to students and colleagues became asking them about their "why?" People set goals, but values determine why they want to achieve their goals. In a medical setting, patients use values as motivation to achieve healing goals. In a school setting, students use values to keep looking forward as they set life goals. Through it all, we own our stories. David (2016) asks, "which truth do you hold on to? Your story is your story. You need to own it, rather than it owning you, and to honor it with compassion" (p. 79). By honoring narratives, we acknowledge experiences, celebrate accomplishments, mourn losses, and find the courage to write the next chapter.

DESCRIPTION OF BOOK CHAPTERS

Each chapter tells its own narrative, but read in order, the book tells a larger narrative of using writing for healing. All of the chapters contain activities, ideas, and strategies to use both during and after the pandemic. I begin each title with the word "reflections." The song of the same title by The Supremes describes how life used to be, a feeling experienced by numerous people during the pandemic. If one cannot reclaim the life lived before the pandemic, how does it become possible to envision a new life after the pandemic ends? During the pandemic, life slowed down, leading to opportunities for reflection.

Reflections of Writing Narratives serves as an introduction to writing as healing in a variety of settings, including my classroom, a hospital, and a church. *Reflections of Technology Narratives* discusses the pros and cons of extensive technology use. Too much technology causes stress; yet, technology became a lifeline when people could not see loved ones in person. *Reflections of Health Coaching Narratives* describes how physical therapist Eric Wanner and I introduced health coaching to physical therapy patients in a hospital. I describe the emerging medical field of health coaching and why it helps both patients and healthy people interested in setting goals. *Reflections of Leadership Narratives* provides examples of why I needed to become a transformative leader in my classroom. I share strategies leaders in all fields can implement to practice self-care while serving as role models for others. *Reflections of Teaching Narratives* tells my story of implementing innovative teaching methods. I explain how methods I teach in my classroom adapt to other fields. *Reflections of Emotional Truth Narratives* compares and contrasts fact and fiction writing. I share why writing served as a valuable resource for me when coping with the death of my mom. *Reflections of Curriculum Narratives* provides examples of the PAGES curriculum program and its use in various settings such as schools and hospitals. *Reflections of Anxiety Narratives* presents the research Eric and I conducted about helping college students cope with anxiety, and people of all ages benefit from the resources. *Reflections of Spiritual Narratives* revisits my role as a pastoral care volunteer, health coach and Stephen Minister in a hospital. I apply the life lessons I learned about faith to overcoming obstacles. *Reflections of Healing Narratives* discusses the research Eric and I designed when using an original survey with physical therapy patients at Eric's clinic. I connect my role as a researcher to my role as a patient. In every chapter, I share narratives from my life because, as Crosby (2020) believes, "let's lead with our own imperfect and give others the gift of offering more grace to themselves" (p. 199). May my writing inspire reflection, hope, and healing!

REFERENCES

Boyes, A. (2015). *The anxiety toolkit*. Perigee.

Brown, B. (2020). The gifts of imperfection (2nd ed.).

Cameron, J. (1998). *The right to write*. Tarcher/Putnam.

Crosby, C. (2020). *You are the key*. Zondervan.

David, S. (2016). *Emotional agility*. Avery.

DeVito, D., Shamberg, M., & Sher, S. (Producers), & LaGravenese, R. (Director). (2007). *Freedom writers* [motion picture]. United States: MTV Films.

Doyle, G. (2013). *Carry on, warrior*. Scribner.

Gilbert, E. (2016). *Eat pray love* (2nd ed.). Riverhead.

Goff, B. (2018). *Everybody always*. Nelson.

Goff, M. (2017). *Love lives here*. B&H Publishing Group.

Gruwell, E., & the Freedom Writers. (1999). The Freedom Writers diary. New York, NY: Broadway.

Heard, G. (1995). *Writing toward home*. Heinemann.

Holland, B., Dozier, L., & Holland, E. (1967). Reflections [Recorded by the Diana Ross and the Supremes]. On Reflections [CD]. Detroit, MI: Motown.

Kanold, T. D. (2017). *Heart!* Solution Tree Press.

Neff, K. (2021). *Fierce self-compassion*. Harper Wave.

Pennebaker, J. W. (1997). *Opening up: the healing power of expressing emotions*. The Guilford Press.

Tindle, H. (2013). *Up: How positive outlook can transform our health and aging*. Hudson Street Press.

Acknowledgment

Whenever I write a thank you page, I always hope I don't forget anyone! Thanks to the entire team of people who made this project possible.

Thanks to designer Tori Parks, and the publishing team who helped with this book. I have edited previous publications with IGI and it was wonderful to return for this one.

This book is dedicated to the kids in my family: Mia, Jackson, David, Colton, and Braylon. You give me hope every day that the future will be beautiful.

Every day I feel blessed to belong to my amazing family who supports my dreams and makes me feel I can do anything. Much love to Dann Bird, Diane McLoughlin, Susie DeBeck, Bill DeBeck, Robin Newkirk, Derrick Newkirk, David Bird, Patricia Bird, Melissa Bird, Derek Bird, Gabrielle Bird, Barbara Harbin, Marsha Bird, Sandy Bridges, Joanna Claridge, Carl Claridge, Erica Younkvich, Margaret Bridges, Michael Schafer, Cher Schafer, Benjamin Schafer, Crystal Schafer, Arthur Bruggisser, Brian Bruggisser, Amanda Bruggisser, and the O'Connor family. And to Marilyn Kepler Bird, my mom and guardian angel.

I write these words now because of the support from my friends, colleagues, and students throughout the years. The names are too numerous to mention in this space, but please know I thank you for being part of my life and appreciate all of you.

Chapter 1
Reflections of Writing Narratives

ABSTRACT

Writing becomes a catalyst for healing. When people transfer thoughts and feelings to paper or a computer, stressful emotional events in the mind and physical tension in the body often improve. While writing cannot take the place of a medical expert's evaluation, it can help the healing process. This narrative focuses on how students in a classroom, patients in a clinic, and anyone coping with uncertain times can use the writing process to share ideas, track symptoms, vent frustrations, compose prayers, or reflect on life.

I JUST WANT YOU TO KNOW WHO I AM

How can writing help people heal? This question served as motivation for research and led to discoveries in my roles as a high school English teacher, Stephen Minister at my church, and health coach. While writing cannot take the place of an evaluation by a trained medical expert, it can help the healing process. When a patient writes about symptoms in a journal to share with a medical professional, a high school student writes about the day's events in a journal to deal with emotions, or an adult writes a prayer in a journal to cope with uncertainty, the process of writing serves as a valuable resource. Regardless of the circumstances which motivated the writer to pick up a notebook and pen or type at a computer, writing releases thoughts and emotions from the mind to the page. When people transfer ideas to paper, stressful emotional thoughts in the mind and physical tension in the body often improve. Writing therefore becomes a catalyst for healing.

This chapter uses narrative inquiry to share stories and apply artistic methods, such as writing in journals, to the practice of healing. The theory of narrative inquiry invites writers to own their writing voices by using the first person pronoun "I" to make stories accessible. Clandinin and Connelly (2000) explain, "questions of form for a narrative inquirer are with us from the outset of an inquiry. Even as we tell our own research stories prior to entering into the midst of the field stories, there is a tentative sense of plot. As we engage with research participants and live and tell stories with them, the plotlines under composition are restoried, that is, they are relived and retold. All of these tellings and livings prefigure the narrative forms of our research texts" (p. 165). Narrative inquiry, as a qualitative interpretive form of research, focuses on stories and the finding of narrative threads, or themes, in the stories. Narrative

DOI: 10.4018/978-1-7998-9051-5.ch001

inquiries may include objective data, such as a tally of the number of times events occurred; however, a narrative inquiry also includes subjective data, such as the stories of participants. Consequently, the researcher in the field of narrative inquiry may choose to participate as a participant observer instead of only observing other people. Clandinin and Connelly (2000) discuss, "narrative inquiry has the compelling, sometimes confounding, quality of merging overall life experiences with specific research experience, realms of experience often separated in inquiry" (p. 115). If the researcher chooses the role of a participant observer, attention must be paid to the dual roles. Heifetz (1994) describes the dual roles by using the extended metaphor, "consider the experience of dancing on a dance floor in contrast with standing on a balcony and watching other people dance" (pp. 252-253). Narrative inquirers alternate between the balcony perspective of observation and the dance floor perspective of interacting with participants.

My research into writing as healing focused on studying the stories of others during my doctoral dissertation, and included my own story about the death of my mom. I didn't want to interview others about the narratives which shaped their lives without also including my own transformative narrative. My research consequently transformed into having a larger purpose. DeSalvo (1999) explains, "the writing process, no matter how much time we devote to it, contains a tremendous potential for healing" (p. 73). My experiences of how I used writing as healing meant as much to me as the stories of the people I interviewed. The research for this chapter exists as observational research and reflections of previous research projects. It serves as a qualitative interpretive analysis as well as an introduction to writing as healing for anyone looking to explore the concept in their lives.

This narrative connects writing methods to the practice of education and medicine with the goal of helping people heal. This section's title, *I Just Want You to Know Who I Am*, is a line from the song *Iris* by the Goo Goo Dolls. It describes how patients feel when seeking help: They want someone to know their stories. When seeking medical treatment, a patient wants to feel like his or her story is being heard and the medical provider sees a person, not just a name on a chart. Rankin (2015b) advises that despite demands from a sometimes frustrating medical system, those practicing medicine need to take the time to look their patients in the eyes and not stand with a hand on the door to the exam room because, "just as healers must stand up and reclaim the lineage of their professions, patients must reclaim their own power, standing up with their autonomy, their intuition, their willingness to question and participate in changing the system from within, and their vote. It all starts with change at the level of the healer-patient relationship" (p. 238). Whether a patient talks to a health coach, receives prayers from a Stephen Minister, or writes in a journal, the important thing is that the patient feels the story is heard. Encouraging the students in my classroom to practice journal writing provided a foundation for me to apply similar methods to the medical field.

PANDEMIC NARRATIVES

Who am I now in this pandemic? I suspect others ask this question of themselves as everyone searches to reinvent themselves and their lives. Every day, the news about the virus seemed worse. Wasn't the year 2020 supposed to represent optimism, clarity, and new vision? Wasn't 2021 supposed to be different? What is happening in the world? I knew I needed to return to writing, because writing always provides the clarity I need to survive difficult situations. Writing helps me make sense of the uncertainty and chaos. It captures my experiences so that years from now I will look back at what I survived during this time in my life.

"Write in your journal," I tell my students, "transferring thoughts from your mind to the page helps relieve stress." I say the words to my students when we all meet in my classroom, transition to all meeting online, and then return back to the classroom with the enhanced precautions of masks and social distancing. Our reality in these coronavirus infested times means that regardless of whether we gather online thanks to the amazing videoconferencing system, gather in the classroom behind plexiglass on the desks, or gather with students in a hybrid of both modes, our journals travel with us. Dalebout (2016) explains the writing process in words relatable to teenagers as, "journaling is basically texting your feelings to the most nonjudgmental friend you could ever have" (p. 11). I constantly hear stories from students that writing eases their stress and helps them organize their thoughts. I know from my research as well as my personal experiences that writing makes a difference in helping people heal both emotionally and physically. Life coach Beck (2012) argues that people who experienced traumas in life make a difference for others since, "all these people can help others back from hell because they've found their own way back from internal, infernal experiences" (p. 244). Writing helped me process my thoughts and emotions as I grieved the loss of my mom. Surviving this trauma instilled in me a desire to share my knowledge with others and teach them how to use writing to help make a positive difference in their lives.

In rereading and reflecting on my previous research, I realize it still relates to modern online society as the pandemic unfolds. In fact, as at the time of this writing, as an increasing number of people follow government orders to stay home to prevent the virus from spreading, I argue that people need journal writing more than ever. The more people stay at home with their thoughts, the more they need a way of processing such thoughts and emotions. Writers live stories once, and relive the stories when writing about them. Or as Goldberg (1986) states, "writers live twice" (p. 48). Life is a series of stories that everyone lives once, but writing enables the writer to relive the story and attach meaning to it. Cameron (1998) explains, "because writing is a practice of observation as much as invention, we can become curious as much as frightened in the face of change. Writing about the change, we can help it along, lean into it, cooperate. Writing allows us to rewrite our lives" (p. 31). I can't change the pandemic, but I can change how I react to it and how I rewrite that part of my life story. I vent about the negative moments and release those thoughts while simultaneously finding positive moments of gratitude in the midst of uncertainty.

Research illustrates that stress makes people sick. Rankin (2015a) explains, "when exposed to stress, the body tends to whisper before it yells. Stress often manifests through less immediately life-threatening physical symptoms, such as backache, headache, eye strain, insomnia, fatigue, dizziness, appetite disturbances, and gastrointestinal distress" (p. 35). If you find yourself experiencing any strange health symptoms, check the stress level in your life and call your doctor, since emotional stress can manifest physically in your body. Writing remains an almost free method of coping with stress. All anyone needs to start writing is a piece of paper and a pen or pencil. Patients might write about symptoms to share with a medical professional, especially if there is concern over what symptoms mean and questions about whether a symptom could indicate the coronavirus. Children and adults might write about the day's events and find moments of joy despite a scary news cycle. Members of a religious community who can't gather in person to worship might write prayers and share them with each other to still feel connected. All these practices allow writing to become a catalyst for healing. DeSalvo (1999) writes, "I use my writing as a way of fixing things, of making them better, of healing myself" (p. 7). Writing can't fix events beyond our control, such as a pandemic, but writing does provide insight into how to cope and make life better.

Taking a trip to my garage reveals that since I was old enough to hold a crayon, I wrote in a journal. Stories about the kitten I had as a child transitioned into accounts of family vacations and teenage drama of worries about boys and grades. I didn't realize how writing could truly save me until my mom died unexpectedly when I was in graduate school. I didn't use writing as a replacement for either sessions with a therapist or the antidepressant my doctor prescribed at the time, but writing became an effective way for me to cope, especially in the middle of the night when I couldn't sleep. Most of the writing got added to the box of old journals in the garage or destroyed when I felt like ripping up pages; the rest became my doctoral dissertation. I became a woman on a mission. I couldn't save my mom's life, but I could maybe save other people by sharing my experiences. This writing as healing odyssey led to finding other people who shared my vision, completing research studies illustrating the benefits of writing for physical therapy patients and college students, achieving the success of publications, and most importantly making a difference in the lives of others. I would trade all the things I just mentioned to hug my mom one more time, which is why when a friend asked me how I felt about the pandemic my honest reply was, "it's not the worst thing that ever happened to me."

WRITING AS HEALING

While a story can be spoken, writing enables the author to capture additional details of a narrative. Pennebaker (1997) theorized from his research as a psychologist, "if my experience was any indication, writing about upsetting issues must work in ways similar to talking about them" (p. 30). Any patient who has ever walked out of a doctor's office with the realization of forgetting an important question may benefit from writing notes to remember experiences. Brown (2015) summarizes, "Pennebaker's research, combined with what I've learned in my own work, has convinced me that even brief engagements with writing can lead to significant results" (p. 88). Patients therefore do not have to write a long narrative for their medical practitioners or themselves; a short series of notes or freewriting of a few sentences serves as enough information to share the story.

Journal writing may be relatively new to the medical field, but for years English teachers have used journal writing in their classrooms. Anderson and MacCurdy (2000) advise English teachers, "we are, however, arguing what we know to be true – stories about painful, traumatic events in the lives of students do appear in our classrooms, they have always appeared, and they will continue to appear, not because we want or don't want them to, but because writing is quite simply the medium in which, for many people, the deepest, most effective, and most profound healing can take place" (pp. 8-9). Writing in journals gives students a space to explore their thoughts and feelings. While some students do choose to write about painful events, students may also choose to write in their journals about other topics, such as their feelings about an inspirational quote or work of literature. By writing, students transfer emotions out of their minds and onto the page. Gruwell (2007), whose students became known as the Freedom Writers, states, "I, like my students, realized that it would take more than just writing to feel better – but at least it was a start" (p. 148). The purpose of journal writing is for students to trust themselves and their first impressions while they write. Students have a short amount of time, such as five or ten minutes, to write their first impression on a topic. As Conner (2008) writes, "first thought is a precious gift. It is an impetus from deep within your soul that wants to be seen and heard. Honor it" (pp. 92-93). The time limit is to capture the writer's first impression about an idea before self-criticism creates any doubt or second guessing.

Journal writing helps students discover their writing voices. Lamott (1994) shares, "so I sit for a moment and then say a small prayer – please help me get out of the way so I can write what needs to be written" (p. 117). Writing what needs to be written serves as a form of self-expression through writing practice that leads to the discovery of writing voice. Romano (2004) states, "voice is the writer's presence on the page" (p. 5). English teachers encourage students to use the power of their unique writing voices. As Cameron (1998) states, "when we just let ourselves write, we get it 'right'" (p. 8). When students write in their journals, no right or wrong answers exist. The only answers students need to find become the ones which help them speak their truths and live authentic lives.

CLASSROOM JOURNAL WRITING

When I teach, I like rituals. Rituals provide stability amongst the ringing bells and constant traffic in high school hallways. When the high school where I teach moved to online teaching, I practiced different yet similar rituals. I greeted my students and reminded them to write. I used to give students a quote to explore though writing, but now I tell them to write about whatever they are thinking about at that moment. I also offer them the security of not reading their writing, while reminding them that if they find themselves writing something that concerns them to tell their parents, the school psychologist, or me. Sometimes the school psychologist will meet with a student and will then ask me if I have concerns about a student's writing. Cameron (2002) believes, "as mental-health experts are quick to point out, in order to move through loss and beyond it, we must acknowledge it and share it" (p. 129). Journals gave students an outlet to share all their losses from the pandemic. Some students experienced large losses, such as the death of a family member from the coronavirus. Other students experienced smaller yet still important losses such as the cancellation of traditional school events. Writing about the losses acknowledged and honored them.

Because I don't read every word my students write, I realize the possibility exists that students may grab a writing utensil and compose in poetic verse about their English teacher who annoys them with large amounts of writing, but I live with that. At the end of each quarter, I hold individual conferences with students where they discuss what they learned from journal writing. During the pandemic, I find that I don't have to wait until the end of each quarter to discuss writing, since students who need reassurance that life will be okay want to discuss their writing more often.

BACKGROUND OF WRITING AS HEALING

Writing helped me through difficult situations by bringing clarity to my life. I echo the sentiment of DeSalvo (1999) that "writing has helped me heal. Writing has changed my life. Writing has saved my life" (p. 3). As a National Board Certified Health Coach, I advocate a holistic approach to healing. Writing helps me manage my stress most of the time, but it does not exist as the only option or a magic cure. A couple times in my life, losses such as the death of my mom caused my stress to transform into anxiety; I needed therapy and medication, and no shame exists in either option or in asking for help. Consequently, none of my words serve as a good alternative for a conversation with your doctor if you experience anxiety or any other health issue. Writing, however, may help relieve some symptoms of stress and anxiety.

Research exists to support the theory of writing helping people heal, beginning with the work of psychologist James Pennebaker. Pennebaker and Smyth (2016) discuss Pennebaker's original study, which led to the discovery, "people who wrote about their deepest thoughts and feelings surrounding traumatic experiences evidenced enhanced immune function compared with those who wrote about superficial topics" (p. 21). They continue with the observation that improved health continued after the writing experience and elaborate, "people who wrote about their deepest thoughts and feelings related to stressful or traumatic experiences had reliable improvements in health in the two to three months after writing" (p. 25). Additional studies on wellness and writing followed. Evans (2010) summarizes the literature and reports, "wellness and writing are connected in ways yet to be fully researched and exploited, but the literature of several disciplines declares that for many people wellness and writing are connected in ways useful for emotional, physical, and spiritual health" (p. 3). In the years since Evans reported that the connections had yet to be fully researched, Sandberg and Grant (2017) report, "more than a hundred experiments have documented the therapeutic effects of journaling. It has helped medical students, patients with chronic pain, crime victims, maximum-security prisoners, and women after childbirth" (pp. 62-63). Sandberg and Grant continue, "writing about traumatic events can decrease anxiety and anger, boost grades, reduce absences from work, and lessen the emotional impact of job loss. Health benefits include higher T-cell counts, better liver function, and stronger antibody responses. Even journaling for a few minutes a few times can make a difference" (p. 63). Furthermore, people do not have to write about traumatic events to receive the benefits of writing. Brown (2015) described the participants in her research as, "many of them worked through their emotions in letters they knew they would never send but needed to write" (p. 87). The writing process possesses the potential to help anyone who feels willing to explore self-discovery. Fallon (2020) elaborates, "when there are no safe places in our lives for us to disclose an event, or when we aren't sure who or where those safe places are, writing is an incredible tool that gives us the freedom language brings. Writing can help us break the control that our stories often have over us" (p. 165). Writing provides a safe space to explore ideas and the freedom to share stories because the page won't offer an opinion or judge the writer.

Mindfulness expert Cameron (2018) explains, "whether you write for five minutes or 60 minutes a day, journaling helps you gain perspective and deepen self-awareness – revealing your thoughts, habits, strengths, and ways of interpreting the world" (p. 45). Cameron continues, "although journaling is an excellent practice for self-awareness, insight, and clarity, it has also proven to be a tremendous tool for navigating times of change, uncertainty, and dealing with difficult emotions" (p. 45). She encourages anyone interested in practicing journaling to use either prompts to explore ideas, or to open a notebook and put pen to paper as an act of mindfulness.

As a high school English teacher, I know life as a high school student can be difficult. It can be even more difficult when adding a pandemic to the equation. The words English teacher Johnson (1998) wrote over twenty years ago remain true today when she gives teachers the advice, "don't belittle your student's concerns. Acknowledge their feelings, accept their right to have a bad day or a worry, just as adults do" (p. 174). Students appreciate when teachers treat them with respect. Journal writing provides an outlet for describing feelings when students may not want to discuss something. If you want to begin a writing practice, pick up a pen or open a blank document on your computer to receive the benefits of writing. Romano (2013) observes, "the work is the writing. The writing can be healing" (p. 176). Indeed it can.

WRITING AND TEACHING

As soon as the bell rings, my students and I have a ritual: We reach for our journals. At the beginning of most of the high school English classes I teach, I allow about five to ten minutes for journal writing time. I give students three options: Write about the quote I have on the board, write about the current work of literature we are reading, or write about whatever happens to be on their minds that day. At the end of each quarter, I hold individual conferences with each student where I flip through the journals to make sure they are writing, but I do not read their writing unless they request it. I tell students that if they write something which concerns them to share it with a trusted adult. Interestingly, by giving the students the freedom not to share, sometimes they want to share more. It soon did not surprise me to see students arrive early to class to show me a journal entry and ask for my opinion. While I look through the journals, I ask students how they feel about writing. The majority of students tell me it helps them process thoughts and feelings. Several students tell me it helps manage stress. Students also describe that journal writing serves as practice, or warm-ups for formal essays. According to Carter (2015), "shoot for a perfect first draft and you are screwed, though; most people are paralyzed by the impossibility of that task" (pp. 204-205). I don't believe there is such a thing as a perfect first draft, but the imperfect first drafts that may not meet the requirements for a formal essay work perfectly for expressive writing in journals. Gruwell (2009) writes of her students, "they realized that everyone has a story; they just needed the opportunity to be heard and an entrée to the healing power of writing" (p. xviii). I want my students to know that their stories matter.

Journal writing encourages the writer to complete expressive writing. Writing teacher Romano (2013) describes, "expressive writing is where we start when we pour forth first words, seeking to make meaning from fragmented, chaotic inner speech. Expressive writing is writing closest to our speaking voice, the seedbed from which all other writing grows" (p. 189). Expressive writing focuses on the first thoughts before the voice of the internal censor starts questioning the words on the page. I want my students to feel like Lamott (1994) when she describes her process as, "so I'd start writing without reigning myself in. It was almost just typing, just making my fingers move" (p. 24). Some students prefer to type their journals, and they receive just as much as benefit as they process day to day issues in their writing. Sandberg and Grant (2017) believe, "turning feelings into words can help us process and overcome adversity" (p. 62). When adversity appears in the lives of my students, it becomes essential for me to honor their stories.

Students sharing stories leads to transformation. I love the work of teacher Erin Gruwell and her students, The Freedom Writers. My classes read *The Freedom Writers Diary* and discuss the philosophy of Gruwell (1999), who describes of her students, "the students continued to write and began to forge stronger identities and to create a sense of community and an outlet for expression" (p. 275). My classes develop into strong communities where students care about each other and support each other. That outlet for expression enabled them to share their past experiences as well as future dreams with each other to enact change in their lives and the lives of their community. While I do not require them to share their writing during group discussions, when students do choose to share their writing with their classmates or me, they learn that others in the class share their feelings and they are not alone in their experiences.

While I choose not to share the writing of my students in this narrative to maintain the confidentiality I promised them, to give you an example of student writing I include a journal entry I wrote as a junior in high school. I keep my old journals and occasionally revisit them to reflect on my experiences.

Okay, I'm a junior. Let me see...what does that mean....more cafeteria food for one thing. Just kidding. For one thing, I'm not afraid of the school now, I know my way around (for the most part). I don't have to worry about graduation for another year. I guess I'm somewhere in the middle. I'll probably take ACTs and SATs this year, but I'm good at standardized tests so I'm not too worried. I do worry a lot though.

While it seems that my sixteen year old self wrote about surface things, at the end of the entry I started to process my thoughts and emotions about worrying. That insight comes from the writer years later after research and experience; my teenage self just enjoyed writing!

My students tell me writing in their journals at the beginning of class helps reduce the anxiety they feel during the school day. Medical doctor Rankin (2015a) describes, "anxiety is an emotional feeling of nervousness, unease, dread, or apprehension" (p. 11). As someone who has experienced anxiety, I relate to the students and feel grateful that writing helps me sort out the stress in my life. Writing becomes part of a balanced wellness plan including exercise, nutrition, and perspective. Unlike the novel *The Scarlet Letter* students read, anxiety should never feel like a scarlet letter worn by anyone who experiences it. Szabo and Hall (2007) offer the encouragement, "it's time we all learned that each of us has a right – and a responsibility – to face our issues, be honest about our needs and emotions, and most importantly, to ask for help when we need it" (p. 221). Each day when the bell rings and my students pick up their journals, I know the writing process helps them.

THE PROCESS

If you are a teacher or other educator and want to use journals in your classroom:

- Give students a choice of whether to write in a notebook or type their journals.
- Allow time for writing. A minimum of five minutes works well. Less than five minutes means students may not have the time to process their ideas.
- Maintain silence in the classroom so students can be alone with their thoughts and not distracted by classmates.
- It is your choice whether or not to read the writing, but make sure students know in advance if you will be reading their writing. Students do not want to be surprised if you tell them later you will be reading their personal writing.
- I recommend either not grading the writing or taking a participation grade. Students write differently when they know the content will be graded.
- You may have administrative tasks to complete, but take the time to write in your own journal when students are writing so they can see you as a writing role model.

WRITING AND EMOTIONAL PAIN

I first studied the field of writing as healing for my doctoral dissertation at Miami University in Oxford, Ohio. The topic of writing helping people heal emotionally became my purpose in life due to unexpected circumstances. My mom died in the middle of my graduate program, transforming me into not only an observer in my research study, but also a participant. Whenever my thoughts started racing or I missed my mom with an intensity which made me want to curl up on the floor and not get up again, I reached for my journal or my computer. My personal experiences with the transformative power of writing redefined my career and my life. I would trade all I have learned about writing as healing to be able to pick up the phone and call my mom again, but since I can't I choose to use my experiences to help other people with their journeys.

While interviewing teachers about how they used writing to process their experiences, I also used writing to help with my grieving process. Zimmermann (2002) believes, "writing allows you to access your wider mind, a wiser, more encompassing place deep within. Your story will unfold and through the writing of it, you will honor and embrace your sorrows, grow from them, and arrive at a place where life is more full and more joyful than you ever thought possible" (p. 19). Some days it became hard to feel when the emotional pain became too intense, but writing became my coping mechanism. Looking back at the writing, I see my anger, devastation, and even moments of hope. This is an excerpt from my journal six months after my mom died when I traveled from Ohio to Delaware and Florida to visit my aunts, uncles, and cousins.

If the life you want isn't possible because of various circumstances, how do you piece together another life that may not be what you want but can still provide you with a little happiness? I think of all my dreams and my future plans that involved my mom. As I return from two weeks of visiting different cities and flying across the country on planes, I can't help but think that she would have been the first person I would have told of my adventures. I told her anyway; I know she was still part of my trip even though not in the way I wanted her to be.

After graduation, I decided to move from Ohio to Florida to make a new start and live closer to my family. Conner (2008) explains, "writing works amazingly well. If you want to engage in a vibrant conversation with the wisdom that dwells just a hair below your conscious awareness, write" (p. 57). In addition to helping me process my grief, writing helped me set new goals and dreams. By getting everything from my mind to the page, I gained clarity about my experiences. Sometimes when thoughts swirl around in a person's mind, the truth of the narrative becomes distorted. Social worker Brown (2017) elaborates, "the brain's self-protection mode often ramps up the stories we tell ourselves about what's happening, creating stories that are often not true or exaggerate our worst fears and insecurities" (p. 55). For weeks after my mom's death, I existed in survival mode and my subjective perspective of my life didn't always match my objective reality. My mind attempted to protect itself by processing pieces of the traumatic event at a time and when my thoughts couldn't focus, writing became a lifeline. Writer Heard (1995) believes, "a first memory is the first story embedded on the soul" (p. 72). Through a combination of writing and therapy, I refocused the first memory of the trauma and remembered the happy memories of my mom. I do not want to give the impression that writing solved everything for me during this difficult time; I also saw a therapist once a week to talk about my experiences and took an antidepressant at the advice of my doctor. Nevertheless, writing helped me on the days between therapist visits and especially the nights when I couldn't sleep and had already woken up my friends with phone calls. My journal and computer became reliable and constant companions who never gave advice and let me vent my emotions.

I could have stopped there; I did enough work on myself to not only survive but thrive. Still, I wanted to do more. Handler (2013) writes, "the passage of time between the event that caused grief and when the writer feels ready to pick up a pen or open the laptop is one place where your story is found. The person you were then, and the person you are now, create the voices that combine to tell the story" (p. 165). Immediately after the experience, my main focus was of course helping myself, but as time passed, I realized I wanted to share my story to help others. Along my journey I met people who cared about the topic as much as I did and we wrote together. When my words make a difference in someone else's life, that is my mom's legacy, and my legacy too.

THE PROCESS

If you are going through a difficult time emotionally and want to write about it:

- Remember no one has to see your writing except you.
- Stop writing if it is too difficult.
- Your writing and computer won't judge you, so don't judge yourself for anything you write.
- If you would be upset if someone else read your writing, keep your journal in a locked file cabinet or other safe place.
- If you find yourself writing about something that disturbs you, it's time to share with a trusted friend or professional therapist.
- It is not a sign of weakness if you need therapy or medication. Don't be afraid to ask for help if you need it.

WRITING AND PHYSICAL PAIN

While I knew writing could help people heal emotionally, another serendipitous moment on my journey led me to research how writing helps people heal physically. I found myself in physical therapy for neck pain and kept a journal to try to make sense of why I felt little pain one minute and intense pain the next. I couldn't make any sense of it, but fortunately for me my physical therapist used my writing to help make a diagnosis and help me heal. I felt grateful for his compassion and creative thinking, since not all medical practitioners would feel enthusiastic about a new idea. After my treatment ended, we continued to work together and research how writing helps patients heal. An enjoyable interdisciplinary collaboration led to research results that made a difference in the lives of patients.

In designing our research and implementing our survey, physical therapist Eric Wanner, research professor Claudia Jayne Brahler, and I wanted to answer the question if there was a relationship between a patient's positive outlook when writing down his or her feelings and the patient's recovery process. Our initial study revealed that patients who used more positive language when responding to short answer writing prompts on the survey we designed showed higher objective improvements on existing physical therapy measurements such as the DASH (Disabilities of the Arm Shoulder Hand), LEFS (Lower Extremity Functional Scale), NDI (Neck Disability Index), and Modified Oswestry (for back pain). (Wanner, Bird, and Brahler, 2016).

When we asked patients to respond to short answer survey questions, we asked for their first impressions. Writing teacher Goldberg (2013) shares, "practice is not for something else. Practice is the practice of being here with your life and pen now. Go, across the page – or your computer screen – what are you thinking of? Put your life on the line" (p. 22). The process of trusting first impressions in writing not only works for high school English students in a classroom, but also physical therapy patients in a clinic. When I designed my pain journal, I needed to share my first impressions in order to have the most accurate information to share with my physical therapist. When patients responded using their first impressions, they shared the most accurate impression of how they felt before the self-censor could take over their thoughts. As Bernstein (2010) writes, "let your pen flow across the page and allow your mind to release its thoughts" (p. 23). When I shared my journal, I needed to trust my physical therapist to keep my information confidential and also use it to help me. I'm sure at times my writing entertained him while he read my thoughts about my neck pain!

Most of us will be patients sometime in our lives. While writing cannot heal physical pain on its own, it can contribute to healing. When people write and release their emotions, the decrease in emotional stress leads to a decrease in muscle tension. Enayati (2015) argues, "in a way, extreme stress is self-fulfilling. The key is to switch the focus of both our perceptions and stories to post-traumatic growth" (p. 72). Even if the patient has no control over the physical pain, the patient does have control of how he or she feels about the pain. Beck (2021) explains, "physical pain comes from events. Psychological suffering comes from the way we deal with those events" (p. xviii). Writing can switch the mental focus of the pain narrative from helplessness to achieving growth. Duckworth (2016) defines, "it was this combination of passion and perseverance that made high achievers special. In a word, they had grit" (p. 8). While this definition of grit applies to a variety of situations, passion and perseverance become important during the recovery process from physical pain.

Pain may lead to frustration, but a positive attitude makes a difference. Beck (2008) explains, "in other words, the negative reaction cluster – the stress reactions, the emotional pain, and the physical weakness that are wired together in your brain and body – can be rewired. The associative learning that makes us feel depressed, anxious, and old can be unlearned" (p. 11). Writing holds us accountable by revealing our thought patterns. Once we illuminate our thought patterns, we find the power to change them. Dalebout (2016) observes, "journaling allows you to stop identifying with your negative beliefs or thought patterns and instead see yourself as separate from them. You start to move from judging yourself to simply witnessing your thoughts, cozying up with them, learning from them, and ultimately letting them out" (p. 12). Letting out thoughts in the form of journal writing allows the page to worry about an issue while simultaneously serving as a stress release.

Another way writing helps with physical pain is by creating a journal to show medical professionals. How many times does the best question get thought of as soon as the doctor leaves the room? A pain journal or symptom journal ensures that all questions are asked and all information is conveyed to the person in charge of the patient's care. The most important quality of a pain or symptom journal is honesty. A doctor best helps a patient when he or she has all the information. Brown (2015) believes, "we can't get to our brave new ending if we start from an inauthentic place. So give yourself permission to wade through the sometimes-murky waters of whatever you're thinking and feeling" (p. 88). At times it may feel difficult to act vulnerable and authentic in front of someone in the medical field. Brown (2012), provides the reminder, "vulnerability is the core, the heart, the center, of meaningful human experiences" (p. 12). Remember, most clinicians are compassionate professionals who will walk with you on your health journey. Medical doctor Rankin (2013) explains, "being unapologetically who we are – not just at work, but at home, in the schoolyard, at church, wherever – soothes the mind, halts the stress response, induces the relaxation response, and heals the body. Authenticity, in work and in life, can be medicine for the body" (p. 117). When a patient demonstrates a willingness to show vulnerability and articulate needs, clinicians appreciate knowing all the information to best help the patient.

Despite my love of television medical dramas, I have no desire to observe a surgery. I did, however, have a desire to learn more about the health care field, so I earned my health coach certification from Duke University Integrative Medicine. According to Caldwell, Gray, and Wolever (2013), "health coaching entails a specific structure and provider relationship that reinforce each other. The coach-patient relationship is specifically centered on the patient's health goals and supporting the patient in those goals" (p. 55). Health coaches partner with the patient's medical team to align the patient's personal goals with the treatment goals and help the patient stay motivated to achieve the goals. Writing does not eliminate pain, but may become part of the health plan. Writing about moments of success or moments of challenge helps determine the next best steps, as well as illustrate progress. Whether writing down goals, keeping a pain journal, or processing feelings about pain, writing exists as a resource for the healing process.

THE PROCESS

If you are sick or in pain and want to write about it:

- Obviously, if you have severe pain or illness, don't write. Seek medical help immediately.
- Be honest in your writing. Your medical team can best help you if you tell the truth about your symptoms and feelings.
- Members of your medical team want to help you. Don't fear that they will judge you for writing the truth.
- Try to keep a positive attitude. Healing is a journey, and small steps still equal progress. A great lesson my physical therapist, Dr. Eric Wanner, told me when I wanted my neck pain to heal immediately is to "think like a turtle" and make slow and steady progress. Turtles travel at a slow pace, but eventually reach their destination.
- An excerpt of my pain journal is below; feel free to use it as a model for your own pain journal.

WRITING AND SPIRITUALITY

On a beautiful Florida winter afternoon, my students and I sit outside by the lake on the high school's campus. We discuss the poetry of Walt Whitman. Whitman (1855) writes in his poem *O Me! O Life!* "That you are here – that life exists and identity, that the powerful play goes on and you may contribute a verse" (p. 341). This leads to a conversation about the difference between spirituality and religion. My students give insightful answers. In their words, religion is what people practice while spirituality is how people feel. I explain that everyone has a right to his or her own religious beliefs, yet together as a class we have a spiritual moment sitting by the water in silence as we write in our journals and read poetry.

Religious institutions may choose to use writing with members of their congregations; furthermore, anyone may choose to use writing as a reflection and form of prayer. Niequist (2016) believes, "whatever it is that you clutch onto with angry fists, that you grab like a lifeline, when you release that thing, when you let it go, that's when you'll hear the notes between the music" (p. 97). Reflection and prayer allow for silence so the noise of a busy life becomes silent. Sometimes when life seems uncertain, people turn to destructive habits; writing serves as a healthy alternative to coping with a situation and provides a

Table 1. The author's neck pain journal

Fri 3/30	Right Side Pain Low = 2, High = 4, Average = 3	Best right after leaving physical therapy. Worst when looking down at notes and stressing about summer teaching schedule. Spend time with family today which leads to laughter.
Sat 3/31	Right Side Pain Low = 2, High = 4, Average = 3	Best when doing exercises. Going for a mellow experience and listening to Taylor Swift this time.
Sun 4/1	Right Side Pain Low = 3, High = 5, Average = 4 Was going to play an April Fool's joke on you and make the numbers really high so laughed thinking about that.	Best when out to lunch with cousins and laughing. Worst when trying to hold Grandma back and prevent wheelchair escape. Epiphany of day: This is a journey. Keep thinking like a turtle. You'll get there!

reminder that a lifeline to internal strength provides more power than external distractions Enayati (2015) explains, "adversity may or may not be out of our control, but we do have control over our stories: what we tell ourselves and others about our circumstances, and how we choose to respond to them" (p. 51). When we can't control the outcome of a situation, we can still control how we react.

Whatever your religious or spiritual practices may be, writing becomes accessible to all who choose to pick up a notebook and pen or reach for a computer. Does the story you tell yourself about your life and current situation reflect your reality? Is an obstacle a roadblock or an opportunity to learn? Brown (2015) explains, "the most dangerous stories we make up are the narratives that diminish our inherent worthiness" (p. 82). Putting thoughts on paper in the form of journal writing clarifies the difference between the actual truth of a situation compared to our interpretation of it. We remind ourselves of people and things we have for which we can show gratitude and determine what needs to change. As Goldberg (2007) states, "we are finishing the circle, closing the gap, making sense of the senseless" (p. 299). Events which may originally appear as detours taken on the road of life lead to new goals and opportunities.

In addition to my roles as high school English teacher and health coach, I serve as a Stephen Minister at my church. Haugk (2000) defines, "Stephen Ministers are lay Christians carefully recruited, selected, trained, commissioned, and supervised for lay caring ministry" (p. 17). With my role as a Stephen Minister, I use the same skills of reflective listening and partnering with people on their healing journeys as I do as a health coach. The difference with Stephen Ministry is that people may be experiencing a spiritual crisis instead of a health crisis, and I also have prayer as a resource. While I write about Stephen Ministry from the perspective of my experiences, the writing practices I describe are not meant to be seen only from the perspective of Christian faith.

Regardless of a person's views on religion and spirituality, the practice of self-compassion leads to reflection and kindness toward oneself. Often people criticize themselves more harshly than other people ever could. While self-compassion occurs by thinking kind thoughts, writing serves as an affirmation of thoughts of kindness. Neff (2011) suggests, "try keeping a daily self-compassion journal for one week (or as long as you like). Journaling is an effective way to express emotions and has been found to enhance both mental and physical well being" (p. 103). A daily self-compassion journal reminds the author to practice kindness and self-forgiveness. Whenever life seems challenging, we enjoy the journey more by showing ourselves and others kindness and compassion. Mistakes happen as part of life, but since we cannot recapture the past like the main character in *The Great Gatsby* longs to do, writing can help us move forward. Germer (2009) shares, "keeping a journal is itself a contemplative practice and a self-compassion exercise" (p. 242). Contemplation shares characteristics with the practice of mindfulness, which promotes self-awareness and living in the present moment. Tindle (2013) explains, "the main difference between mindfulness and contemplation is that at its core, contemplation is a practice in which the contemplator seeks to come closer to a higher spiritual power" (p. 108). Some people may choose to practice mindfulness and remind themselves to refocus their attention to the present moment, while others may choose to pray as a form of contemplation.

While prayer exists mainly through spoken words, they may also appear in the forms of thoughts or written ideas. Cameron (1998) states, "it is my belief that all of us are naturally intuitive and that writing opens an inner spiritual doorway that gives us access to information both personally and professionally that serves us well" (pp. 206-207). Often, when a decision needs to be made, writing provides insights to the solution or peace about the process. Matousek (2017) believes, "like all forms of awakening practice, writing requires mindfulness. Just as we bring our attention back to the breath during meditation, you learn to observe the wandering mind without excessive control, and gently return your focus to the question at hand" (p. 5). Whatever question may bring the writer to the page, writing about it may provide the answer.

As a Stephen Minister, I often give short prayers when I visit someone in need in the hospital or pray with someone at church after the service. During such times, I begin speaking and trust I will say the words the person needs to hear. Bernstein (2016) believes, "we change the world when we shift spiritually – when our attitudes become more loving, when we forgive, when we heal our wounds from the past, and when we embrace the present moment" (p. 172). Just like it helps people heal emotionally and physically, writing helps people heal spiritually. The journal serves as a safe space to explore thoughts and feelings for self-forgiveness, or a place to work through a difficult conversation if it would help to forgive someone else. If the person who needs forgiveness is not willing to have a conversation or longer alive, forgiving may still take place for the writer in journal pages. Bernstein (2018) explains, "putting pen to paper is a prayer. It's an offering. You humbly look at your judgment, choose again, and then pray for that judgment to be replaced with love" (p. 186). By writing, we acknowledge our pasts, remind ourselves to remain mindful in the present, and share hope for the future.

My research and writing became part of my life's purpose. By writing about my experiences, I saw the connections between the moments that happened to me. It's a magical feeling when ideas weave together like threads of a tapestry. If my mom hadn't died, would I still feel that research and writing exist in my life as part of a larger purpose? I do know that helping other people makes me feel that I use the pain of my life experiences to make a meaningful contribution to the world. I understand that some people may see everything as coincidences, but my spirituality leads me to believe in what Rushnell and DuArt (2017) call Godwinks, which they define as, "Godwinks are those little events that defy human understanding. In the beginning you were tempted to call them coincidences, but inwardly you sensed there was something more going on – and that God had something to do with it" (p. ix). Whatever you believe, I hope writing helps you discover your personal gifts. I then encourage you to share your gifts with others who may benefit from the knowledge.

THE PROCESS

If you are a church leader or anyone who wants to use writing as a spiritual resource:

- If you are contemplating a question or need to make a decision, start writing and see what answers your intuition discovers.
- If you find yourself being your own worst critic, practice self-compassion and write about your strengths in your journal.
- Create a gratitude journal and make a list of things for which you are grateful. Use daily, weekly, or as often as you need.
- If you feel discouraged by acts of hate in the world, shift the focus to love and create an observation journal of random acts of kindness that you practice or witness others practicing throughout the day.
- Write a prayer for yourself or someone else.

THE ART OF WRITING IN A PANDEMIC

Throughout this narrative, I cite research studies illustrating the healing benefits that happen with writing. Even with the technical dimensions of research, creativity drives the artistic writing process. I view writing as an art form, where self-expression becomes essential for the writer. Sharing the story with oneself in the pages of a journal provides healing benefits, while sharing writing with a supportive reader builds trust and provides additional support for the writer. Romano (2015) describes of sharing stories, "it's been good to write about it and give it to readers" (p. 21). The writer decides who to trust; finding the right reader leads to a source of encouragement and helps the writer build resilience. Writing serves as a coping mechanism for life's fragile moments and transforms negative thoughts into positive ones by reframing the stories.

So how does writing reframe a pandemic narrative? Duckworth (2016) references grit and argues, "the hope that gritty people have has nothing to do with luck and everything to do with getting up again" (p. 169). Getting up again and finding meaning after loss feels difficult. Requirements to stay at home to stay safe cause days to blend together. To reframe my present pandemic narrative and focus on a (hopefully not too distant) future where life has more freedom, I revisited one of my pandemic journals from summer 2020 in the middle of the pandemic.

I'm nervous about going back to school in person. I want my family to be ok. I have to remember to breathe and that flexible is going to have to become my mantra this year. I have no idea when I will ever be on an airplane again. Anxiety is increasing not knowing what the school year will bring and being tired of the virus. Not knowing what risk is involved just by going to the store. Missing my family. Wondering how long I will have to wear a mask. I need to remember to breathe. The world won't always be like it is today.

Looking back in the summer of 2021 almost a year after writing those words, I notice I keep reminding myself to breathe, which I find interesting since patients who have the coronavirus complain of a lack of breath. I experienced challenges during the school year, but I found the strength to deal with each obstacle and motivate my students to experience the best year possible considering the circumstances. I somehow avoided catching the virus, and receiving a vaccine for the virus gave me hope. As I write these words now, the pandemic has not reached its conclusion, but the world seems on a path to get there soon.

One day in class before the pandemic, I discussed pain journals with my students and the importance of setting goals. I brought my black and gold sequined journal with me to discuss how I felt when experiencing neck pain. When looking over my notes, I realized I wrote my symptoms, pain levels, and how I felt. However, I had not written my goals. Bernstein (2019) advises, "affirm in your journal how you want to feel" (p. 29). While I learned from research how setting specific goals helps the healing process, I forgot this step when I became a patient. Following Bernstein's advice to "write your affirmation in your journal" (p. 29), I wrote:

I am in pain.
I want to get back to 100% pain free.
I believe I can get better with the help of my physical therapy team.
After I wrote my intention in my journal, was I suddenly pain free? No.
After I wrote my intention in my journal, did I still need to do my exercises? Yes.
After I wrote my intention in my journal, I articulated my goal, which helped me.
After I wrote my intention in my journal, I finally believed I would heal from pain.
My current pandemic affirmation is:
I am a resilient survivor.
I feel a myriad of emotions, which is okay.
I believe it is okay not to be okay.
I want to hug my family again, and I will soon.
I need to practice self-care during this pandemic.
After I wrote my affirmation in my journal, I felt better.

Just as a painter glides across a blank canvas with a paintbrush, the writer glides across a blank page with a pen. Heard (1995) writes, "when I return to writing, the lessons from art guide me. Painting and writing are both about relationships. In painting, paint thickness, brush strokes, image, canvas texture, color, and outline all work together. In writing, the words, images, rhythm, voice, and meaning must work together as well" (p. 119). In the stories captured in the pages of a journal, the writer may search for meaning instead of starting with a specific destination in mind. Journal writing focuses on the journey. During the process, the writer's voice, as unique as a speaking voice, shines through on the page. Trusting first impressions gets the writer closest to the truth of what is on the mind and in the heart. Cameron (1998) explains, "yes, writing is an art, but 'art' is part of the verb 'to be' – as in 'Thou art truly human.' To be truly human, we all have the right to make art. We all have the right to write" (pp. 232-233). Writing means connecting with the self and painting a picture with words.

THE PROCESS

If you want to begin your own writing story:

- Use writing to illuminate your narrative. Trust the words that appear on the page to capture the truth of your thoughts and feelings.
- Show yourself some compassion. No one is perfect. It's okay to feel what you feel.
- Take turtle steps. Whatever your personal journey may be, change takes time.

- Be authentic. No one else is you. Don't feel you need to pretend to be someone else on the page. It won't comment on your writing.
- Show grit. Passion and perseverance will help you achieve goals you set for yourself.
- Track progress. You do not have to reread previous writing, but it can help you see patterns and appreciate accomplishments.
- Share your story. You do not have to share your story, but a supportive reader can offer support and encouragement on your journey.

MY STORY

In my high school English classroom, I encourage my students to write in journals. This happened before the pandemic, happens during the pandemic, and will happen after the pandemic. I stand in front of teenagers who sit in their bright blue chairs as I show my own black and white composition book and give the instruction to just keep writing. I ask my students to show me their best writing, meaning there are pages I never read. I feel fine with that; students tell me the practice of writing helps them relieve stress, process their ideas, and become better writers. Fallon (2020) believes, "where we get unstuck in our writing, we get unstuck in our lives" (p. 34). One of my favorite teaching moments happens when I conference with each student about his or her writing process. Not only do students reflect on their writing during these conferences, but they also reflect on their lives. I notice that writing often shows me the path of where I need to go and what I need to do in my life.

Soon after my mom died, I never could have imagined my experiences of using writing to cope with grief would become something positive. Handler (2013) believes, "distance from the event that caused your grief can shed light that's necessary when you're writing about the tough stuff. What caused your grief is in the past, and your perspective has changed naturally as you've continued to survive" (p. 16). Not only did I survive, I used my pain to help other people.

I agree with writer Katie Dalebout (2016), who elaborates, "by putting these deep thoughts and fears down on paper, I acknowledged their presence – and was one step closer to releasing them, along with each of my failed attempts at control" (p. 9). Getting thoughts on paper transforms fears from the mind to the page and gives the writer the chance to let them go. Cameron (1998) compares writing to healing by stating, "writing is medicine. It is an appropriate antidote to injury. It is an appropriate companion for any difficult change" (p. 31). The simple act of putting pen to paper remains effective. Lamott (1994) writes, "there was a part of me that believed that my journal could be a gift for others" (p. 188). But if writing in a journal leads to healing, it also serves as a gift to the person writing it.

It did not prove as difficult as I thought it would to write about my mom's life. Bernstein (2016) believes, "true healing occurs when you give yourself permission to feel whatever feelings live below the triggers" (p. 44). Time provided comfort and fun nostalgia instead of tears when I wrote about my mom. Pennebaker and Smyth (2016) describe this as, "writing about emotional topics is more than learning how to put a story together. It is a way for us to learn more about our own emotions, relationships, and thought patterns" (p. 162). I linked my mom's story with mine to explore my own thoughts and feelings about both our experiences. Like Strauss (2010), "I wrote and wrote and listened close for whatever the past was trying to say to me" (p. 177). Getting to know my mom again through writing about her makes me proud to be her daughter.

As writer Anne Lamott (1994) observes, "you don't even have to know how or in what way, but if you are writing the clearest, truest words you can find and doing the best you can to understand and communicate, this will shine on paper like its own little lighthouse" (p. 235). May my writing serve as a lighthouse for others to find their way and may I continue to live a life that would make my mom proud of me.

YOUR STORY

Writing helps students in a classroom, patients in a hospital, and readers of this narrative who want to pick up a pen and write a new chapter. Sharp (2000) offers anyone wanting to write the encouragement, "someone who takes the time to sit down, perhaps with pen or pencil in hand, and express themselves in their own words – this is a person who has something to say and the commitment to say it" (p. 133). Everyone has a unique writing voice, so let your writing voice shine. Goldberg (1996) provides the reminder, "when you finish a piece, you're refusing to be silenced or ignored. Writing is brave" (p. 201). I encourage you to find the courage to share your story, whether you share it with yourself or a larger audience.

Practicing the art of expressive writing leads to emotional, physical, and spiritual healing. Cameron (2018) shares, "you direct your attention to the page, open your mind, and make the invisible visible by seeing what comes through on the page" (p. 45). She adds, "the greatest discoveries of your life could appear on those paper or on-screen pages" (p. 48). To begin your writing practice, start by writing whatever comes to your mind and see where it takes you. Hopefully by the time you read these words, the pandemic will be, if not over, closer to ending. The next chapter in your life is yours to write. Each day offers a chance to fill another blank page with your hopes and dreams. May you make the most of it.

ACKNOWLEDGEMENT

The preceding chapter contains excerpts from the following previous IGI publications:

Bird, J.L. (2020). Narratives of journal writing. In *Using narrative writing to enhance healing*. (pp. 269-294). Hershey, PA: Information Science Reference.

Bird, J.L., & Wanner, E.T. (2020). Narratives of research design. In *Using narrative writing to enhance healing*. (pp. 40-72). Hershey, PA: Information Science Reference.

Bird, J.L., & Wanner, E.T. (2020). Narratives of writing as healing. In *Using narrative writing to enhance healing*. (pp. 295-338). Hershey, PA: Information Science Reference.

Bird, J.L. (2019). Narratives of writing as healing. In *Healing through the arts for non-clinical practitioners*. (pp. in press). Hershey, PA: Information Science Reference.

Bird, J.L. (2017). Writing healing narratives. In *Healthcare community synergism between patients, practitioners, and researchers*. Hershey, PA: Information Science Reference.

REFERENCES

Anderson, C. M., & MacCurdy, M. M. (2000). Introduction. In C. M. Anderson & M. M. MacCurdy (Eds.), *Writing and healing* (pp. 1–22). National Council of Teachers of English.

Beck, M. (2008). *Steering by starlight*. Rodale.

Beck, M. (2012). *Finding your way in a wild new world*. Free Press.

Beck, M. (2021). *The way of integrity*. The Open Field.

Bernstein, G. (2010). *Add more–ing to your life*. Harmony Books.

Bernstein, G. (2016). *The universe has your back*. Hay House.

Bernstein, G. (2018). *Judgment detox*. North Star Way.

Bernstein, G. (2019). *Super attractor*. Hay House.

Brown, B. (2012). *Daring greatly*. Gotham Books.

Brown, B. (2015). *Rising strong*. Spiegel & Grau.

Brown, B. (2017). *Braving the wilderness*. Random House.

Caldwell, K., Gray, J., & Wolever, R. Q. (2013). The process of patient empowerment in integrative health coaching: How does it happen? *Global Advances in Health and Medicine: Improving Healthcare Outcomes Worldwide*, *2*(3), 48–57. doi:10.7453/gahmj.2013.026 PMID:24416672

Cameron, J. (1998). *The right to write*. Tarcher/Putnam.

Cameron, J. (2002). *The artist's way* (2nd ed.). Tarcher/Putnam.

Cameron, L. (2018). *The mindful day*. National Geographic.

Carter, C. (2015). *The sweet spot*. Ballantine.

Clandinin, D. J., & Connelly, F. M. (2000). *Narrative inquiry*. Jossey-Bass.

Conner, J. (2008). *Writing down your soul*. Conari.

Dalebout, K. (2016). *Let it out*. Hay House.

DeSalvo, L. (1999). *Writing as a way of healing*. Beacon Press.

Duckworth, A. (2016). *Grit*. Scribner.

Enayati, A. (2015). *Seeking serenity*. New American Library.

Evans, J. F. (2010). Introducing wellness & writing connections conference papers. In J. F. Evans (Ed.), *Wellness & Writing Connections* (pp. 3–10). Idyll Arbor, Inc.

Fallon, A. (2020). *The power of writing it down*. Zondervan.

Fitzgerald, F. S. (1925). *The great Gatsby*. Scribner.

Germer, C. K. (2009). *The Mindful path to self-compassion*. The Guilford Press.

Goldberg, B. (1996). *Room to write*. Tarcher/Putnam.

Goldberg, N. (1986). *Writing down the bones*. Shambhala.

Goldberg, N. (2007). *Old friend from far away*. Free Press.

Goldberg, N. (2013). *The true secret of writing*. Atria.

Gruwell, E. (2007). *Teach with your heart.*

Gruwell, E. (2009). *Teaching hope.*

Gruwell, E.Freedom Writers. (1999). *The Freedom Writers diary.*

Handler, J. (2013). *Braving the fire*. St. Martin's Griffin.

Haugk, K. C. (2000). *When and how to use mental health resources*. Stephen Ministries.

Hawthorne, N. (1955). *The scarlet letter*. Washington Square Press. (Original work published 1850)

Heard, G. (1995). *Writing toward home*. Heinemann.

Heifetz, R. A. (1994). *Leadership without easy answers*. The Belnap Press of Harvard University Press.

Johnson, L. (1998). *Two parts textbook, one part love*. Hyperion.

Lamott, A. (1994). *Bird by bird*. Anchor Books.

Matousek, M. (2017). *Writing to awaken*. Reveal Press.

Neff, K. (2011). *Self compassion: The proven power of being kind to yourself*. HarperCollins.

Niequist, S. (2016). *Present over perfect*. Zondervan.

Pennebaker, J. W. (1997). *Opening up: the healing power of expressing emotions*. The Guilford Press.

Pennebaker, J. W., & Smyth, J. M. (2016). *Opening up by writing it down*. The Guilford Press.

Rankin, L. (2013). *Mind over medicine*. Hay House.

Rankin, L. (2015a). *The fear cure*. Hay House.

Rankin, L. (2015b). *The anatomy of a calling*. Rodale.

Romano, T. (2004). *Crafting authentic voice*. Heinemann.

Romano, T. (2013). *Fearless writing*. Heinemann.

Romano, T. (2015). *Write what matters*. Zigzag.

Rushnell, S., & DuArt, L. (2017). *The Godwink effect*. Howard Books.

Rzeznik, J. (1998). Iris [Recorded by Goo Goo Dolls]. On City of angels soundtrack [CD]. Burbank, CA: Warner Brothers.

Sandberg, S., & Grant, A. (2017). *Option B*. Knopf.

Sharp, C. (2000). *A writer's workbook*. St. Martin's Press.

Strauss, D. (2010). *Half a life*. Random House.

Szabo, R., & Hall, M. (2007). *Behind happy faces*. Alegra.

Tindle, H. (2013). *Up: how positive outlook can transform our health and aging*. Hudson Street Press.

Wanner, E.T., & Bird, J.L. (2013). *The Wanner Bird healing survey for pain recovery*. Academic Press.

Wanner, E. T., Bird, J. L., & Brahler, C. J. (2016). Bring out your patient's inner writer for a better experience. *PT in Motion*, *8*(1), 62.

Whitman, W. (1993). O Me! O Life! In *Leaves of grass* (p. 341). Random House. (Original work published 1855)

Zimmermann, S. (2002). *Writing to heal the soul*. Three Rivers Press.

KEY TERMS AND DEFINITIONS

Anxiety: Different clinicians have different definitions of anxiety, and a person who lives with anxiety will describe it from a different point of view than a clinical definition in a textbook, but the general definition of anxiety is chronic fear or stress that can result in panic attacks and a person feeling an inability to cope with life's stresses.

Expressive Writing: Writing that is exploratory and focuses on meaning and first impressions.

Journal Writing: The process of responding to prompts and writing about thoughts and feelings. While journal writing is typically associated with writing classrooms, writing teachers including Julia Cameron and Natalie Goldberg advocate that journal writing can be done by anyone, anywhere.

Medical Professionals: People in the medical profession such as primary care doctors, specialists, physical therapists, and emotional therapists. Medical doctors Hilary Tindle and Lissa Rankin discuss that patients experience improved health when they have a positive outlook and a willingness to share their stories with their doctors.

Narrative Inquiry: Described by F. Michael Connelly and D. Jean Clandinin, narrative inquiry is a qualitative interpretative form of research which focuses on the telling, retelling, and sharing of stories.

Pain Journal: A journal describing symptoms designed to be shown to a medical professional.

Self-Compassion: The act of demonstrating the same kindness for oneself that one would demonstrate for other people.

Spirituality: Regardless of religion, spirituality and a belief in a higher power can lead to increased health and provide both hope and strength.

Writing as Healing: Numerous studies have been conducted investigating the influence of writing on physical and emotional health. James Pennebaker is a leader in the field which explores the health benefits of writing.

Writing Prompts: Questions used as starters to encourage writers to develop ideas.

Chapter 2
Reflections of Technology Narratives

ABSTRACT

This narrative explores the changing role of technology during the pandemic while simultaneously offering strategies for managing stress caused by the overuse of technology. Technology brings people together who cannot see each other in person, such as families who live in different locations and students who attend online classes. Technology serves the dual role of keeping people connected, especially during events such as a pandemic, and making people feel disconnected due to distraction caused by devices.

CONSTANTLY CONNECTED

It feels amazing how quickly time can change things. A few years ago, I wrote about how technology creates stress and why people don't need to feel constantly connected to their phones and other forms of technology. In the current uncertain pandemic era, I feel differently. Now, more than ever, people need technology and crave constant connection.

TECHNOLOGY REFLECTIONS (2020)

As the virus COVID-19 alters the way people live, technology becomes a valuable resource of comfort and connection. The high school in Florida where I teach taught the teachers a new platform for online learning on a Wednesday and five days later on Monday morning, the school closed for in-person learning. Instead of talking to the students in my classroom, we all turn on the cameras and microphones on our laptops to chat with each other. As of this writing, I feel fortunate. My school and the families of my students have the technology to implement this idea, while other schools scramble to find resources. I overbought paper products at a sale two months before businesses began to close, but now thank my past self for having the insight (or perhaps impulsive shopping habit) to stock up on necessities. I feel sad that I cannot take my planned trip to Texas to meet my cousin's newborn son, but thanks to technology

DOI: 10.4018/978-1-7998-9051-5.ch002

my cousin takes pictures on her phone and sends them to me. In a moment, all I write about now can change again. Will I long for this March moment a few weeks from now? Is this only the beginning to more life changes? I don't know the answers to the questions I ask on a daily (sometimes hourly) basis, but I do know that writing helps me find clarity.

TECHNOLOGY REFLECTIONS (2021)

March again. Almost a year since I wrote the words in the previous paragraph. A year since the pandemic began and life changed. My school began meeting back in person in September, in a world where everyone wears masks and everyone in the building surrounds themselves with plexiglass. My teacher's desk contains a large bucket of cleaning wipes and an assortment of hand sanitizers. The television in the back of my classroom connects to the technology platform Teams to welcome students whose families choose to keep them home. At least students at my school have a choice; some schools have not yet reopened for in-person instruction. I now live in a world where I visit my dad and stepmom who live less than an hour away and meet for "social distance visits" in their driveway because I don't want to touch them and risk getting them sick. I still wait to travel to Texas to meet my cousin's son, who just celebrated his first birthday. Thanks to FaceTime on my iPhone, I felt connected when my cousin helped him open the gifts I sent. I co-taught a class at my church on the online platform Zoom while joking that it was the first class I ever taught where I didn't need to wear shoes. I feel gratitude for the smallest moments which give me hope that life can and will change. My phrase "constantly connected" now means something different; it means using technology to stay connected to family, friends, teaching, and other people during an era when people truly need each other.

PANDEMIC DIARIES

As a writer, I capture this moment in time with my words. I write prayers and email them to the members of my church. I write lesson plans to ease the anxiety my students face. I conduct research and send the highlights to my friends in the medical field. I write a letter to my cousin's son and tell him about the first month of his life which thankfully he won't remember. I write to make myself slow down and breathe.

And I can thank technology for all of it. I still have electricity and a working laptop. I have a phone which keeps me updated on however much of the news I feel able to endure at any given moment. I use the same phone to text my friends and family to check on them. The technology I once described as causing stress now causes serenity.

Nevertheless, I don't regret writing the words I did in my previously published chapter from a few years ago where I critiqued technology. My mom used to tell me that if people knew how their life stories ended, they wouldn't take the journey. Ortberg (2014), believes, "for much of our lives, we live in the shallows. Then something happens – a crisis, a birth, a death – and we get this glimpse of tremendous depth. My soul becomes shallow when my interests and thoughts go no further than myself. A person should be deep because life itself is deep" (p. 57). Looking back, critiquing technology when all along I had the power to control that technology seems shallow, especially given the new social distancing society that is 2020. The depth exists in revisiting, reflecting, and perhaps even refuting old arguments. That chapter felt perfect at the time I wrote it, but now I find myself with a new perspective and more to say. Romano (1995) writes, "to write words that stick with readers you must have – or develop – faith in the validity of your feelings. You must be fearless in writing the words that emerge in your mind when you focus to compose" (p. 31). In writing with faith and fearlessness, I admit that the emerging circumstances of the pandemic caused me to see technology from a different perspective.

It feels surreal to think that this moment in time will appear in future history books. Someday we will look back and share stories and memories of this time. Look on the internet and find numerous organizations encouraging people living in this pandemic era to share their stories of how they coped so future generations will understand the life we led. Hale (2014) writes, "it is my hope that my story will inspire you to go out and live your own story a little more boldly and fearlessly" (p. 11). Time will tell if years from now a student in a classroom reads a story from the pandemic era and feels inspired. I believe, however, that it shouldn't matter what others think of our words as long as the writer finds meaning.

2018

It is not yet five in the morning. My alarm goes off, and as I reach over to shut it off, I grab my iPhone from my bedside table. I check the texts I received since I went to sleep, then check my email. I haven't even been awake for two minutes, but already I am typing a reply to a coworker that can certainly wait until I've had breakfast. My mind is racing thinking of my endless to do list before my feet even hit the floor. The tone has been set for the day, and I'm not sure it's a good one.

2020

It is not yet five in the morning. My alarm goes off, and as I reach over to shut it off, I grab my iPhone from my bedside table. I check the texts I received since I went to sleep, then check my email. I haven't even been awake for two minutes, but already I am typing a reply to a coworker that can't wait until I've had breakfast because online school will soon begin. I check the news headlines to stay informed. My mind is calm with gratitude for all I still have in my life before my feet even hit the floor. The tone has been set for the day, and I become determined to make it a good one.

2021

It is not yet five in the morning. I am lacing my Nikes for a walk around the neighborhood before getting ready for school. In the past week I joined friends for a Zoom brunch (where we all made our own food at home and ate together while meeting on the online platform), taught classes online using Teams (another online platform), and connected with my family through FaceTime on my iPhone. The large amount of screen time makes me determined to focus on my mental health and not become overwhelmed by pandemic fatigue. Someday I will hug my family again. In a time when it becomes easy to become disconnected, it becomes even more essential to use technology to stay connected. I possess the power to set the tone for the day, my classroom, and my life.

2021 (A Few Months Later)

In May, on my birthday, I finally hugged everyone in my family for the first time in over a year because all of us received our vaccines. I will never take hugging people for granted again.

TECHNOLOGY AND STRESS

Technology makes the world a better place by connecting people. My out of state relatives are only a text message away, and we send each other pictures on our phones to bridge the distance between us. It makes my life as a writer and researcher easier to know a wealth of information awaits only a mouse click away when I type key words into a search engine. The flip side of the advantages of technology, however, is that we as a society are constantly connected. This constant connection may bring a feeling of stress.

When my parents were my age, they had a landline to call people. Before the invention of answering machines, if someone wasn't home, a call was missed. Even with an answering machine, my parents had to wait until they got home to know who called them. Their dinners at restaurants and trips to the movies were not disturbed by phone calls. Granted, they were difficult to reach if there was ever an emergency, but true emergencies are few and far between. My parents could actually look into each other's eyes at dinner. How many times have my friends and I been at a restaurant and everyone is looking at their cell phones instead of each other?

When my parents were my age, if they were gone when a favorite television show was on, they missed it. Thanks to the invention of the VCR, they could record their favorite shows, but only one show at a time. Members of my generation tend to get overwhelmed by the volume of television shows and all the recording options.

When my parents were my age, it may be difficult to fathom they lived in a world without social media or email. My mom wrote handwritten letters to her family and friends. My dad left work at the office and the only inbox he ever had to check was the paper one on his desk. Email brings people together while simultaneously making it difficult to disconnect. How many times have I been distracted by the ping of an email without seeing the consequences of my inability to focus? Technology itself is not stressful; it's the reaction by people to the technology that often creates stress.

STAYING CONNECTED

Technology has made the world a better place by keeping people connected during difficult times. My out of state relatives, as well as my relatives who live near me but who I cannot visit because of the quarantine, are only a text message away and we send each other pictures on our phones to bridge the distance between us. I love research, and as much as I love the feeling of books in my hands, it is comforting to know a wealth of information exists only a mouse click away because most of my books are not with me but still in my classroom at school. I once wrote that the fact we as a society are constantly connected may bring a feeling of stress. Now, I feel people would feel more stress if unable to keep the constant connection to each other as a lifeline.

I relate to Niequist (2016), who writes, "I bet it all on busyness, achievement, being known as responsible, and escaping when those things didn't work. What I see now is that what I really wanted was love, grace, connection, peace" (p. 63). How many times did I refer to my life as crazy busy when talking to other people and wear the label of accomplishment as a badge of honor? I don't know what the future will bring, but I know I don't want the crazy busy life I led before the pandemic back again. Brown (2012) believes, "one of the most universal numbing strategies is what I call crazy-busy. I often say that when they start having twelve-step meetings for busy-aholics, they'll need to rent out football stadiums. We are a culture of people who've bought into the idea that if we stay busy enough, the truth of our lives won't catch up with us" (p. 137). When I feel disconnected, I avoid that feeling by staying busy. Staying connected offers more value for me than staying busy. I need to learn silences are okay and I actually achieve more if I have time to reflect instead of being in constant motion. And if I don't achieve at all, that's okay too.

Based on my previous research, I of all people should know how stress affects health. Soukup (2016) explains, "reducing our exposure to the things that cause stress is something that each of us can and should begin to work on. Our health depends on it" (p. 181). Stress results in negative effects on health; emotional stress often results in physical symptoms. Lyons (2017) observes, "most of us carry chronic stress for so long we no longer recognize the weight of it" (p. 165). Only after researching stress and its consequences did I realize I needed to heal myself before I could teach others the lessons I learned. Over and over again, I return to the lessons I learned when I feel stressed. I'm not perfect at managing stress but I now know my triggers and can deal with them sooner. I know when I need to take a break and rest and when I need to move my body by taking a long walk. Leonard (2018) learned, "it wasn't just my body that needed rest; my soul needed it as well" (p. 224). I go to my doctor for physical health checkups and learned to go to my therapist for mental health checkups. I nourish my body with healthy food, so remind myself to nourish my soul with things which bring me joy.

One strategy that helps manage stress involves awareness of thought patterns. Hollis (2019) explains, "You have to choose to be positive, to see possibility, and to see the blessings in your life each day. You choose your thoughts, and there isn't one thing running through your mind that you don't allow to be there" (p. 200). While some days I feel happier than on other days, I remember I always have a choice with my outlook. If I feel sad, I need to let those emotions out too, whether by crying, talking to someone, or writing in my journal. Hollis (2018) elaborates, "our words have power, but our actions shape our lives" (p. 17). If I write something in my journal which concerns me, I need to ask for help. If my words indicate I feel stressed, I need to take action to manage it. I say I want to control technology, but need to take action to put away my phone for awhile or temporarily turn off the news. I make a list of all the things I want to do once the pandemic ends, but still need to take steps to achieve my dreams and goals.

When choosing outlook, writers choose how to best share their narratives. Tindle (2013) writes, "aspects of outlook can be contagious, and just as one person can serve as ground zero for the spread of disease, a single person with a healthy attitude can have a halo effect on friends, family, neighbors, and coworkers…and you see where it can go from there." (p. 217). If the experiences which surround us, such as the current stress of dealing with a worldwide pandemic, seem beyond control, the thing still within control becomes the method of coping with stress. Brickman (2015) provides the reminder, "there is a good chance you're stressed if you walk around caught up in your own head and don't really see much around you" (p. 3). Just now, writing these words, I look up from the computer screen and out the window at the yellow flowers on the tree in my neighbor's yard. We find things of beauty and moments of peace even in the midst of stressful times. Hopefully by the time you read these words, I will have finally gotten on a plane to visit my out of state family.

LETTERS TO TECHNOLOGY (THEN AND NOW)

2018

Dear Technology,

I love you, but we need to take a break. I am not a person anyone would describe as mellow, but my stress level has been increasing recently. I am feeling like I have no downtime and feeling that I always have to be on without any breaks. Even now as I write this I am checking my phone for text messages. People know how to find me, so why I am I so concerned that I am going to miss something? This has to stop.

Best wishes until we meet again,
Jen

2020

Dear Technology,

Two years after I wrote that somewhat amusing breakup letter, I feel I can relate to the character Elizabeth Bennet in the novel "Pride and Prejudice" after she initially rejected Fitzwilliam Darcy. Fortunately, they gave each other another chance, just as I must show willingness to give you another chance. Now I appreciate the ability to check my phone for text messages to know the people I love are okay. And when I described the feeling of having no downtime? Since spending a significant amount of time at home lately with more downtime than I ever imagined, I realized that, while you became complicit in my actions, I take ownership for causing my own stress.

Best wishes and sincerest apologies,
Jen

INFORMAL TECHNOLOGY EXPERIMENTS (2018)

I decided to complete informal technology experiments because my life was becoming consumed by email. I would check my email periodically throughout the day, only to stop whatever activity in which I was currently engaged to answer the email. As you probably already know, email is a wonderful resource. The reality is that most people do not have the time to pick up a pen and write a handwritten letter, but they do have time to type a few lines from their phone or computer keyboard. Information can be transmitted quickly, and an entire conversation takes place in a matter of minutes if both people are checking their email.

However, email should not be used in place of real conversations. Several of my friends eventually found true love on dating websites, but sitting at a computer sending emails back and forth wasn't going to make a true connection. That could only be done in person. The same applies for work issues. Emails can't convey writing voice or subtle nuances. If your colleagues work down the hall, consider chatting in person occasionally. If your colleagues work across the country, consider picking up the phone and calling them. Email is an incredible technological tool, but not when it takes the place of in person conversation.

ADDITIONAL REFLECTIONS (2020)

I laugh now as I read my writing from two years ago. In this current moment in today's sequestered society, I can't walk down the hall to chat with a colleague in person; our contact is limited to contact through videoconferencing and email. Email is an incredible technological tool, especially when in person conversation cannot take place. I also learned I can send emails and write handwritten letters without having to choose one or the other.

Back in 2018, I completed two informal technology experiments. I recount them here as originally written and then share my commentary.

INFORMAL TECHNOLOGY EXPERIMENT #1: NOT SENDING EMAILS TO MY PHONE

I stopped sending my email to my phone for a month. It feels weird. Now whenever I want to check email I have to go to an actual computer. No more grabbing my phone as soon as I open my eyes in the morning. I have to admit it also feels kind of nice. I wake up, feed my two cats, go for a workout, eat breakfast, get ready for work, and then check emails. I'm not missing much. In fact, there isn't anything in my email inbox that couldn't wait while I was sleeping. Sure, I know the information a few hours later, but if someone needed an instant response they have my phone number and can call me. No one called me about a work issue and now that I've eased into my day I feel that I deal with things easier. I like this.

One Month Later.....

I confess I couldn't keep it up. Despite the peacefulness of easing into my day, I started sending emails to my phone again. I just felt like I was going to miss something. But is reading emails before I do anything else in my day really how I want to live my life? There is a time and a place for everything, and like I learned the past month, emails become a part of life without consuming it.

Two Months Later.....

I have managed to find a balance in my life; just because an email goes to my phone doesn't mean I have to read it as soon as it arrives. If something is important, I will receive a phone call or text. Most email is not urgent and will wait until I have time to read it. I now save designated times during the day to check email.

INFORMAL TECHNOLOGY EXPERIMENT #2: LEAVING MY PHONE AT HOME

I confess I am guilty of needing to know the constant whereabouts of my beloved iPhone. Too often I look down at my phone when I should be looking up at my surroundings. So for a month I decided not to bring my phone to church with me. Granted, my church is within walking distance of my home and I have a large group of friends who attend my church. If I had car trouble, I could walk home. If I needed help, numerous people would volunteer. I sing in the choir at my church, so I have a limited of amount of things I carry with me anyway, and why do I need to have my phone with me when I am trying to concentrate on the minister's inspirational message? This worked for about three weeks. One week the choir director asked us all to pull out our cell phones for a special musical number. I hurried home to get my phone. I now bring my cell phone to church, although it is turned off during the service.

So what did I learn from my informal technology experiments? With both of them, it became about finding a balance between using helpful technology and not letting that technology consume too much of my time. While email and the apps on my iPhone enhance my life, they are not a substitute for interaction with other people. During a conversation, I need to look other people in the eyes instead of talking to them while looking at my phone. There are also times when it becomes beneficial to put my phone away with the knowledge that time spent with others is more meaningful than any content that might appear on my phone screen.

As previously mentioned, taking this advice is not easy. I admit that while writing these paragraphs, I have paused to check my email several times because of fear of missing something. I have also responded to several texts and admit it took me a short time after each one to regain my train of thought for this chapter. I am reminded I need to get better at setting boundaries with technology and realize that understanding people will wait for a response.

2020 VISION

Several popular clichés exist to describe the current year, such as hindsight is 20/20 and 20/20 vision. In the case of my informal technology experiments, hindsight does indeed provide additional clarity and perspective. When looking at email all the time on my phone, that became my own decision. Even though the technology existed, I always had the choice to use it or not to use it. I became better when setting boundaries, and now the emails on my phone seem almost like a nonissue because I, not the phone, will decide when to read them.

As for not taking my phone to church, I wish I had that option now as my church has gone to online services only. Someday I will sing with the church choir again, but it remains a comfort to know I hear an inspirational message and powerful music while watching on my phone from the confines of my living room couch.

In the play *Our Town*, Wilder (1938) has the character Emily say, "It goes so fast. We don't have time to look at one another" (p. 100). I felt that way about life before the pandemic, and one unexpected benefit of life slowing down out of necessity is the time to look at people and things with more time and detail. My favorite line from the play *Our Town* is when the character Emily asks the Stage Manager, "do any human beings ever realize life while they live it? – every, every minute?" (p. 100), to which the Stage Manager replies, "no. The saints and poets, maybe – they do some" (p. 100). Sometimes I let the little moments in life pass me by while thinking of something else. Bernstein (2019) shares the valuable advice, "there are many ways to make appreciation a habit. A great way is to begin your day with it! Write three to five pages of appreciation in your journal every morning" (p. 161). I started following this advice only I decided to write in my journal in the evening instead of the morning. Every evening, I get out a pen that writes in pink neon ink to write about things which made me feel grateful during the day or moments I enjoyed. I appreciate the moment of gratitude and reflection before I sleep.

ADDITIONAL REFLECTIONS (2021)

Last fall, my beloved cat Andy lost his battle with cancer and I put away the gratitude journal and the pen that writes in pink neon ink. I felt grateful that Andy blessed my life for sixteen years. I felt grateful that my cat Lucy comforted me as much as I comforted her. I felt guilty because people I knew lost a loved one to the coronavirus while I grieved the loss of a cat. I felt angry because my loss felt important to me. For once, I didn't want to write anything even though I endlessly tell people about the value of writing as healing. Technology helped me in the form of old pictures and videos on my phone which showed Andy healthy, happy, and playing with Lucy. I have yet to pick up my gratitude journal again, but feel thankful I took the time to slow down and write in it. The enforced free time due to the lockdown and change of lifestyle caused by the pandemic gave me the strength to cope with another loss. Life changes; coping methods change with life.

DISCONNECTED (2018)

It is the middle of the week, and I am finished with work for the day. My family members have other plans on this weekday evening, and I am too tired from a busy day to call friends and go out for the evening. So I send some emails and text a few friends. Even though I have communicated with them, I feel restless and disconnected. Texting someone is not the same as looking a person in the eyes or sharing a hug. I open the YouTube app on my iPhone and discover that old television shows from my childhood are only a few clicks away. I watch a few clips, but don't feel the same happiness I did when I originally watched the shows years ago in the living room of my childhood home with my family. I talk to my cats, Lucy and Andy, just to be able to hear the sound of my own voice and know someone is listening even if they can't reply with anything other than a meow. I have difficulty sleeping and wake up the next morning tired, completely defeating the purpose of a quiet evening at home.

CONNECTED (2020)

It is the middle of the week, and I am finished with my online work for the day. I wish I could go out for the evening, but stores (except the grocery) and restaurants remain closed. I text my family members and enjoy the communication, knowing I feel grateful and connected. Texting someone is not the same as looking a person in the eyes or sharing a hug, but it is the only option I have right now. I open the YouTube app on my iPhone and watch a few clips of silly pet tricks, laughing because I know my two cats, Lucy and Andy, would never let me set up an obstacle course in the living room and film them. Even though chaos exists in the world and I will face more stressful news headlines in the morning, I feel calm as I fall asleep immediately.

STILL CONNECTED (2021)

March arrives again. My family and friends enjoy the group text messages we created. We send pictures to each other. Distance doesn't feel as far. Chaos still exists in the world, but hope exists too. I tell my students to find things in the world for which they feel grateful. It forces me to find things which make me feel grateful.

I JUST HAD TO CHECK THAT TEXT MESSAGE (2018)

I am at the doctor's office in the middle of an appointment. The doctor has left the room for a moment to check on another patient. My phone is on silent, but I hear it buzz. What is in that text message? I debate for a moment. I am in a doctor's office. I have greater priorities at this moment in time other than the content of that text message, such as making sure I ask my doctor all the medical questions I have written down so I don't forget anything. But what if something has happened to someone in my family? What if there is important information in that text that cannot wait until I leave the doctor's office? I probably have a couple minutes before the doctor returns, so I quietly creep over to my purse and steal a glance at my phone. The pharmacy is informing me that I have a prescription ready. It was nothing that couldn't have waited. Even though no one saw me, I am embarrassed. Why did I think that text message was so important that I had to interrupt something even more important to check it? I am reminded of the billboards I see on the interstate urging drivers that text messages can wait, that nothing in that phone is worth a life. At least I wasn't driving. I make a mental note to be more mindful, to perhaps even turn my phone to off and not silent when I am involved in something serious such as a doctor's appointment, or when I am involved in something fun such as a meal with family or friends where we all put our phones away and take the time to look at each other.

WAITING TO CHECK THAT TEXT MESSAGE (2020)

As I walk into my doctor's office for bloodwork which cannot be postponed, I observe all the medical practitioners wearing masks and gloves. Chairs in the waiting room face the wall, forcing people not to sit next to each other. It doesn't matter; appointments have been scheduled so I am the only patient in the waiting room. I choose not to sit and stand looking out the window. When my name is called I walk back to the lab, watching as the chair is disinfected in preparation for my arrival. The team still jokes with each other and maintains a sense of humor. No way am I even thinking of checking for text messages, not only because my arm has a needle in it while blood is drawn, but also because I refuse to touch my phone until I use the hand sanitizer I have in my purse on the walk to my car, get home to wash my hands for the required minimum of twenty seconds, disinfect my purse with an alcohol wipe, and wash my hands again.

I would love to be able to have the things I worried about two years ago, or even two weeks ago, be my biggest concerns.

TIRED OF TEXTING (2021)

Each writer has a voice. Romano (2004) believes, "our voices are shaped by the places where we learned language – in our parents' arms, at our school desks, in the neighborhood, on playgrounds and streets" (p. 6). Text messages, a valuable part of technology, have their own language. The sender of the text message attempts to capture voice and tone, although sometimes confusion results for the reader. Fletcher (2013) explains, "voice in writing has to do with a unique personality-on-paper" (p. 78). Voice also relates to a unique personality on a screen in the form of a text message. But sometimes I need a break from typing. As another form of connection, and because I need to hear the speaking voice of someone instead of reading a writing voice, I dial the phone.

VOICE LESSONS

Usually when people think of voice lessons, music comes to mind first. Writing voice shines through when writers follow the advice Goldberg (2007) gives, which is, "say what you want to say, not what you think you should say" (p. 2). Goldberg (2013) tells writers the same words in another publication, and they are worth repeating because you need to "say what you want to say, not what you think you should say" (p. 22). Voice also influences how writers share their stories, such as how I choose to tell this one in a series of short narratives. In order to write what is truly on our minds and in our hearts, Goldberg (2013) gives the advice, "in the face of all inner – and outer – resistance and opposition, just write. Pick up the pen and face yourself" (p. 179). Through writing, I face myself, I face my fears, and I face my life lessons.

I use the pronoun "I" to own my stories and share my writing personality. Heard (2002) believes, "the more you include yourself in the piece and are able to tell your unique story, including your particular details, the more we, as readers, can experience it too" (p. 54). It becomes possible to write first person narratives while simultaneously including research and the citation of sources as part of the stories; therefore, you are reading narratives with a scaffold of research as the objective research frames the subjective narratives. This type of research is called narrative inquiry. Clandinin and Connelly (2000) explain, "voice, and dilemmas created by the consideration of it, are always sorted out by the exercise of judgment" (p. 147). Each writer makes the judgment call of how to present his or her story. Clandinin and Connelly (2000) write, "when narrative inquirers are in the field, they are never there as disembodied recorders of someone else's experience. They too are having an experience, the experience of the inquiry that entails the experience they set out to explore" (p. 81). In her research about vulnerability, Brown (2012) used a form of qualitative research called grounded theory and explains, "stories are data with a soul and no methodology honors that more than grounded theory" (p. 252). Clandinin and Connelly (2000) acknowledge the similarities between grounded theory and narrative inquiry and elaborate, "narrative inquirers tend to begin with experience as lived and told in stories" (p. 128). We skate a thin line on the ice between artistic narratives and technical research as we let our voices sing.

When a writer's voice shines through in a composition, it is like the writer is in the room having a conversation with the reader. Goldberg (2000) discusses voice in writing and explains, "if I had consciously looked for a writing voice, I might have missed it" (p. 143). If writers try too hard to find a voice, their true personalities often don't appear. Just like people sometimes silence their speaking voices, they similarly silence their writing voices. But listening to one's voice leads to acceptance of the present moment. Lamott (1994) describes writing voice as, "and the truth of your experience can only come through in your own voice" (p. 199). Seeing words on a page encourages action because the writer can no longer ignore the truth of life experiences.

By not censoring ourselves, we illuminate what we truly need and want. We start making plans for how to get to where we are in the present to where we want to be in the future. It gives a person hope that the present situation won't always be the way it is now. Connelly and Clandinin (1988) explain, "narrative unity is a continuum within a person's experience and renders life experiences meaningful through the unity they achieve for the person" (p. 74). Reflecting on the past helps the writer determine how to move from the present to the future by finding the unity in a life narrative.

Often writers ask themselves questions such as: What do I say? How do I say it? Heard (1995) encourages writers to speak and shares, "as I walk, I write. Words circle my head. I speak lines out loud to see how they'll sound" (p. 32). Sometimes writing happens in the mind before a writer ever puts pen to paper or fingers to computer keyboard. This prewriting process, often called percolating to capture the image of an idea brewing just like coffee before it can be shared, is valuable. Nevertheless, an idea will forever remain in the writer's mind unless he or she finds the voice to speak it or write it. Lamott (1994) advises writers, "you need to trust yourself, especially on a first draft, where amid the anxiety and self-doubt, there should be a real sense of your imagination" (p. 112). That self-trust is how we as writers find our voices that always remained with us; we just need to find the courage to share.

FINDING BALANCE BY EMBRACING A CURRICULUM OF CHANGE

I witness both sides of technology. On the one hand, one piece of technology, my computer laptop, enables my fingers to fly over the keys and make my ideas reality. On the other hand, another piece of technology, my iPhone, keeps distracting me from this writing. Yet, my beloved iPhone has made my life easier and better with all its apps, from the map app that keeps me safe and keeps me from getting lost, to my photo apps that allow me to preserve my family's memories.

To integrate technology into our lives without letting it overwhelm us, it helps to borrow a page from the playbook of curriculum design and integration. Beyer (1996) explains, "the belief that significant educational and social change is possible has been fueled by a number of forces – both theoretical and practical" (p. 16). Even though twenty years have passed since that statement was written, the sentiment remains the same. Both theoretical and practical forces fuel change. For example, in theory it would be nice to tell people to only use cell phones at certain times of the day if they are going to be a distraction. But in practice, people remain attached to cell phones and depend on them. The compromise, therefore, is to find a balance and that balance will be different for everyone. For example, my family has agreed to put the cell phones away during dinner so we have time for conversation with each other. Other families may have different boundaries for technology. With technology and stress, answering some questions helps set and maintain boundaries. Does using this technology at this moment in time make me happy and enhance my life, or does it bring me additional stress?

Continuing with the theme of curriculum integration, Beane (1997) provides the information, "the ideas that people have about themselves and their world – their perceptions, beliefs, values, and so on – are constructed out of their experiences" (p. 4). Past experiences provide insight for how to help live in the present moment as well as set goals for the future. For example, my informal technology experiences such as not sending my email to my cell phone made me more present in each moment and overall more relaxed. Remembering that feeling will help me integrate that strategy into my life. Connelly and Clandinin (1988) believe, "from the point of view of curriculum the idea is that the curriculum a person has experienced is found in that person's overall past record of experiences in private life as well as in professional life" (p. 20). When maximizing technology use in your life while simultaneously minimizing stress, design your curriculum of a personal philosophy and live it.

STRESS RELIEF STRATEGY #1: SELF-COMPASSION AND CONNECTION

Whether caused by technology or another source such as life during the pandemic, stress may feel overwhelming. Perhaps from the tone of my writing voice in the last passage, you could infer that I wasn't being too kind to myself. It would have helped if I practiced self-compassion and did not mentally beat myself up for what I thought was a wasted evening of my life watching YouTube videos. Neff (2011) describes self-compassion as, "if we can compassionately remind ourselves in moments of falling down that failure is part of the shared human experience, then that moment becomes one of togetherness rather than isolation" (p. 65). I am certainly not the first person to use technology to waste time, and I will certainly not be the last. Therefore, the fact that I am willing to share my story in this chapter will perhaps cause you as the reader to smile, relate to it, and know that you are not alone either. Germer (2009) concurs, "self-compassion is the foundation for kindness toward others. When we're accepting of our own idiosyncrasies, we become more accepting of others" (p. 87). And kindness and connection with others leads to less stress.

Even though I attempted to connect with friends through text messages, I didn't feel as happy as when I see them in person. I needed more connection than a text could provide. Rankin (2013) discusses the value of community and explains, "chronic social isolation can lead to loneliness, and multiple studies demonstrate that loneliness can trigger stress responses in the body, the same kind of fight-or-flight responses fear of bodily harm can elicit" (p. 93). Being part of a strong community helps reduce both loneliness and stress. Used well, technology brings people together. A text message reminds a person that a loved one is thinking about him or her. Skype enables people across the country and even around the world to see each other. But there is a time for technology and a time to get out of the house and get together with people in person. During the pandemic, when people may not have the opportunity to leave the house and see loved ones in person, technology builds a bridge.

Some people find strength in spirituality and their community in churches. Spirituality provides comfort in times of need. Hale (2013) believes, "just like a puzzle, it takes time for all of the pieces in your life to come together" (p. 142). It feels disappointing when a story doesn't have the ending you want, but that means it becomes time to write another story and have faith in the new narrative. Interestingly, while writing these words, the puzzle I put together on my dining room table has a piece missing. I suspect my cat Lucy knocked it on the floor. The puzzle still looks beautiful with a missing piece. Life still looks beautiful, even with missing puzzle pieces.

Furthermore, while some people find their community in a church, a church is not the only place to go for community connection. It is possible to find community in a gym, in a classroom, or around a table in a restaurant. No one needs to experience social isolation and there are numerous opportunities to reach out and connect with others. Germer (2009) believes, "connecting with others is another form of self-care – to stop isolating" (p. 108). He explains that this is important because "a sense of isolation can turn even ordinary unhappiness into despair or minor anxiety into dread" (p. 108). Technology brings people together in the form of a community of practice, where a group uses technology as a platform to share their ideas and collaborate on projects.

Whether it is directed toward self or others, compassion becomes essential for increased health and happiness. Neff (2011) shares, "one of the most robust and consistent findings in the research literature is that people who are more self-compassionate tend to be less anxious and depressed" (p. 110). She discovered that self-compassionate people had lower levels of the stress hormone cortisol and concluded, "self-compassion gives us the calm courage needed to face our unwanted emotions head-on" (p. 124).

Remaining calm lowers stress while helping people assess a situation and take ownership of their emotions. The next time you make a mistake or feel isolated and lonely, try to be kind to yourself and rely on your community where others will demonstrate kindness toward you. Self-compassion becomes especially essential during the pandemic. We're all in this together, so give yourself grace.

STRESS RELIEF STRATEGY #2: FOCUS ON YOUR HEALTH

Concerned about something you looked up on an internet search engine or worried about a friend's post on social media? It may influence your health. Tindle (2013) reports, "anxiety, self-doubt, and related thoughts and feelings are associated with increases in blood pressure, heart rate, and stress hormones such as adrenaline and cortisol, all of which pound our organs like waves on the beach" (p. 100). Tindle discusses that a positive outlook leads to better health, and one way to change outlook is through exercise because "physical activity can temporarily catapult you out of the territories of depression, relapse, and other unsavory outlook addresses long enough to get your bearings and steer yourself in a different direction" (p. 138). For specifics about the right exercise plan for you, consult a physician or physical therapist. Rankin (2013) provides additional insight from a doctor's perspective and elaborates, "there's something powerful that gets set in motion when we believe, without a doubt, that we will get well and are supported by clinicians who share our optimism" (p. 17). A positive attitude cannot cure the coronavirus or any other illness, but a positive attitude from the patient and the medical team can make a difference during the patient's recovery process.

If you are experiencing stress, meditation helps. Beck (2008) provides the reminder, "remember, you can't force this kind of calm; pressuring yourself to feel no anxiety merely creates more anxiety" (p. 101). It becomes very easy to focus on what you don't have, but stopping for a moment to think about gratitude and what you do have is an effective method of relaxing and relieving stress. Beck (2001) advocates facing fears and addressing anything that may be creating stress, and she describes an experience where writing down her anger at a situation helped with her back pain because "as soon as I wrote it down, I felt a tingle along my own spine, and the pain in my back relaxed significantly" (p. 195). As you will read in the next section, writing serves as a valuable resource for stress management; however, before you continue reading take a deep breath and give yourself permission to let go of any stress you may be feeling today. Tindle (2013), a doctor of internal medicine, also refers to mindfulness and explains, "this is called the triangle of awareness, in which we remain mentally centered in the midst of our thoughts, feelings, and physical sensations, each of which represents a point on the triangle" (p. 104). You can't control a pandemic, but you can choose to exercise, eat nutritious food, and get enough sleep in order to deal with the stress life may bring.

STRESS RELIEF STRATEGY #3: WRITE YOUR STORY

Stressed? Pick up a pen and put it to paper or let your fingers roam over the keyboard of your computer. Cameron (1998) elaborates, "writing gives us a place to say what we need to say, but also to hear what we need to hear" (p. 83). Writing, whether handwritten or typed, enables expression because a piece of paper or the computer screen won't criticize the writer. Pipher (2006) discusses the value of blogs because "writing a blog is instant self-publication, which is its own special kind of creativity" (p. 200).

While technology allows blogs to be shared with a large audience, writing does not have to be shared if the writer does not wish it to be. Nevertheless, some writing needs sharing. During the pandemic, my commitment to write included handwritten notes sent to family and friends as another way of staying connected.

While value exists in sharing written words, writing has healing benefits even if no one sees the words except the writer. Brickman (2015) believes journaling is a great method of self-exploration because, "it is a wonderful way to explore your life and figure out what's working and what's not. You'll also find reviewing your journal at the end of the year a great way to explore your accomplishments and figure out what you want to do over again" (p. 104). Writing helps reveal the stories we are telling ourselves. We choose the path our writing takes. Goldberg (1990) states, "think of something now that you sincerely want to tell and go ahead and tell it" (p. 7). We might share our writing with a trusted medical professional who can see patterns to our pain. We might publish our writing in a blog and share it with readers we may not even know. Or we might keep the writing private in a journal, letting the page worry about an issue so we experience a little less stress and perhaps a little more sleep. Heard (1995) believes, "the task of every writer is to dig beneath the surface and find complexity in each situation" (p. 45). Life can be complex. Stories can be complex. Your story is your story. Sharing it, even with only yourself, helps you heal physically, heal emotionally, and relieve stress.

Sometimes people don't want to share their writing because it makes them feel vulnerable. Cameron (1998) elaborates, "vulnerability requires that we contradict ourselves. It requires that we change our minds. It requires that our perspective shifts" (p. 148). Reflecting on thoughts and feelings means being vulnerable. The script in a person's head may read: What if someone doesn't like the real me? What if I don't like the real me? Heard (1995) believes, "memories darkened by ages of forgetting are still inside somewhere hiding, waiting for the right smell or touch to unlock them" (p. 86). Writing reveals the memories lurking in the corners of my mind, and if the script in my head annoys me, writing helps me rewrite it to remind me that I still like myself even if other people don't. Fallon (2020) elaborates, "but that's what writing will do, again and again. It will call us back to ourselves. It will make us the strongest, most resilient, most beautiful versions of ourselves – the truest "us" that's been there all along" (p. 76). Writing reminds us who we are, what we want, and how we can find a path to get there.

STRATEGIES FOR MANAGING TECHNOLOGY

Technology enhances people's lives. Cameron (1998) describes that technology enhances writing, "because it is instantaneous, email tricks people into evading their censor" (p. 33). While the use of email, like other technology, enhances people's lives, too often people abuse the technology. Carter (2015) asks the questions, "Do you check your email, texts, voicemails, Facebook, Instagram account, or Twitter feed within an hour of waking up or going to sleep? While you're in line at the store? During dinner with your family? Would you check it at church while waiting for a funeral to start? If so, ya ain't alone" (p. 97). Carter explains that there is a reason for such behavior. She elaborates, "there is something gratifying about constantly checking our email and social-media feeds. The distraction is pleasurable because it gives us what researchers call 'variable ratio reinforcement.' In other words, we are drawn to our smartphones in the way we are drawn to slot machines. We never know when we'll get a satisfying message on Facebook or an email with good news, so we just keep checking" (p. 97). Even though people rationalize their actions, it doesn't mean their actions lead to healthy behavior. Brickman (2015) observes, "so far, I haven't missed any career or life-changing moments by not facing the morning with a first-thing phone fling" (p. 20). He recommends easing into the morning before checking technology.

Brown (2012) discusses research on anxiety and elaborates, "when it comes to anxiety, we all struggle. Yes, there are different types of anxiety and certainly different intensities. Some anxiety is hardwired and best addressed with a combination of medication and therapy, and some of it is environmental – we're overextended and overstressed" (p. 143). Brown observed differences between two groups of people and discovered, "participants from both groups often used today's dominating technology as an example of an anxiety-producing source during the interviews" (p. 143). While both groups shared the experiences of anxiety from technology, one group found ways to manage the anxiety while the other changed behaviors that led to anxiety. Brown provided the example that the first group constantly checked emails and made sure they were all answered although sometimes at the expense of sleep, while the second group asked people not to send unnecessary emails and indicated it might take several days for a reply. Brown concluded, "when we asked that group about the process of setting boundaries and limits to lower the anxiety in their lives, they did not hesitate to connect worthiness with boundaries. We have to believe we are enough in order to say, 'Enough!'" (pp. 144-145). Because abuse of technology possesses the potential to cause anxiety, it helps to set boundaries for technology use.

Carter (2015) concurs that there is a connection between technology and anxiety with the explanation, "even though our brain tends to seek that variable ratio reinforcement, which suggests pleasure, usually we aren't consciously checking our email for fun or recreation. We check constantly to abate our anxiety that we are missing something" (p. 98). Carter offers suggestions such as disabling push features that provide instant alerts on phones and computers, designating spaces in which technology will be used, and deciding on times when not to use technology. She concludes, "what all this means is that unless we want to feel overwhelmed and exhausted, we need to unplug. A lot" (p. 99). Following this advice may not seem easy, but it becomes necessary for a life filled with less stress.

Enayati (2015) discusses the connections between technology and stress and explains, "the effects of stress are compounded by the fact that we are rarely turned off and are always connected. Stress in its various forms has access to us at all times. In the old days people got up and were able to go for a walk to get away. Now we are never far from all sorts of bad news. The solution: turn it off! Go on technology fasts" (pp. 158-159). Enayati concludes, "we can choose narratives that help us reframe stressors, thereby strengthening our ability to withstand (or avoid) the stress coming our way and to counter it with positive emotions" (p. 159). Choosing and reframing a narrative changes a person's perspective on stress and anxiety.

REVISING A TECHNOLOGICAL LIFE

At the high school where I teach, technology is integrated into the curriculum and every student has a laptop. As I reflect on potential obstacles and opportunities, I know students look to me to set the tone of the classroom. My motivation involves helping students by making their lives a little bit easier. Connelly and Clandinin (1988) believe, "program implementation may be done in heavy-handed ways or in very subtle ways" (p. 148). In my classroom before the pandemic, I designed subtle transitions between asking students to handwrite their ideas in a journal, type essays on their laptops, put down the computer screens for a conversation about literature, and then asking students to conduct internet research. It becomes possible for all of these teaching methods to coexist in a creative classroom. In the era of online learning, I embrace the numerous resources which enable students to download a writing prompt, type the essay on their computer, and upload their final draft. I read students' compositions on my screen without worrying about collecting physical papers.

My classroom, like my life, will have both goals and boundaries for technology, which I will continue to reflect on and revise. Much like writers revise their compositions, people have the opportunity to revise the lives they compose. Welch (1997) states, "we become, as we write and revise, exposed to competing ideas of ourselves and to competing social forces that would shape our voices and beliefs" (p. 50). I know now to reconcile the competing forces of my love for technology and the stress I sometimes feel when overwhelmed by it.

Through reflection on the words I wrote two years ago compared with the words I wrote last year as well as the words I write today, I realize that even though technology causes stress if used excessively or inappropriately, it provides a source of solace during uncertain times. Hale (2015) offers the encouragement, "we often reach for the 'sure things' in life because they seem easier. More convenient. Less scary. But I urge you to save some room for the unexpected" (p. 194). In the years 2020 and 2021, when every news story brings more uncertainty about the future of society due to the coronavirus, technology becomes the sure thing which unites people with each other.

As Zimmermann (2002) discusses, "write about ways you can light a candle. You can learn from your sorrow and somehow help others to better endure their own. You can grow from the pain you have experienced and share with others what you've learned" (p. 180). Before the pandemic, on the first day of every new class I taught, I gave each student a candle and reminded them they can be the light in the lives of others and if they are going through a difficult time a little bit of light is all they need until life gets better. During the pandemic, everyone needs that reminder. Handler (2013) also uses the light metaphor and writes, "many writers have gone across that bridge before you. Their experiences and the ways in which they chose to write about their loss shine a light on your path" (p. 5). Through writing, we use our experiences to reach back across the bridge and light the way for others to follow, even when, during online learning, the light which shines the way beams from a computer screen.

FINAL REFLECTIONS (2021)

As I write these words, the pandemic has lasted over fifteen months, from March 2020 to the current time in June 2021. The pandemic appears close to the end, but news stories still show people suffering around the world. I wonder what lessons I will ultimately take with me from my experiences and what pandemic narratives I will ultimately tell. I know I do not want my life after the pandemic to become a mirror image of life before the pandemic. I want to take more time for self-care, less time for stress, less time for text messages, and more time for actual conversations. Through everything, I remain grateful for the technology that, while sometimes becoming a distraction, also helped keep me sane and connected with other people.

ACKNOWLEDGEMENT

The preceding chapter contains excerpts from the following previous IGI publications:

Narrative Inquiry: Described by F. Michael Connelly and D. Jean Clandinin, narrative inquiry is a qualitative interpretative form of research which focuses on the telling, retelling, and sharing of stories.

Self-Compassion: The act of demonstrating the same kindness for oneself that one would demonstrate for other people.

Story Sharing: By sharing a story with a supportive audience, either in conversation or in writing, it frees the storyteller of unneeded physical and emotional stress caused by holding the story inside and worrying about it. Brene Brown explains that it helps people to share stories instead of numbing pain with unhealthy choices.

Writing as Healing: James Pennebaker is a leader in the field which explores the health benefits of writing. Numerous studies have been conducted by researchers investigating the influence of writing on physical and emotional health.

Writing Voice: Voice in writing describes how a writer uses word choice and tone to reflect the unique personality of the writer. Just like each person has a unique speaking voice, each writer has a unique writing voice.

Chapter 3
Reflections of Health Coaching Narratives

ABSTRACT

This narrative focuses on a health coach collaborating with a physical therapist and working with the emotional needs of physical therapy patients, but anyone looking to improve health can use the strategies presented. Integrative health coaching incorporates vision and values into a person's goal-setting process. Health coaches provide resources such as journal writing to assist the healing journeys of patients as well as strategies for healthy people who want to make wellness behavior changes.

HELP FROM HEALTH COACHES

During the pandemic era, numerous patients suffer from the coronavirus. Visitors and family members no longer crowd hospital waiting rooms awaiting news of loved ones. Instead, patients experience procedures and treatments alone except for their caring medical team. Medical teams wear personal protective equipment (PPE) as they work long hours saving lives. Some patients recover quickly, while others need a long rehabilitation. Whether they recover from the coronavirus, another illness, or injury, patients need a supportive team after they leave the hospital. Health coaches have the potential to make a difference for patients recovering from the coronavirus because health coaches play an essential role in helping patients maintain optimism and focus to achieve healing goals.

BACKGROUND OF INTEGRATIVE HEALTH COACHING

Integrative health coaches (IHCs), such as the ones trained at Duke University Integrative Medicine where Jen received her training, focus on an eclectic approach to healing. The Wheel of Health from Duke Integrative Medicine (2010) encourages patients to reflect on multiple dimensions of health including movement, exercise and rest; nutrition; personal and professional development, physical environment;

DOI: 10.4018/978-1-7998-9051-5.ch003

relationships and communication; spirituality; mind-body connection; and mindful awareness (p. 5). This makes health become a comprehensive plan that focuses on the person, not just the disease.

Health coaching and conversations about the responses to both written and numerical subjective questions help patients illuminate the health stories they tell themselves. Health coaching builds a bridge between helping patients decode complex medical terms and comprehending their treatment plan. When patients feel that their medical practitioners and health coaches earn the right to hear their stories, the sharing of narratives leads to healing conversations. Health coaches are not psychologists; if a patient wants to share a painful story about the past, the health coach will make a referral to a psychologist. Instead, health coaches help patients maintain forward momentum for achieving their goals by providing encouragement, suggestions for completing a prescribed treatment plan, translation of potentially confusing medical terms, and a supportive person to listen.

Since health coaching is a new field in medicine, there is not a large amount of previous studies to share. Simmons and Wolever (2011) report, "broadly defined, health coaching is a method of working with patients that utilizes thoughtful inquiry, accountability, goal clarification, goal setting, identification of obstacles, use of support systems, and connection to intrinsic motivation, vision, and values to improve health through positive behavior change" (p. 1). Simmons and Wolever summarize the existing research and elaborate,

Despite the infancy of the research, several studies have demonstrated that coaching does improve health outcomes. The strongest findings have been in cardiovascular health, where coaching has been shown to improve total cholesterol, body mass index, stress, exercise, diet, and smoking cessation. Studies of cancer patients have demonstrated decreased pain severity and increased pain control. Studies of coaching for patients with diabetes and related kidney disease have shown increases in health promoting behaviors like physical activity and diet, as well as decreases in fasting blood glucose, hemoglobin A1C, hospital admission rates, and amputations. A coaching intervention also improved outcomes in obese patients (BMIs >30), including decreased waist circumferences and increased functional health status. (p. 1).

Heath coaches inspire patients to become educated about a diagnosis and treatment plan as well as collaborate with the medical experts who want to help with the healing process.

FROM THEORY TO PRACTICE

To best help people, health coaches practice active listening and ask questions to know more about the narratives people tell themselves and others. Narrative insights provide as much valuable information as numbers on a patient's chart. Helldorfer and Moss (2007) believe, "we are players on a hallowed stage, writing our own lines as we perform" (p. 182). Health coaching requires the strength of listening to people's stories and finding themes in the narratives. Patients complete a combination of numerical subjective and written subjective questions about their current and desired states. They rank numerically on a scale of 1 (low) and 10 (high) how they feel about different aspects of health and respond to a corresponding writing prompt explaining why they assigned that number. The health coach needs to read the writing, pull together the narrative threads, and connect them into a cohesive theme. The following technique and observation section is written in general terms to protect patient confidently.

Eric, a physical therapist, and Jen, a health coach, worked with staff members at a hospital who had a physical health issue such as back pain, knee pain, or neck pain. Several staff members at the hospital wanted to use health coaching to enhance their physical therapy sessions, so Eric would complete a physical therapy evaluation followed by Jen's health coach evaluation. Eric gave the patients specific exercises to complete or performed appropriate manual techniques after diagnosing their condition, while Jen talked with them to assess the importance of the treatment plan to them and their confidence in completing the treatment plan. This helped us see the patient's barriers to the recovery process so we could help the person overcome those barriers. This process made a positive difference in patients' healing and has been very rewarding for us as practitioners.

Because health coaching is individualized for each patient, Jen adjusted the questions she asks based on the patient responses. Some questions that health coaches ask include the following:

Describe your future health vision. What does it look like to you? How does the treatment plan that your physical therapist gave you connect to that vision? Rate on a scale of 1-10 (1=low, 10=high) how important the treatment plan is to you. (Questions then diverge depending on patient responses. The purpose of the questions is to align the treatment plan with the patient's value system). Sample question for low number response: What are some things you could do to make the treatment plan more important to you (listening to music during exercises, writing in a journal, setting goals, etc.)? Sample question for high number response: Now that I know this is really important to you, tell me on a scale of 1-10 (1 = low, 10 = high) how confident you are accomplishing this treatment plan. (Questions then diverge depending on patient responses. The purpose of the questions is to provide the patient with a vision of success). Sample question for low number response: Tell me more about a past success you had when you achieved a goal. Sample question for high number response: Are there any obstacles we haven't addressed that would prevent you from achieving your goal?

At the conclusion of the health coaching session, Jen offered suggestions for the patient based on the patient's response, but the purpose of health coaching is not to tell the patient what to do; the purpose is to empower the patient to take ownership of his or her own health. Jen provided resources as needed, such as giving the patient a notebook if he or she wanted to write in a journal.

JEN'S PERSPECTIVE

I'm sitting in an exam room reviewing a patient's responses to short answer writing prompts while Eric completes a physical therapy evaluation on the same patient. The patient has responded to the prompts before the combined physical therapy/health coach session. As the patient answers Eric's evaluation questions, I write notes on the writing prompts. I'm studying voice and tone as well as pulling out themes from the writing in a similar manner to how I study the essays written by the college students I teach. The responses align. The diagnosis Eric makes with his medical evaluation aligns with my observations from the patient's writing responses. It's all connected.

ERIC'S PERSPECTIVE

It is very helpful to listen to the patient during the evaluation process in take in how they are truly feeling. Most of the time they lead you down the correct path for their diagnosis. Listening to patients allows for more accurate diagnoses and better outcomes. If the patient can tell that you are truly listening to them they might be more compliant with your treatment intervention you design for them. Patients can become more motivated if they feel they are doing the right thing to get better and more enthused to reach their goals. Health coaches act as a catalyst to the patient's healing process helping them overcome barriers or obstacles in their way. They help the patient come up with ideas for how they can become more compliant with their home exercises and have them set goals to add to their accountability. I think this is a key component for all types of patients, especially ones that have had chronic pain. Those are usually the most difficult to treat since there can be many different things that developed over time, and on top of that the patient usually develops a psychological component thinking that they will never get better. This only makes things worse. Health coaches break down that barrier and let them know that they can have that ability and it might just be that staying compliant with a treatment intervention including consistency with their recommended home exercises is that missing component. This is a new thing in the health field and very exciting seeing the results.

OBSERVATIONS AND INSIGHTS

Visualization makes a difference. Jen led one patient through a visualization exercise while the patient completed Eric's prescribed exercises. The patient's leg lifted higher when visualizing a calm nature scene as opposed to talking about something stressful. Visualization techniques also help people imagine what they want to achieve. Hanging a picture or symbol of a past accomplishment on the wall is a method not only to celebrate past success, but also to envision future success.

People appreciate accountability. Clients who are not receiving physical evaluations but have health goals they want to work on appreciate checking in to give updates on their progress. It makes Jen smile when people find her for a quick check in to report success with their goals. While one of the purposes of health coaching is for people to feel self-empowerment, it always helps to have a health coach to celebrate progress. In sports, the coach motivates, but it is the individual or team who runs plays and scores points. The same applies to health coaching. The health coach motivates, but it is the individual who completes a personalized health journey.

There is value in making progress. As a baseball fan, Jen loves using the extended metaphor that baseball players can hit the ball a little over three out of every ten times and receive a batting average that still lands them in the hall of fame. Progress is not an all or nothing journey. If someone has what feels like a setback on one day, there is always tomorrow to make progress. Health coaches can't wave a magic wand like a fairy godmother in a children's story and make everything go away. Change takes time, and progress, even a small amount, can eventually lead to large changes. Jen has a necklace with two charms, an elephant and a turtle. It's symbolic meaning? Always remember to slow down.

Coaching increases enthusiasm. The word excited has been mentioned frequently as people feel empowered to take control of their lives. Additionally, coaching gives people permission to take time for themselves without feeling selfish. People in helping professions often selflessly give to others without taking time for self-care. Several 'aha' moments happened when practitioners receiving coaching realized they cannot control others, such as a patient who won't get out of bed, but they can control their reactions. If practitioners feel happy, the happiness becomes a ripple effect that leads to happy patients.

Health coaching focuses on vision and values to help people build bridges and make connections between where they are now and where they want to be. Health coaches work with people who are mostly healthy but want to make lifestyle changes such as getting more sleep or eating healthier. Health coaches also work with patients by helping them align their vision and values with the treatment plan prescribed to them by a medical practitioner such as a physical therapist. Cameron (1998) believes, "we need to decide that we will, one, write no matter what and, two, share that writing no matter what" (p. 135). Health coaches frequently ask people questions to guide them to their goals, ask them to write their goals, and then share the goals to achieve ownership of the accomplishments. However, once a patient finishes a session with a health coach, it becomes his or her responsibility to take the necessary steps to achieve the goals. Family members who are willing to act as cheerleaders for their loved ones during the process serve as an additional source of support during the healing journey. Like pages being turned in a book, health coaches encourage patients to write the next chapters in their health stories.

It may be physical pain that causes a patient to walk through the doors of a physical therapy clinic for treatment, but the patient's emotional outlook contributes to physical healing. In addition to talking to a health coach, writing encourages patients to share their narratives, which may help physical therapists make a diagnosis and adjust a treatment plan as needed. Even though a session with a health coach cannot heal physical pain or take the place of a treatment plan prescribed by a physical therapist, it helps patients discuss their narratives and help them eliminate emotional barriers that may impede physical healing.

HEALTH COACHING AND PHYSICAL THERAPY

Health coaches work in settings such as clinics, private practice, and hospitals; their purpose is to encourage patients to envision success and set goals to accomplish results. Caldwell, Gray and Wolever (2013) elaborate, "the major tenets of the health coaching process, then, are patient-centeredness and patient control focused around patient-originated health goals that are accomplished within a supportive coaching partnership" (p. 56). Due to health coaching's success in other medical fields, it has the potential to be successful with physical therapy patients.

According to the American Physical Therapy Association (APTA) (2021), "as we continue to live with COVID-19, many outpatient physical therapy providers could see a surge in 'long COVID,' which the National Institutes of Health now refers to as post-acute sequelae of SARS-CoV-2 infection, or PASC" (https://www.apta.org/patient-care/public-health-population-care/coronavirus/management-of-patients). During and after the pandemic era, while physical therapists focus on physical healing, health coaches focus on emotional healing. In addition to goal setting, health coaches help with stress management and healthy behavior as patients deal with lifestyle changes in addition to pain.

Health coaches work with both physical therapists and patients to ensure the accomplishment of goals. Bezner (2015) discusses the value of the emerging field of health coaching and explains, "the American Physical Therapy Association (APTA) has recently undertaken an effort to identify and create resources to support physical therapists and physical therapist assistants to incorporate approaches that promote health and enhance wellness into physical therapist practice" (p. 1436). Resources include health coaches to focus on the emotional side of healing and goal setting for patients. While some physical therapists and physical therapist assistants are also health coaches, more frequently physical therapists are partnering with health coaches so the patient has another supportive person on his or her team during the healing journey. Due to the large number of patients that physical therapists and physical therapy assistants treat in a day, they may not have time for lengthy conversations with patients about motivation. A supportive medical team consisting of a physical therapist, health coach, and other compassionate caregivers provide encouragement and accountability.

PARTNERSHIP WITH PATIENTS

Patients bring their own vision of a healthy life as well as their personal values into their narratives of experience. Health coaching focuses on aligning a person's vision and values to goals so the person develops ownership. The goal, therefore, becomes something the person wants to do (intrinsic motivation) instead of something the person is told to do (extrinsic motivation). Illuminating values leads to encouragement; health coaches consistently connect a patient's goals to vision and values in order for people to see connections to the goals in their lives and feel excited about achieving them.

As they begin a treatment plan, patients want to feel better, but how do they get there? Sometimes the road ahead may seem long and overwhelming. The process is following the road to healing in small, manageable, yet productive steps. If the treatment plan a clinician provides is not important to a patient, the patient will be less likely to want to accomplish it. It therefore becomes the role of the health coach to determine what the patient values and how the patient will align the treatment plan with his or her values to achieve improved healing gains. If the patient is not confident he or she can accomplish the treatment plan, the patient will also be less likely to comply with it. Once patients become non-compliant it is not possible for them to get satisfactory results. The health coach provides a vision of past success for the patient to build momentum in order to achieve future success.

Numerical subjective questions focusing on a number scale and written subjective questions featuring open ended short answer prompts assess importance, confidence, and expression of priorities to present a snapshot of patient motivation. If an exercise treatment plan is not important to a patient, if a patient is not confident in completing the plan, or if a patient expresses other emotional barriers, the health coach will partner with the patient to develop an action plan for overcoming obstacles and accomplishing goals. Increasing patient motivation through importance, confidence, and expression leads to behavior change. Behavior change and a transformation in outlook possess the potential for increased patient compliance of a treatment plan.

While each patient will most likely have a series of treatment goals set for them, such as a plan of exercises to complete at home designed by a physical therapist, a health coach will encourage a patient to align that treatment plan to personal goals, as well as align the treatment plan to vision and values. A patient may not want to complete exercises as part of a treatment plan prescribed by the physical therapist, but the patient may want to go on a family vacation. By asking open ended questions as well as summarizing and reflecting the patient's statements, the health coach helps the patient find connections between the value of spending time with family, the vision of a pain free vacation, and the treatment plan. The patient realizes how the goals set by the physical therapist (a certain number of exercises per day) relate to the personal goal of a vacation (more quality time with family). Writing down a goal also leads to accountability. Beck (2001) advises, "forming a goal, especially if you write it down and visualize it, creates a search image that programs your brain to focus on anything resembling or leading to that objective" (p. 303). Whether they are short term goals of being pain free or long term goals about health and life, capturing them on paper and displaying them in a prominent place becomes a powerful reminder to stay motivated.

Health coaches serve as another member of the team for both patients and clinicians. Steele (2009) encourages medical teams "to develop the tools and systems needed for effective and consistent patient education and expectation setting" (p. 99). Such tools, according to Jones, Brady, and Gaunt (2009), include "a diary showing type of surgery and progress" (p. 100) and "homework sheets that contain exercises and assignments for patients outside scheduled PT sessions" (p. 100). Health coaching provides patient education for patients. As Helldorfer and Moss (2007) explain, "one important component in the way many medical facilities measure success is by the degree of patient satisfaction. How patients feel about the care they are receiving starts with first impressions. Taking the time to look a patient in the eye, say hello, and ask them how they feel is an ongoing challenge when we are busy" (p. 275). Health coaches follow up with patients about how they are feeling and provide a continual assessment for clinicians of how important each patient feels about the treatment plan and his or her confidence in achieving it. An example of continual assessment would be a physical therapy patient who tells the story that they have no time to complete their at home exercise plans. The patient may develop an initial plan of completing exercises at home in the evening before falling asleep. However, the competing priority of the need for sleep at the end of the day wins and that plan doesn't work. The health coach helps the patient develop the idea that it makes sense to complete exercises during an uninterrupted time instead of trying to fit exercises in during the day and adjusts the plan to complete exercises first thing in the morning.

BE SMART AND SET GOALS

Goals provide people with something to strive for in life. Whether a teacher teaches a lesson plan, a physical therapist designs a treatment plan, or an individual sets a personal goal, the acronym SMART can be used to describe the goals. Soukup (2019) explains, "it's basically the idea that your goals should be Specific, Measurable, Attainable, Relevant, and Time Bound. Meaning you should know exactly what you are trying to do; your goal should be quantifiable in some way; it should be something you can actually accomplish; it should be meaningful to you; and it should have a deadline" (pp. 102-103).

Health coaches trained at Duke University Integrative Medicine encourage clients to think SMART (specific, measurable, action oriented, realistic, timed) when setting goals. Professors at Florida Atlantic University encourage students training to be teachers to think SMART (specific content, measurable outcome, attainable action verb, resources, timeframe) when planning a lesson. Physical therapists use a similar goal setting procedure for their patients as well. Randall and McEwen (2000) elaborate, "we define functional goals as the individually meaningful activities that a person cannot perform as a result of an injury, illness, or congenital acquired condition, but wants to be able to accomplish as a result of physical therapy" (p. 1198). While the SMART acronym is not explicitly stated in the discussion of functional goals, the procedure is implicitly described as patients are encouraged to collaborate with their physical therapist in goal setting. Randall and McEwen advise therapists,

Often the best way to identify patient-centered functional goals is simply to ask the patient, 'What are your goals for therapy?' In our experience, patients seldom focus on impairments and rarely say, 'I'd like my range of motion to be within normal limits' or 'I'd like to have 5/5 strength.' They are likely to respond with a focus on functional limitation or disability: 'I want to return to work,' 'I need to be able to take care of myself at home,' 'I want to play in the game on Saturday,' or 'I want to do what the other kids do at my school.' These statements can become the starting point for writing measurable patient-centered functional goals. (p. 1199).

Furthermore, health coaches use a similar approach as physical therapists for encouraging patients to set their goals. When talking to a health coach, patients also tend to focus on a personal vision instead of the treatment plan, such as perhaps not valuing the exercises but wanting to go on a cruise in a couple months. The health coach helps the patient make the connection that the exercises provided by the physical therapist will help accomplish the goal of going on the cruise. Health coaches encourage patients to dream big but also be realistic to avoid disappointment. Coates (1999) emphasizes, "goals must be realistic in terms of patients' situations and expectations, their likely length of contact with health professionals, the available resources and the abilities of the educators" (p. 84). Goals also give patients a sense of control. Kolt (2003) discusses goal setting with athletes and explains, "by having a sense of control over their rehabilitation programs, athletes can increase commitment and adherence to the behaviors required for successful rehabilitation" (pp. 176-177). The same philosophy that applies to athletes applies to any patient recovering from an injury or any individual looking to create change in their lives. Brown (2012), a professor of social work, believes, "hope is a combination of setting goals, having the tenacity and perseverance to pursue them, and believing in our own abilities" (p. 240). The biggest gift health coaches and physical therapists give their patients is the gift of hope.

Health coaches, just like physical therapists, use reflective listening to identify themes in a patient's story. Croft (1980) provides the example that "because of the frequency and intensity of therapist-patient verbal and nonverbal interaction, each therapist must consider the potential therapeutic or destructive power of his every response. An effective response is one that fulfills one or more of these processes: clarification, reflection, interpretation, facilitation, or silence" (p. 1035). Such conversations lead to what Randall and McEwen (2000) call writing patient-centered functional goals because "after the therapist and the patient have decided on general outcomes of physical therapy, measurable goals leading to achievement of the outcomes should be identified" (p. 1200). With health coaching, patients set personal goals for themselves in addition to the treatment goals set by the physical therapist. The purpose is that if a patient becomes empowered to feel both extrinsic (external) motivation from the physical therapist as well as intrinsic (internal) motivation from within, there will be a stronger ownership of the goal. Randall and McEwen continue, "we also believe this approach to writing patient-centered functional goals will make therapy more effective and meaningful for patients, and perhaps for the therapist as well" (p. 1202). The encouragement from physical therapists, health coaches, and other medical practitioners on the team lead the patient to feel supported and not alone on the healing journey.

Sometimes when patients experience pain, they can't picture what it feels like to do the things they love again; therefore, the power of visualization helps patients set goals. Beck (2001) discusses how visualization helps people achieve what she calls Wildly Improbable Goals (WIGs) and elaborates, "the thing was that, even though I didn't really think I could attain these goals, from the day I wrote them down I had something in my little brain that scientists might call a 'search image.' A search image is a subconscious alertness toward something you hope to find" (pp. 302-303). Writing a list of goals or using a form of artwork such as a dream board collage helps people picture what they wish to accomplish. Beck continues, "forming a goal, especially if you write it down and visualize it, creates a search image that programs your brain to focus on anything resembling or leading to that objective" (p. 303). Of course, simply visualizing a goal without taking any action won't lead to results. As Beck advises, "try to visualize every step you must take to realize the WIG you've got stuck on your planning board.

If you don't know exactly – and I mean exactly – what you must do to achieve your WIG, your scheme still needs elaboration" (p. 309). The key to setting a successful goal means thinking about what you want to achieve, not what anyone else in your life thinks you should accomplish.

According to Caldwell, Gray, and Wolever (2013), "health coaching entails a specific structure and provider relationship that reinforce each other. The coach-patient relationship is specifically centered on the patient's health goals and supporting the patient in those goals" (p. 55). Health coaches partner with the patient's medical team to align the patient's personal goals with the treatment goals and help the patient achieve the goals. Beck (2001) advocates, "today, take one turtle step toward your goal. Just one" (p. 323). A turtle step is a little step that, taken with numerous other little steps, leads to success.

Granted, patients often have healing goals set for them, such as when a physical therapist makes a goal for a patient to be able to ambulate independently throughout the community for up to 300 feet to be able to safely get groceries after two weeks of treatment. If patients set their own goals which align with the prescribed treatment plan, they will be more likely to comply with that plan. And if patients need help setting personal goals in addition to the treatment goals set for them by the physical therapist, a health coach guides the patient through the goal setting process. Arterburn (2011) believes, "whether it is a physician, a health practitioner, a counselor, or a trusted friend, the need to connect during the pain-to-healing process is profound" (p. 104). When a patient feels encouraged by a strong health care team, everyone celebrates the progress toward goals regardless of the speed at which those goals are achieved. "Thinking like a turtle," or making slow and steady progress, leads to elite results. So celebrate the small victories; turtles make slow progress, but they eventually arrive where they need to go.

HEALTH COACHING: THE MISSING LINK IN COMPASSIONATE CARE

As anyone who has ever been a patient can tell you, being a patient is not easy. Helldorfer and Moss (2007) elaborate, "patients enter a hospital with many unspoken fears. Most of the time they don't say a word either because they're not in touch with their feelings or they're embarrassed to express them. Some do not want to make waves. For the most part, they have an underlying belief in the technical proficiency of the professional taking care of them, yet most of them secretly yearn to be reassured anyway that they are in good hands and that we care as much about their well being as they do. We can take our profession to the next level by understanding our patients' needs beyond the unspoken" (pp. 50-51). As much as medical professionals such as doctors, nurses, and physical therapists want to be able to have long conversations with their patients, health care frequently has to focus on productivity with doctors needing to see a certain amount of patients in any given hour due to continual reimbursement cuts from insurance companies. Rankin (2013) reformed her own medical practice after learning the value of nurturing care instead of always having her hand on the door when talking to a patient and elaborates, "I now firmly believe that positive belief and nurturing care turn off the stress response, trigger the relaxation response, and return the body to its natural state of psychological rest so it can do what it does best – heal itself" (p. 79). While Dr. Mark Greene was a character on the medical drama *ER* and not a real life doctor, his advice to colleague Dr. John Carter describes today's real hospitals as well as fictional television ones: the staff of the hospital sets the tone for how patients feel about their treatment.

Furthermore, taking time to talk to patients is not contradictory to efficiency. Jones, Steele, and McClennan (2009) explain, "improving patient satisfaction and patient outcomes while reducing costs will create more value in our healthcare system" (p. 28). A patient feels happier when he or she feels a medical professional sees a person, not just a description on a chart. To do this, Jones, Steele, and McClennan continue, "we must tap into their values and preferences as much as possible" (p. 32). Vision and values are the additional piece of the healing process that health coaching provides. As summarized by Smith and Wroth (2011) the integrative health coaching process begins with vision and values, then proceeds with assessment, focus, readiness to change, goal setting, preparation for action, action, and maintenance (p. 59). Most treatment plans begin with a medical practitioner setting goals for patients. The patient is more likely to accomplish the goals if he or she feels ownership and that the treatment plan aligns with his or her vision and values. Jones, Steele, and McClennan (2009) add, "in addition, patients appreciate being made part of the solution" (p. 34). Health coaching encourages patients to set their own goals in addition to goals prescribed for them. While compassionate clinicians provide patient education and empathy, health coaches become an additional person on the patient's health care team. Health coaches assist patients by helping them frame their goals in easy to comprehend language while being an empathetic presence in the patient's life.

Health coaches provide patients with the gift of being present by practicing mindful awareness to remain focused on the present moment. Helldorfer and Moss (2007) state,

"to be a healing presence, we must be genuinely present to the other person in need" (p. 170). This means the focus must be on the current patient, not on the long to do list that needs to be accomplished. Even within the fast pace of a hospital, it becomes important to slow down. Helldorfer and Moss explain, "within health care, our mission is to foster the health and healing of our patients. It is easy to forget that before we can bring a healing presence to others, we first have to slow down to be present" (p. 180). In fact, health coaches refer to the people they help as clients instead of patients to provide a different connotation to the professional relationship that implies a partnership instead of a doctor issuing a prescription. Health coaches partner with their clients to facilitate the change process. Pipher (2006) explains, "with our presence and attention, we suggest that honest exploration of issues is healing and that hiding from them is toxic" (p. 86). While psychologists help patients process past experiences, health coaches focus on the present moment to help clients build a vision for the future.

Narratives also enable health coaches to better understand their patients. Clandinin and Connelly (2000) introduce the theory of narrative inquiry by explaining, "for us, life – as we come to it and as it comes to others – is filled with narrative fragments, enacted in storied moments of time and space, and reflected upon and understood in terms of narrative unities and discontinuities" (p. 17). They continue, "in narrative inquiry, people are looked at as embodiments of lived stories" (p. 43). Learning a patient's narrative means the health coach helps determine the life vision and values which will motivate the patient. While health coaches use psychological theories in their practice, the difference is that psychologists use narratives to help patients understand the past, whereas health coaches use narratives to help patients set goals for the future. Psychologist Clark (2018) discusses the value of both writing and talking to someone as, "journaling talking with a friend, and attending talk therapy all share the common thread of identifying and understanding one's experiences" (p. 343). While not psychologists like Pipher and Clark, health coaches are trained in psychology and provide patients with a safe space to explore issues and obstacles that may prevent them from reaching their healing goals. Pipher (2006) continues, "facilitating a change process in clients or readers often involves orchestrating situations that allow for aha experiences" (p. 101). This is why health coaches listen more than they talk during a session and use reflective responses so a client hears his or her own words and perhaps have an 'aha' moment. Health coaches partner with patients to advance their health and accomplish this by reviewing patients' health narratives, assisting patients in setting goals, promoting positivity, helping patients rewrite their health story, and supporting patients on their healing journey.

PROMOTING POSITIVITY

When Jones, Brady, and Gaunt (2009) speak of coaches, they are talking about family members instead of health coaches as they advise, "one of the coaches' responsibilities is to come to post-op group therapy classes, where they act as assistant physical therapists. Coaches encourage their loved ones and are shown and taught the dos and don'ts by the physical therapist. Many times, coaches are equipped with digital counters to ensure completion of the activities. If no family member is available, hospital volunteers often take up the coaching role" (p. 102). Family members as coaches serve as an additional source of encouragement for patients as they complete their physical therapy treatment plan. Throughout the family coaching process, health coaches provide education and support for the families of patients. While family members will have the best intentions when serving as coaches for their loved ones, it is easy for the family to become emotionally involved because the outcome of the patient's progress affects the entire family. Health coaches provide encouragement, while providing objective distance often missing when family members coach their loved ones. Health coaches care about their clients, but they are not attached to the outcome like family members are and will provide observations family members are sometimes unwilling or unable to see unfolding due to being too close to the situation.

Health coaches also share resources for family members to take care of themselves as they take care of their loved ones. Most importantly, health coaches work with physical therapists to "teach the teachers," the family member who will take over the patient's care once the patient returns home. The importance of this is once the patient goes back home there will be a continuity of care for the patient while he or she is awaiting home physical therapy and then outpatient physical therapy. This may lead to quicker recoveries for patients. And if everyone, from the health coach to the family to the patient to all the members of the medical team work together, the beneficiary is the patient. Helldorfer and Moss (2007) share, "and, if we think through the domino effect of our work, the life we save or extend impacts families almost beyond comprehension" (p. 191). Health coaching starts or continues a positive ripple effect; drop a pebble into a pond and see how far the water spreads. As teachers know, students remember their words long after classes end. Brady and Vega (2009) observe, "the best way to learn is to teach" (p. 128). Nevertheless, as Brady and Vega continue, "most places lack a teaching and learning culture, because no one has organized it" (p. 128). Health coaches do not give lectures like professors in classrooms, but they provide teachable moments for patients. Just like coaches of sports teams, health coaches intertwine education and encouragement to help patients keep a positive attitude while shifting motivation from the extrinsic of doing something just because a doctor says to the intrinsic of doing something because of a sense of personal accomplishment.

Maintaining a positive attitude helps patients heal. Medical doctor Lissa Rankin (2013) describes the medical science behind the connections between positive attitude and healing as "when our beliefs are hopeful and optimistic, the mind releases chemicals that put the body in a state of physiological rest, controlled primarily by the parasympathetic nervous system, and in this state of rest, the body's natural self-repair mechanisms are free to get to work fixing what's broken in the body" (p. 29). She elaborates, "if, however, the mind thinks negative beliefs, the brain perceives these as a threat" (p. 29). While a positive attitude leads to healing, a negative attitude leads to a stress response in the body. Rankin concludes,

"It's not enough to focus solely on the body without taking into account the health of the mind" (p. 74). She changed her patient intake form and added questions about life issues as well as medical ones. Tindle (2013) concurs, "Why should outlook matter more for people who are medically 'down'? A big part of the answer, as we've seen, is that our outlook naturally influences the way we care for ourselves. Thus the associated benefits of looking up have to do with the fact that a brighter disposition goes hand in hand with better self-care and making healthier choices" (p. 199). Healthier choices influence a patient's life long after a hospital stay concludes. As Helldorfer and Moss (2007) write, "that is what being a healing presence means – leaving others a little better as a result of our care" (p. 206). Health coaching means empowering patients to take ownership of their own health stories.

REWRITING A HEALTH STORY

Regardless of whether a person is a patient needing inpatient physical therapy after surgery or a mostly healthy individual looking to make a few adjustments to improve health, each person possesses the power to write his or her own health story. Connelly and Clandinin (1988) explain the value of believing in the power of our own narratives by providing the reminder, "narrative is designed to be thought of as an overall life study. As such it encompasses a person's past, his or her current state of mind, and his or her personal knowledge, which shapes teaching work in the future" (p. 34). Health coaches love exploring narratives. Clandinin and Connelly (2000) discuss, "formalists begin inquiry in theory, whereas narrative inquirers tend to begin with experience as expressed in lived and told stories" (p. 40). Traditional narrative inquiries focus on past, present, and future, but health coaches meet the patient in the present.

Health coaching brings a contemporary addition to the traditional field of medicine, but in order to best serve patients, change becomes necessary. Helldorfer and Moss (2007) explain, "having the freedom to implement new ways of doing things is critical if we want to become the organization we envision" (p. 274). A hospital with a health coach adds an additional compassionate professional to its team while simultaneously being on the cutting edge of medicine.

Health coaching empowers patients to control and rewrite their narratives. Sometimes we can't control the things that happen to us, such as a scary health diagnosis. We can, however, control our reaction to the events and also control how we make meaning from the story. The advice Brown (2012) gives to herself and others is, "own the story! Don't bury it and let it fester or define me" (p. 80). No matter what has happened in the past, health coaches help their clients believe change is possible in the future. Through conversations where the health coach reflects a client's words, a person hears his or her own story and gain new insights. When people hear the stories they tell themselves, they may reflect how the meanings they give the stories may change with a different interpretation of the narrative.

Changing one's health story occurs whether a client is an overall healthy person looking to make behavior changes or a patient recovering from an illness. Arterburn (2011) believes, "every illness provides us with choices. In the context of healing, the greatest choice is the decision to pursue healing! When people make that choice, they typically improve" (p. 52). Healing takes place as a physical therapy patient follows through with a treatment plan to return to normal activity. Healing also takes place when a healthy person makes minor lifestyle changes in order to achieve major health benefits. Clandinin and Connelly (2000) describe the process of using narratives to shape a life as, "we tell remembered stories of ourselves from earlier times as well as more current stories. All of these stories offer possible plotlines for our futures" (p. 60). For everyone, the future remains unwritten with opportunities for healthy decisions.

NARRATIVE MEDICINE IN PHYSICAL THERAPY CLINICS

Experts in the medical field illustrate that narratives are not limited to the English classroom. Charon (2006) explains, "I use the term narrative medicine to mean medicine practiced with these narrative skills of recognizing, absorbing, interpreting, and being moved by the stories of illness" (p. 4). Charon studied the genre of writing in a medical chart and made the connection that, "whatever the specialty of the writer, his or her chart note carries information in its form as well as its content. As is true for novels, plays, or poetry, the news one gets from a hospital note is transmitted by the words written as well as by the formal characteristics in which it is written" (p. 142). While she acknowledges that medical practitioners need to practice clinical detachment, it also helps them to know a patient's story as well as a diagnosis.

Greenfield, Jensen, Delany, Mostrom, Knab, and Jampel (2015) advocate the use of narratives in physical therapy education and practice. They elaborate, "highlighting context, characters, and plots allows a narrative to carry meaning, to potentially counter a reliance on objective measures of practice, and to build a bridge or create dialectic that connects the objective and subjective in clinical practice experience to help therapists iteratively move between these 2 essential aspects of human experience" (p. 925). A patient's narrative provides a clinician with additional information that, connected to the data from existing objective physical therapy measures, can lead to a diagnosis. Physical therapists use evidence from objective measures such as the DASH, LEFS, NDI, and Modified Oswestry to help categorize patient pain and design a treatment plan. While written responses by a patient cannot diagnose a patient's medical condition, writing does show contributing factors for what the diagnosis may be. Physical therapists put subjective aspects such as writing responses into the clinical prediction rule to predict what the chances are that a patient has a specific diagnosis.

In addition to traditional diagnostic reasoning, Greenfield and Jensen (2010) encourage clinicians to use narrative reasoning. They explain, "narrative reasoning involves understanding the patient's story – his or her illness experience and its context and his or her beliefs and values. This strategy involves an interpretive paradigm, similar to phenomenology, focusing on context-dependent and subjectively constructed knowledge (about phenomena)" (p. 1194). Narratives are subjective, as each patient views his or her story through the lens of experience. Clandinin and Connelly (2000) believe, "as narrative inquirers we work within the space not only with our participants but also with ourselves. Working in this space means that we become visible with our own lived and told stories" (pp. 61-62). The combination of actively telling the stories of others while reflecting on their own stories enables researchers to relate to the story. By learning the patient's story, the clinician views the narrative from the patient's perspective.

Greenfield, Jensen, Delany, Mostrom, Knab, and Jampel (2015) reference Charon's work and elaborate, "narrative medicine provides the clinician an opportunity to listen carefully to and reflect upon a patient's experiences with illness, representing that experience in a story or narrative, and ultimately providing the clinician insights that foster a strong commitment in caring for that patient. These ideas are particularly relevant for physical therapist practice, where therapists form close bonds with their patients and depend on their patients' cooperation and active engagement in their rehabilitation" (p. 928). When a patient writes a narrative, it helps both the patient and the physical therapist.

Activities a patient engaged in to cause pain at the beginning of the week may be forgotten or misinterpreted by the time the patient tells the story to the physical therapist at the end of the week's physical therapy session; therefore, writing helps the patient remember. Greenfield, Jensen, and their colleagues (2015) continue their discussion of narratives by stating, "based on our experiences with students and clinicians, writing narratives is a skill that needs to be taught, learned, and practiced in the same way that problem solving and other forms of clinical reasoning require practice and explicit instruction" (p. 928). Patients feel more comfortable during treatment if a compassionate clinician demonstrates willingness to listen to their stories. In a study measuring communication between physical therapists and patients with back pain, Roberts and Bucksey (2007) concluded, "once the content of a physical therapy encounter is established, the next challenge is to use communication skills that maximally enhance treatment outcomes" (p. 586). While one study certainly cannot capture conversations between all physical therapists and their patients, it does raise awareness of the value of using narratives to enhance communication between therapist and patient.

INCORPORATING THE THEORY OF NARRATIVE INQUIRY AND THE PRACTICE OF HEALTH COACHING

It benefits physical therapists to know their patients' narratives that illuminate emotional barriers to physical healing. Linton and Shaw (2011) argue, "the application of psychological knowledge in physical therapy might range from providing reassurance to setting goals or inquiring about the functional consequences of pain. However, there is an apparent lack of knowledge and tools to adequately apply this knowledge" (p. 700). Due to the large number of patients that physical therapists must see a day, even though the physical therapist may want to have a long conversation with a patient, it may not be possible due to time restrictions. This is where a health coach helps. While health coaches use conversation to learn patients' stories, they may also use journal writing methods that reflect strategies English teachers use with their students. Regardless of whether they use conversation or writing to have patients talk about their answers to questions, health coaches learn the narratives of the people they serve in order to best provide encouragement and support as a new chapter in each person's story is written. This narrative focuses on using health coaching with physical therapy patients, but health coaches benefit patients in other medical settings as well.

Asking questions and finding themes in stories involves inquiry. Narrative inquiry is the qualitative interpretive field of research where researchers find narrative threads in stories that reflect themes. Like a physical therapist finds a narrative thread in a patient's story which may help explain physical symptoms, a health coach finds narrative unity in a patient's story which may help explain emotional barriers to adhering to a treatment plan and accomplishing goals. By rereading previous writing and interpreting the narrative thread that runs through their stories, writers rewrite narratives. Medical professionals such as physical therapists help patients rewrite narratives by reframing a negative perspective into a positive one. Connelly and Clandinin (1988) elaborate, "this ongoing reflection-on-action on a daily basis begins to provide insight into personal knowledge when you reread entries over several days and weeks. What connecting threads are apparent over time? Are there events or ideas that recur?" (p. 35). From this perspective, one narrative becomes placed in a larger context to show how the puzzle pieces of a person's story fit together.

Often people have value conflicts which prevent them from making changes in their lives. A patient may want to complete a home exercise plan from a physical therapist, but that will take away time from watching a favorite television show with family. The strategy of motivational interviewing helps patients identify such barriers and potential solutions. Bezner (2015) believes, "applying health behavior change theories and using motivational interviewing will enable physical therapists to effectively counsel and support the patient or client to adopt healthy behaviors" (p. 1441). Or, if due to needing to see a large number of patients, the physical therapist is unable to provide the counseling, a health coach shares the responsibility. Caldwell, Gray, and Wolever (2013) discuss how health coaching is similar yet different from motivational interviewing and explain, "first, there is a more directive element in MI that is usually not seen in health coaching. Second, MI often helps patients target a social or provider-determined goal (eg, abstinence from substance use) as much as a patient-driven goal. Third, while in MI, the central focus is on overcoming ambivalence to change, the overarching aim of IHC is broader, though elements of MI may be used in the process" (p. 55). Health coaching uses motivational interviewing as one of its foundations. Grant (2021) describes motivational interviewing as, "motivational interviewing starts with an attitude of humility and curiosity. We don't know what might motivate someone else to change, but we're genuinely eager to find out. The goal isn't to tell people what to do; it's to help them break out of overconfidence cycles and see new possibilities. Our role is to hold up a mirror so they can see themselves more clearly, and then empower them to examine their beliefs and behaviors" (p. 147). By asking open ended questions, practicing active listening, and using reflective statements, motivational interviewers provide a mirror to what is and a window to what could be. In motivational interviewing, Miller and Rollnick (2002) argue, "the implication is that there are at least these three critical components of motivation: readiness, willingness, and ability" (p. 10). Are we willing to change? Do we feel we have the ability to change? Are we ready to change?

Integrative Health Coaches see the patient as a person, not just a diagnosis. Smith, Lake, Simmons, Perlman, Wroth, and Wolever (2013) elaborate of integrative health coaching, "while coaches may have a wide knowledge base of medical issues and diverse healthcare resources, their area of expertise is not medicine – it is specifically in building motivation for behavior change" (p. 69). Health coaches don't tell people what to do; they ask questions and serve as a supportive presence until people find the solutions to their problems.

While physicians, physical therapists, and other medical professionals provide a diagnosis and treatment plan, health coaches partner with both medical teams and patients to build bridges between where the patient is now and where he or she wants to be. Smith, Lake, Simmons, Perlman, Wroth, and Wolever (2013) explain, "often in collaboration with clinicians and educators who design and clarify treatment plans, IH coaches work with each patient's whole situation – from his or her spiritual beliefs to exercise aversions – to foster an environment where their plans can take hold" (p. 69-70). Health coaches have a variety of backgrounds but must receive specific training to become a certified health coach and partner with patients on their healing journeys.

PATIENT NARRATIVES

Every patient has a story. Recent trends in physical therapy focus on patient narratives. Greenfield, Jensen, Delany, Mostrom, Knab, and Jampel (2015) explain, "an initial goal of introducing narrative, therefore, is to demonstrate how narrative can be meaningful and relevant to physical therapy practitioners" (p. 928). To learn more about writing narratives, physical therapists may adapt methods from English teachers. English teachers encourage students to write in journals because first drafts of writing capture the writer's truest thoughts. Writing teacher Goldberg (1986) explains, "first thoughts are present. They are not a cover-up of what is actually happening or being felt" (p. 10). Writing opens a window to the stories people tell themselves, which becomes beneficial for helping not only students in a writing classroom but also patients in a physical therapy clinic. By having insight into a patient's thoughts, the medical practitioner learns insights about the patient's narrative that will enhance the development of a successful treatment plan.

Journal writing provides an outlet of expression, thus allowing for the emergence of writing voice. Greenfield and Jensen (2010) discuss the value of patients' voices and elaborate, "imagine what we may find out about the work of physical therapists if we developed clinical case knowledge that is based on understanding the patient's voice? How could we better hear that voice?" (p. 1195). English teachers hear their students' voices through writing as well as speaking, so writing provides information for physical therapists that patients may forget to share during a conversation. Writing teacher Tom Romano (2004) describes, "one of the great things about writing is that by doing it, we can construct a persona. We can craft an authentic voice" (p. 218). When students share their authentic voices, writing teachers help them discuss their emotions; similarly, when patients share their authentic voices, physical therapists help them discuss their symptoms.

WRITING NARRATIVES

How much about a patient's story does a clinician know? Patients may feel like the doctor doesn't have enough time to spend with them. Rankin (2013) explains things from a doctor's perspective and states, "nobody intends for this to happen. Health-care providers have often sacrificed so much for their patients that they stop being mindful about why they're doing what they were called to do" (p. 48). She continues, "it's time to put the care back in health care" (p. 48). In conducting research about outlook and aging, medical doctor Hilary Tindle (2013) reports, "our outlook, which colors our reaction to everything, can set in motion a physiologic chain reaction that we may not even be aware of, a process that ebbs and flows constantly. In medical terminology, this process is called the 'neuroendocrine response to stress' where stress is essentially any stimulus that engages us" (p. 15). Tindle discovered only one percent of people achieve ideal cardiac health and one of the questions she included on a list that existing research has yet to answer was, "what is the script going on inside their heads, if there is one?" (p. 24). For years, English teachers have used writing to learn about the script going on inside people's heads. Writing teacher Julia Cameron (1998) explains, "when we are telling the truth about how we feel and what we see, we find very precise language with which to do it" (p. 140). Writing provides a method for clinicians to learn about the script in patients' heads.

Pages of a notebook provide a place for patients to process their thoughts and also create a journal of symptoms. If a physical therapist reads the patient's journal, he or she might then make adjustments to the treatment plan if the patient's observations illuminate additional insights. It also provides personal awareness and accountability to the current situation for the patient. Cameron (1998) emphasizes the importance of reflecting on feelings and states, "writing can be done the same way. It can be done by listening to how we feel rather than thinking about how we feel" (p. 156). Health coaches do not have to use journals with patients, but if the patient is willing and able to share thoughts in writing, journals provide an additional healing resource. Writing should not be seen as a required homework assignment, but rather a chance for exploration and insight. To do this, writing teachers such as Natalie Goldberg (1986) recommend writing quickly without thinking too much about the words on the page since "the aim is to burn through to first thoughts, to the place where energy is unobstructed by social politeness or the internal censor, to the place where you are writing what your mind actually sees and feels, not what it thinks it should see or feel" (p. 8). Writing captures a writer's first impressions and truest thoughts, and although health coaches must never pressure anyone to share, often people want someone to know their story. It then becomes the decision of the writer whether or not to share the writing with the health coach, physical therapist, or anyone else.

While writing has healing value for the writer regardless of whether or not it is shared, if writing is used during health coaching, knowing a patient's perspective provides the health coach with additional information to help with goal setting. Goldberg (2000) feels, "but there does come a time – I can't honestly tell you when – that we must step over the line of practice and speak and expect to be heard. But no one's listening, we whine. Then we have to figure out how to make them listen" (p. 180). How many times do patients think of one more question or observation after the medical practitioner has left the room? Even though medical practitioners are trained to hear sensitive health stories, patients may still feel embarrassed to share them which could actually make their situation harder to diagnose. The most eloquent person may still be rendered speechless when needing to ask a personal health question. Brown (2007) describes the feelings many patients have and shares, "there is nothing more frustrating, and sometimes frightening, than feeling pain and not being able to describe it or explain it to someone. It doesn't matter if it's physical pain or emotional pain. When we can't find the right words to explain our painful experiences to others, we often feel alone and scared" (p. 155). Writing captures questions and fears on paper so patients obtain the answers they need.

PAIN JOURNALS

Writing techniques apply to the medical field for patients interested in using writing while in an inpatient or outpatient setting, and for medical professionals interested in knowing more about the healing benefits of learning patients' narratives. DeSalvo (1999) writes, "after I became ill, I began, as many writers with wounded bodies do, to keep a record of my illness in diary form, largely because no matter how sick I was, I could always manage to scratch out ten minutes of writing while propped up on pillows" (p. 200). Processing the emotional pain that often occurs simultaneously with physical pain may lead to decreased stress and increased health. Rankin (2013) feels, "if it's true that the mind's positive beliefs can heal the body, everyone has an equal chance of benefitting from this phenomenon" (p. 10). While a positive attitude assists the patient with the perception of pain, sharing writing with a trusted medical professional can bring additional healing benefits. Writing down a list of symptoms and bringing it to the attention of the physical therapist or physician can help the clinician see patterns and obtain additional insights about a patient's health to adjust the treatment plan if necessary.

Psychologist James Pennebaker conducted significant research illustrating writing can lead to healing. Pennebaker and Evans (2014) discuss how expressive writing leads to improved health and report, "across our first four writing studies, those in the expressive writing condition made forty-three percent fewer doctor visits for illness than those who were asked to write about superficial topics" (p. 2). Pennebaker and Evans continue, "since the first expressive writing studies were published in the 1980s, at least 300 studies about the benefits of expressive writing have been published. While the first studies focused almost exclusively on physician visits for illness, the scope of benefit measures has grown exponentially" (p. 9). Journal writing, a type of expressive writing frequently used by English teachers and often used by health coaches, provides an additional resource for both patients and physical therapists. Fallon (2020) explains, "But do you want to know my favorite part about the expressive writing process? The words we put on the page don't have to stay the same. We get to decide how they transform. We get to expose more and more truth as we go on" (p. 106). Writing helps patients explore the truth about how they feel in order to eliminate emotional barriers to physical pain. The patient reflects on the narrative to rewrite the story of pain into one of healing. From a health coaching perspective, writing does not eliminate pain, but becomes part of the health plan to help patients stay motivated to reach their goals.

Patients do not need to write a long essay in a physical therapy clinic or write a significant amount of words at home in a journal to remember what to tell their physical therapist about their pain levels. Short answer response questions, whether they are on a survey used in a clinic or in a notebook to write out steps for goals, are effective in leading to the processing of emotions. Wilkerson Miller (2017) describes the recent trend of dot journals, also known as bullet journals, as, "a dot journal is a system for writing down all the things you want to remember in a single notebook" (p. 4). Patients may use this method to write down questions or information they want to remember to share with their physical therapist. Physical therapy patients may also apply this method by writing quick notes or observations between sessions to share with their physical therapists of what activities they were doing when they felt pain. A patient may have a low pain level right before a physical therapy session but forget to tell the physical therapist about a higher pain level felt the previous day. A pain journal may assist the physical therapist in modifying the treatment plan as needed based on information revealed in the writing that the patient may forget to mention during a conversation about pain levels. While written responses by a patient cannot cure a condition that requires physical therapy, writing does show contributing factors for the cause of the pain. A patient's narrative provides a clinician with additional information that, connected to the data from existing objective physical therapy measures, can lead to a diagnosis. And with the support of a strong medical team, writing becomes an additional resource in the healing process.

COACHING AS RELATIONSHIP-BASED CARE

Health coaching is a type of Relationship-Based Care. Koloroutis (2004) defines, "Relationship-Based Care (RBC) is comprised of three crucial relationships: care provider's relationship with patients and families, care provider's relationship with self, and care provider's relationship with colleagues" (p. 4). While the primary focus of health coaching is on the care-receiver, it is also essential for the care provider to have strong self-care in order to help others, as well as be part of a team of colleagues working together to provide an integrative approach to medicine and healing. Koloroutis continues, "the care provider knows that each person's unique life story determines how he or she will experience an illness" (p. 5). Health coaches realize that while a person's unique life story leads to the moment when care is needed, it is possible to start from the present moment and add a new chapter where the life story does not become defined by illness. According to Koloroutis, "true healers provide the space for patients to heal themselves" (p. 249). Health coaches, like any Relationship-Based Care practitioner, provide encouragement and empowerment for people to take ownership of their health so they can heal.

Sometimes healing becomes enhanced in a group setting, also known as group coaching. In group coaching, participants sit in a circle and share their goals and dreams. Group coaching may look like group therapy, but it is not. Instead, group coaching more closely resembles a college writing seminar, where participants have the opportunity to respond in writing to a prompt, and then choose whether or not to share. The coach facilitates a safe space where participants motivate each other and encourage each other to succeed. Personal and private health information is never revealed by the coach in group coaching, but by finding common ground participants see they are not alone. Baldwin (1998) discusses the value of calling a circle and elaborates, "the circle can act as a trustworthy group of people who mirror back to us our own unique qualities" (p. 139). Circle time creates a supportive environment for people to share their experiences with others. Health coaches and other clinicians also use intuition and compassion to create a supportive environment for patients, especially during challenging times such as the current pandemic.

How does intuition relate to being a patient? Groopman (2007) explains, "clinical intuition is a complex sense that becomes refined over years and years of practice, of listening to literally thousands of patients' stories, examining thousands of people, and most important, remembering when you were wrong" (p. 20). So for medical professionals, their clinical intuition becomes refined by learning from experiences and listening to patients. Groopman cautions against relying too heavily on intuition, because in the medical world, feelings about a diagnosis must often be supported with factual data.

However, medical professionals place value on both their own and patients' intuition. Rankin (2015a) explains that people often feel fear in life and "although false fear can illuminate areas in your life that need your attention, healthy decisions that guide appropriate behavior never arise from false fear; they arise from intuition and integrity" (p. 51). Inherently, people know what they need to do to make healthy decisions and take care of themselves. And that sense of purpose helps them feel the importance of their actions. Rankin discovered, "the people I interviewed who had cultivated and learned to trust their intuition felt like they were always being guided, and they were supported by this guidance more than they were controlled by their fears" (pp. 142-143). She admits that the busy pace of a doctor's schedule doesn't allow as much time with patients as doctors would like, but she learned that if she partnered with her patients and took the time to listen to their stories, it helped her make a diagnosis and adjust her treatment plan. Rankin (2015b) learned, "my new patient intake form was 12 pages long, and what these questions revealed about my patients' lives shocked me. When combined with the intuitive information I sometimes received from patients, I started to get a sense of the link between their physical health and their emotional health" (p. 120). Her story illustrates how a medical professional trusting her own clinical intuition and the intuition of her patients in the stories they shared with her helped patients heal.

How does compassion relate to being a patient? Tindle (2013) reports that self-compassion "has been linked to better self-care and healthier behaviors" (p. 77). How does this happen? Carter (2015) argues, "self-compassion – being warm and supportive toward ourselves, and actively soothing ourselves – has many benefits over self-criticism. It leads to less anxiety and depression, and greater piece of mind" (p. 219). And since emotional health is linked to physical health, if emotionally we are more compassionate to ourselves, physically we feel less tense from anxiety and stress. Self-compassion provides the insight that a one day divergence need not derail an entire nutrition or exercise plan. Tindle (2013) reminds us, "self-compassion and the deep sense of self-worth that it fosters are at the very foundation of our physical and mental health" (p. 182). Because when people believe they have value, that confidence is reflected in their health. Stories help us find common ground, see life from a different perspective, and remind us that someone knows who we are and cares to let us know we are not alone on our journey.

ACKNOWLEDGMENT

This chapter was co-authored by Dr. Eric Wanner, Director of the Physical Therapy Department at Palm Beach Sports Medicine and Orthopaedic Center. Eric loves research, and I enjoyed collaborating to designing a unique survey featuring both numerical subjective and written subjective questions to assess goal setting for physical therapy patients. Eric and I also conducted research to assess anxiety in college students and recommended effective methods for coping with anxiety, such as exercising, nutrition, writing, and belonging to a supportive community. We continued our collaboration by using health coaching to supplement physical therapy treatment plans for both staff members and patients at a hospital. I feel proud of our lasting contributions to interdisciplinary research that helped numerous people and remain grateful for Eric's talent of condensing my overly wordy first drafts into the most essential ideas.

The preceding chapter contains excerpts from the following previous IGI publications:

Bird, J.L, & Wanner, E.T. (2020). Narratives of health coaching. In *Using narrative writing to enhance healing* (pp. 73-100). Hershey, PA: Information Science Reference.

Bird, J.L. (2020). Narratives of patient care. In *Using narrative writing to enhance healing* (pp. 157-184). Hershey, PA: Information Science Reference.

REFERENCES

American Physical Therapy Association. (2021). *Physical therapist management of patients with or recovering from COVID-19*. American Physical Therapy Association. Retrieved from https://www.apta.org/patient-care/public-health-population-care/coronavirus/management-of-patients

Arterburn, S. (2011). *Healing is a choice*. Thomas Nelson.

Baldwin, C. (1998). *Calling the circle*. Bantam.

Beck, M. (2001). *Finding your own North Star*. Three Rivers Press.

Bezner, J. R. (2015). Promoting health and wellness: Implications for physical therapist practice. *Physical Therapy*, *95*(10), 1433–1444. doi:10.2522/ptj.20140271 PMID:25908523

Brady, L., & Vega, P. (2009). 5 keys to structural success. In Orthopedics and spine (pp. 107-132). Danvers, MA: HCPro.

Brown, B. (2007). *I thought it was just me*. Gotham Books.

Brown, B. (2012). *Daring greatly*. Gotham Books.

Caldwell, K., Gray, J., & Wolever, R. Q. (2013). The process of patient empowerment in integrative health coaching: How does it happen? *Global Advances in Health and Medicine: Improving Healthcare Outcomes Worldwide*, *2*(3), 48–57. doi:10.7453/gahmj.2013.026 PMID:24416672

Cameron, J. (1998). *The right to write*. Tarcher/Putnam.

Carter, C. (2015). *The sweet spot*. Ballantine.

Charon, R. (2006). *Narrative medicine: honoring the stories of illness*. Oxford University Press.

Chulack, C., Crichton, M., Wells, J., & Zabel, D. (1994-2009). *ER* [Television series]. Burbank, CA: Warner Brothers.

Clandinin, D. J., & Connelly, F. M. (2000). *Narrative inquiry*. Jossey-Bass.

Clark, A. H. (2018). *Hack your anxiety*. Sourcebooks, Inc.

Coates, V. E. (1999). *Education for patients and clients*. Routledge.

Connelly, F. M., & Clandinin, D. J. (1988). *Teachers as curriculum planners*. Teachers College.

Croft, J. (1980). Interviewing in physical therapy. *Physical Therapy*, *60*(8), 1033–1036. doi:10.1093/ptj/60.8.1033 PMID:7403279

Duke Integrative Medicine Staff. (2010). *Personalized health plan manual*. Duke Integrative Medicine.

Fallon, A. (2020). *The power of writing it down*. Zondervan.

Goldberg, N. (1986). *Writing down the bones*. Shambhala.

Goldberg, N. (2000). *Thunder and lightning*. Bantam.

Grant, A. (2021). *Think again*. Viking.

Greenfield, B. H., & Jensen, G. M. (2010). Understanding the lived experiences of patients: Application of a phenomenological approach to ethics. *Physical Therapy*, *90*(8), 1185–1201. doi:10.2522/ptj.20090348 PMID:20539020

Greenfield, B. H., Jensen, G. M., Delany, C. M., Mostrom, E., Knab, M., & Jampel, A. (2015). Power and promise of narrative for advancing physical therapist education and practice. *Physical Therapy*, *95*(6), 924–933. doi:10.2522/ptj.20140085 PMID:25524869

Groopman, J. (2007). *How doctors think*. Mariner Books.

Helldorfer, M., & Moss, T. (2007). *Healing with heart*. Moss Communications.

Jones, J., Brady, L., & Gaunt, R. (2009). The philosophy of patient-centric care. In Orthopedics and spine (pp. 81-105). Danvers, MA: HCPro.

Jones, J., Steele, D., & McClennan, C. (2009). Defining and pursuing excellence. In Orthopedics and spine (pp. 11-50). Danvers, MA: HCPro.

Koloroutis, M. (2004). *Relationship-based care*. Creative Health Care Management.

Kolt, G. S. (2003). Psychology of injury and rehabilitation. In G. S. Kolt (Ed.), *Snyder-Mackler, L. Physical therapies in sport and exercise* (pp. 165–183). Churchill Livingstone.

Linton, S. J., & Shaw, W. S. (2011). Impact of psychological factors in the experience of pain. *Physical Therapy*, *91*(5), 700–711. doi:10.2522/ptj.20100330 PMID:21451097

Miller, R. W. (2017). *Dot journaling*. The Experiment.

Miller, W. R., & Rollnick, S. (2002). *Motivational interviewing* (2nd ed.). The Guilford Press.

Pennebaker, J. W., & Evans, J. F. (2014). *Expressive writing: words that heal*. Idyll Arbor.

Pipher, M. (2006). *Writing to change the world*. Riverhead.

Randall, K. E., & McEwen, I. R. (2000). Writing patient-centered functional goals. *Physical Therapy, 80*(12), 1197–103. doi:10.1093/ptj/80.12.1197 PMID:11087306

Rankin, L. (2013). *Mind over medicine*. Hay House.

Rankin, L. (2015a). *The fear cure*. Hay House.

Rankin, L. (2015b). *The anatomy of a calling*. Rodale.

Roberts, L., & Bucksey, S. J. (2007). Communicating with patients: What happens in practice? *Physical Therapy, 87*(5), 586–594. doi:10.2522/ptj.20060077 PMID:17405807

Romano, T. (2004). *Crafting authentic voice*. Heinemann.

Simmons, L. A., & Wolever, R. Q. (2011). *Health coaching: Research summary (report)*. Duke Integrative Medicine / Duke University Health System.

Smith, L., & Wroth, S. (2011). *Duke integrative health coach professional training manual*. Duke Integrative Medicine.

Smith, L. L., Lake, N. H., Simmons, L. A., Perlman, A., Wroth, S., & Wolever, R. Q. (2013). Integrative health coach training: A model for shifting the paradigm toward patient-centricity and meeting new national prevention goals. *Global Advances in Health and Medicine: Improving Healthcare Outcomes Worldwide, 2*(3), 66–74. doi:10.7453/gahmj.2013.034 PMID:24416674

Soukup, R. (2019). *Do it scared*. Zondervan.

Steele, M. K. (2009). Orthopedics and spine. Danvers, MA: HCPro.

Tindle, H. (2013). *Up: how positive outlook can transform our health and aging*. Hudson Street Press.

KEY TERMS AND DEFINITIONS

Behavior Changes: Behavior changes occur when people put forth a conscious effort to make lifestyle changes to improve health. While health coaches can encourage behavior changes, ultimately the choice of which behavior changes to implement belongs to each individual.

Community Development: The process of creating a place where people feel welcomed and supported, whether it is a neighborhood, a classroom, or a network of colleagues who provide support for an individual.

Integrative Health Coaching: Integrative health coaches help people make changes that support their vision and values of optimal health.

Integrative Medicine: A holistic approach to medicine that treats the whole person, not just the disease.

Narrative Medicine: The field of medicine, used by programs such as the one Rita Charon founded at Columbia University, which encourages medical practitioners to use theories from the fields of literature and composition to enhance comprehension of the stories patients share.

Physical Therapy Outcome Measures: Tests used by physical therapists to measure the progress a patient makes when a body part is injured, such as such as the DASH (Disabilities of the Arm Shoulder

Hand), LEFS (Lower Extremity Functional Scale), NDI (Neck Disability Index), and Modified Oswestry (for back pain).

Self-Compassion: The act of demonstrating the same kindness for oneself that one would demonstrate for other people.

Chapter 4
Reflections of Leadership Narratives

ABSTRACT

This narrative focuses on a classroom teacher called to forge a path for students during online learning by using journal writing as well as a variety of other methods including sharing life lessons, discussing time management, and organizing priorities. Transformative leadership requires vulnerability, courage, and innovation. During difficult times such as the recent pandemic, leaders need to demonstrate creativity and resilience. Anyone who wishes to enhance a leadership role can benefit from the strategies presented.

TRANSFORMATIVE LEADERSHIP

How could I make sure my students learned literature and writing while making lessons as enjoyable as possible given the distance restrictions? How could I use writing to manage the anxiety students felt as well as the anxiety I felt? Brown (2018) believes, "at the heart of daring leadership is a deeply human truth that is rarely acknowledged, especially at work: Courage and fear are not mutually exclusive. Most of us feel brave and afraid at the exact same time" (p. 10). Therefore, I could demonstrate courage and resilience for my students while still feeling the fear of the pandemic. Every student in my classroom lived a similar yet different experience during the pandemic. Even though we lived a collective experience of dealing with the coronavirus, each person lived an individual experience too. To begin my role as a transformative teacher leader during this challenging time, I needed to learn my students' narratives and honor them.

EDUCATIONAL NARRATIVES

Each person views his or her narrative through the lens of subjective experience. Asking questions and finding themes in stories involves inquiry. Clandinin and Connelly (2000) argue, "in narrative thinking, interpretations of events can always be otherwise" (p. 31). Narrative inquiry is the qualitative interpretive

DOI: 10.4018/978-1-7998-9051-5.ch004

field of research where researchers find narrative threads in stories that reflect themes. Connelly and Clandinin (1988) elaborate, "try to understand a narrative unity as a thread or theme that runs through the narrative of experience and that provides a way to see how the rules, principles, images, and metaphors relate one to the other as they are called out by the practical situations in which we find ourselves" (p. 75). In other words, when a person shares a story, he or she selects what details to share or not to share. Clandinin and Connelly (2000) describe the process of converting informal field texts into a formal research text by stating, "we find ourselves frequently engaged in writing a variety of different kinds of interim texts, texts situated in the spaces between field texts and final, published research texts" (p. 133). The interim texts of my journal entries don't make those texts any less worthy than the formal research projects I designed and implemented. Connelly and Clandinin (1988) argue that education, especially when it comes to narratives, does not have to take place in the classroom and elaborate, "education, in this view, is a narrative of experience that grows and strengthens a person's capabilities to cope with life" (p. 27). People view their lives through the lenses of narratives of experience, and sharing narratives enables people to own their stories. Brown (2015) discusses the value of owning stories and explains, "I know that it takes more than courage to own your story. We own our stories so we don't spend our lives being defined by them or denying them" (p. 40). When people own their stories and find the strength to share their narratives with others, they find the courage to write new chapters to their stories and change the endings of their narratives.

Furthermore, when presenting narratives, writers can choose which genres best illustrate their ideas. Romano (2000) describes this format as multigenre writing and discusses narrative as a foundation as he explains, "multigenre papers, however, as I conceive them, demand that writers think narratively. Writers must meld the cognitive with the emotional" (p. 24). And writers also connect their artistic narratives with technical research. Romano (2013) writes, "I require students to incorporate research into multigenre papers, regardless of their subject, even if they write from deeply personal experience" (p. 43). Therefore, while I present the narrative information in the creative context of methods I use to help the high school students I teach, my goal remains for readers of this text to find helpful insights for life and leadership embedded within the strategies.

TEACHERS SET THE TONE

Teachers need to meet the needs of students, and teaching during a pandemic requires teachers to demonstrate additional creativity. As Romano (1987) observes, "in a classroom full of opinionated teenagers, the last thing a teacher wants to feel is more vulnerable. The job is tough enough" (p. 39). But when teachers share their stories, students experience the practice of learning instead of only the theory.

I felt proud when a visitor to my classroom commented that I gave students a place to be themselves. Students feel they can be themselves when teachers honor their voices. Just like everyone has a unique speaking voice, everyone has a unique writing voice. Romano (2004) defines voice as "our very personalities shape our voices and determine how and what we put on the page" (p. 6). It involves tone, word choice, and feeling. It's the artistry involved in composing a writing piece that reflects the personality of the writer.

Teachers who give students a classroom that symbolizes a safe space for sharing provide a platform for voices to be heard. Romano (2004) reminds students, "voice will come. Voice will come when you heed passion, push forward with language, are brave on the page, everything else be damned" (p. 51).

Teachers encourage students to share their voices by reminding them they have something to say. Gruwell and the Freedom Writers (1999) discuss the power of writing by "encouraging you to pick up a pen and be a catalyst for change" (p. 277). My students read the narrative of the Freedom Writers and became inspired to pick up a pen and write in their journals. I hope my students continue to use writing as a catalyst for change in their lives.

While anyone, regardless of age, always has the option of picking up a pen and a blank notebook, students need guidance from their teachers. Romano (1987) explains, "the teacher is the first and most convincing example of the kind of behavior she wants in her class. She writes honestly, she shares what she's written, she listens to the writing of her students and respects their voices and visions" (p. 43). An English teacher who feels willing to share his or her own writing with students sets the tone for a comfortable class community where students feel encouraged to explore their own ideas through writing. Sharing writing requires vulnerability. Brown (2012) believes, "rather than sitting on the sidelines and hurling judgment and advice, we must dare to show up and let ourselves be seen. This is vulnerability. This is daring greatly" (p. 2). As a teacher and a leader, I feel willing to show vulnerability when sharing my writing because it motivates my students to view my classroom as a safe space to share.

I value my role as a writing role model for students. Johnson (2005) advises teachers, "here's your chance to provide that role model" (p. 26). I illustrate the writing process by projecting one of my computer typed drafts onto the large screen in the room so students can offer feedback while observing me adding, deleting, and revising phrases. If I want to be a writing role model, I need to provide my students with the same writing opportunities. Lamott (1994) elaborates, "there are probably a number of ways to tell your story right, and someone else may be able to tell you whether or not you've found one of these ways" (p. 163). Sometimes my students think of new ways I can revise my writing, and helping their teacher builds their confidence.

Writing teachers who don't write are like swimming teachers who never jump into the pool; why should teenagers take them seriously? So when teaching a writing workshop for students, teachers need to view themselves as writers. Kearns (1997) argues, "students do not see teachers write enough. They see us talking, reading, viewing, reprimanding, ordering, conferencing, and sometimes listening. They need to see us writing" (p. 83). When teachers share writing with their students, it does not mean sharing personal information that will make everyone in the room uncomfortable. It means modeling a strategy so students feel more confident sharing their writing. Romano (1987) writes, "all along the process it is imperative that the teacher-crafter demonstrates to apprentices all the stages of the writing process" (p. 58). Teachers demonstrate the writing process to students and serve as role models in their classrooms. Too often, students feel the pressure to be perfect in school. Cleary (1991) describes this perfectionism as "students became good-grade junkies, and as they began to work for teachers, they stopped writing for themselves" (p. 67). When teachers become willing to model their writing process, with all the revisions, edits, and drafts, students learn to see writing as a process and a journey with all the risks and rewards that come with it.

Very few first drafts are the final draft of a writing composition. Barbieri (1995) believes, "all writing leads to insight and discovery, and revising offers opportunities to dig deeper, to refine thinking, to follow new trains of thought" (p. 25). Modeling can reframe setbacks as part of the learning process, not a catastrophic event. Connelly and Clandinin (1988) believe, "life's narratives are the context for making meaning of school situations" (p. 27). Leadership, whether a teacher models writing for students or a leader serves as a role model in another organization, empowers people.

WRITING WITH PASSION

Most people can relate to the feeling of being completely absorbed in an activity and getting into the zone where time fades away. Writing helps illuminate what the writer values; teachers use this process to help students achieve goals. Romano (2013) explains, "to capture stream of consciousness, the writer has to let go of control more than usual, trust the gush of language and associations even more" (p. 117). If students trust the gush of feeling and become willing to write about things that bring joy, they start on the path to feeling encouraged to find their passion in life.

Discovering passion leads to purpose. A journal serves as a mirror reflecting goals accomplished, which encourages the writer to persevere. Pipher (2006) elaborates, "by diving into the experience of writing, you will learn what you truly think and who you really are" (p. 44). Sometimes people struggle to figure out who they are, especially if an event such as a pandemic creates chaos in a once stable life. Writing can bring you back to yourself and remind you who you are. Romano (1995) describes seeing students find their passion and writes, "in my experience, passion in students has usually led to strong positions, critical thinking, further analysis, and stirring, often eloquent language" (p. 25). One way to find what will bring passion in the future is to remember what brought passion in the past. According to Goldberg (2007), "writing is your practice as you mow through your memories, the even chord among the highs and lows" (p. 70). Memories of past successes and remembering a time when happiness happened often sets the stage for future dreams. Since eventually the pandemic will pass, I want my students to continue to dream and visualize what their lives will look like in the future.

Once we know what we want to do with the one life each of us has been given, the challenging part becomes following our hearts no matter what others think. Lamott (1994) reminds us to recapture our true desires because "you get your intuition back when you make space for it, when you stop the chattering of the rational mind" (p. 112). Writing can help process feelings and goals; a phrase on paper can make the impossible seem possible if it is broken down into steps. Goldberg (1990) describes a strategy for articulating goals and feelings and advises, "a helpful technique: right in the middle of saying nothing, right in the middle of a sentence, put a dash and write, 'What I really want to say is…' and go on writing" (p. 73). We say what we need to say. We keep writing. We keep living. We welcome the encouragement from others as we set our goals and find the strength to encourage ourselves. As the leader of my classroom, I encourage students to use their journals as a method of setting goals. I also encourage them to draw and create vision boards as another method of visualizing their goals. Beck (2001) states, "miracles really can and will occur when you connect with your dreams, but they're both more likely and less necessary if you do everything in your power to reach your goals" (p. 306). Writing down goals and envisioning them happening is common practice for transforming dreams into reality and visualizing life after the pandemic.

THE PERFECT PROCESS OF IMPERFECT WRITING

As Heard (1995) observes when struggling with a piece of writing, "I had changed the intent of the writing, just as people move a stream by redirecting its banks, hoping the water will obey. It never does. Neither did my writing" (p. 41). The writing process provides opportunities for experimentation with style and ideas. Barbieri (1995) describes the writing process as, "words came onto the page that I had not intended; the whole point of what I had been trying to say became clear to me, and I knew what I needed to write next. Stunned, I thought I had discovered magic" (p. 16). When it leads to discovery, writing does seem like magic. Kearns (1997) counters, "good writing is not the result of a magic wand; it comes from hard work" (p. 16). But when that hard work falls into place it looks effortless, like magic. And teachers can help the magic happen by encouraging students. Cleary (1991) believes, "we need our writing curriculum to reattach students to their souls" (p. 167). Writing can help everyone reattach to their souls.

Writing reminds us to practice self-care. I remind both myself and my students to practice self-care, not just during pandemic times, but all of the time. When students lose sleep completing homework, it causes stress. One decision I made is to ask students to write fewer but more meaningful essays. They take their time with the writing process and I don't feel overwhelmed with essays to grade. I followed the assessment advice of Tovani (2011) who argues, " I began to examine my definition of assessment and embrace it in a way that would not only inform my instruction but also provide useful feedback to students" (p. 2). Instead of standing in the front of the classroom (behind the plexiglass) discussing general strategies of revision, I used the online platform turnitin.com to differentiate instruction by writing individualized comments for each students. Because I assigned fewer, more meaningful essays, I had the time to do this and my students' writing improved. I watched the anxiety decrease (theirs and mine), and all of us felt happier.

Prepandemic, people used the self-care metaphor of the airlines informing people to put on their own masks before helping others. Now that people constantly wear masks, the airline metaphor may seem outdated, but taking time for self-care must remain a priority. This is especially important for caregivers giving time to others. Wade (2018) believes, "it is impossible to truly be there for others without taking care of ourselves first. We take care of ourselves by asking what our needs are. We take care of ourselves by making healthy choices when it comes to our physical and emotional bodies. We take care of ourselves by lightening up and not being so damn hard on ourselves" (pp. 2-3). When discussing how outlook influences health, Tindle (2013) discovered, "how we manage our responses to the world influences our health, both in the short and long term" (p. 17). How do we manage a response to life? Write about it! Cameron (1998) explains, "when we write about our lives we respond to them " (p. 94). We are all the experts of our own lives, and no one can tell our story in the exact same way we can.

Writing doesn't have a right answer, like 2+2=4. We write to find the right answers. Romano (2008) believes, "but I am a teacher. I know that the path toward accomplishment can be a zigzag one, replete with setbacks, wrong turns, and backtracking. That's why I value approximation so much: the flawed attempt, the good intentions gone awry, the achievement of approximately what you were after. For those who participate in good faith, learning is a matter of growth and development" (p. 206). We have faith in the fact writing helps us learn and grow in life. Fallon (2020) explains "I've watched writers get stuck, circle the same block again and again a few hundred times, and eventually give up. It's not all that different from what we do when we're trying to change a habit or a pattern in our personal lives" (p. 16). She continues, "not only did I begin to see these similarities, but I also started to see how the writing process itself has a way of creating change for people" (p. 16). When people persevere in revising their writing, they persevere in revising their lives.

TRUSTING FIRST IMPRESSIONS

Journals provide a private place to explore life's issues. But in order to write honestly, the writer has to ignore the self-censor and write from the heart. Cameron (1998) explains, "acting our way into right thinking is putting pen to the page even when the censor is shrieking" (p. 35). This means writing whatever comes to mind and trusting first thoughts and impressions before censoring anything written out of worry of what anyone else might think. Goldberg (1986) answers the question, "why else are first thoughts so energizing? Because they have to do with freshness and inspiration" (p. 10). Frequently writers ignore first thoughts because they fear what others may think if the writing is read. But not all writing needs to be for an audience.

All writing does not have to be read; there is a time to share but also a time to write for one's eyes only. Goldberg (2013) describes the moment of first thoughts as, "a flash, a moment appears when we fall through and what we are fighting, running from, struggling with becomes open, luminous – or, even better, not a problem, just what it is" (p. 23). I tell my students they need to practice writing just like they practice a sport or an instrument. Freedom to experiment in journals results in stronger writing.

Students in an English classroom become used to writing essays, turning them in for a grade from the teacher, and being evaluated. However, teachers also need to give students time to write in journals without requiring students to share the writing. Romano (2004) elaborates, "students need to pay attention to their deep feeling and thinking. They will waste less time if they put aside the tangential, focus on what needs to be written, and respect the words tearing through the brain. They need to respond to their emotions. They need to move on the images flashing in their minds" (p. 49). This strategy also applies to problem solving in any field. In order for leaders to effectively solve problems, it helps for them to trust their first impressions and take action on the solutions.

WRITING WORKSHOPS

I once sent my students on a writing field trip as part of class. They had to pick a location of their choice and write about a topic of their choice. I never asked them to share their writing with me; their only assignment was to send me an email telling how the experience made them feel. This assignment was part of my normal classroom practices and not part of any research study, but a summary of student comments provides the insight that writing felt peaceful and therapeutic for the students who participated in the activity. Murray (1996) believes, "we all need to tell our stories and our stories need to be heard" (p. 7). During their writing time, my students discovered what they needed to say.

I include writing workshops as a daily part of the curriculum of my classroom. During writing conferences, students tell me that writing in their journals helps relieve stress. Stress can be contagious. Visit a high school or college campus around the time of midterms or finals, and witness students collectively getting stressed because while they are sharing the same community experience; that community experience is one of stress. As Enayati (2015) observes, "we volley emotions back and forth all the time, as part of every interaction – however brief or extended – that we have with each another. We can 'catch' other people's stress, all with amazing speed" (p. 154). One student would walk into the classroom sharing concern about an upcoming exam, and soon most of the students in the classroom were worried. Each class, I attempted to shift the momentum by beginning with a reading/writing workshop. Students had ten minutes to write in their journals about either a topic of their choice or a quote I wrote on the board.

I did not grade the writing in order to encourage students to share their feelings with the pages of their notebooks. If students didn't want to write, they could read a book of their choice. I share the belief of Gruwell and her students, The Freedom Writers (2009), who write, "the greatest lesson the Freedom Writers and I have learned is to validate that everyone has a story" (p. 283). My goal as a teacher, writer, and researcher is for students to share their stories through writing. Gruwell and the Freedom Writers (2019) still share the same belief ten years later and state, "we have found that the most profound way to reach people is through the art of sharing stories" (p. 321). I continued daily writing workshops and journal writing during the pandemic. Former students stopped me in the school hallways telling me that writing helped them deal with the stress of a new learning environment, where they needed to wear masks and couldn't eat in the dining hall with their friends. Occasionally, I take my classes outside for socially distanced writing. Students still need to wear their masks, but on a day of beautiful weather they can find peace by sitting alone under a tree, looking at a nearby lake while watching the ducks and writing in their journals.

TEACHERS AS REFLECTIVE LEADERS

Even though I love writing, I do not write daily long narratives in my journal. Sometimes I write quick notes, phrases, bullet points, or observations I want to remember about my teaching. Writing provides not only a place to reflect, but also a space to develop new ideas to share with others and find ways to implement the goals of an organization. Beck (2012) explains, "Wayfinders, by definition, create paths where there are none and find destinations no one knew were there" (p. 280). Journal writing enables leaders, such as classroom teachers, to envision an idea and then make that vision reality. When rereading my journal from my first year of teaching, I observed my use of writing to wrestle with questions such as: What worked about this lesson? What didn't work? What would I do differently the next time? Writing helped me gain confidence in my leadership skills, something a teacher of teenagers definitely needed!

Using writing as a method of reflection helps leaders rewrite their narratives. Enayati (2015) reminds people to pay attention to the stories they tell themselves because, "there are stories that serve us. And stories that don't. What are the stories that you repeat to yourself over and over again? How mindful are you of your unspoken mantras? What are the threads that run through your everyday and eventually, your entire life?" (p. 8). Writing illuminates narratives to help the author know which stories need rewriting. Ideally, writing should become about the journey, not the destination. But ideas help no one if they stay in the pages of a journal. Eventually the leader must stop reflecting and return to action to implement a new strategy. Heifetz (1994) argues, "leadership is both active and reflective. One has to alternate between participating and observing" (p. 252). By alternating reflection with action, leaders develop a dream and share that dream with others to make it become reality.

Transformative leaders leave an organization better than when they found it. Starratt (1993) states, "transformational leaders enable subordinates to find fulfillment from striving for and achieving the high goals and purposes the leaders set for them" (p. 9). Transformative leaders enable everyone to invest in the community's shared vision and values, while simultaneously establishing goals and a sense of purpose. One example of this is when Sandberg (2013) writes of the Harvard Business School, "they laid out a new, communal definition of leadership: 'leadership is about making others better as a result of your presence and making sure that impact lasts in your absence.' They held students responsible for the impact their behavior had on others" (p. 157). And the ripple effect continues.

THE PROCESS OF WRITING NARRATIVES

Advice that follows is designed for teachers interested in using writing in their classrooms with their students, as well as anyone interested in completing the writing process to help with personal stress relief during the pandemic or to organize professional leadership ideas.

To begin, writing doesn't have to be kept in a journal or be a long narrative. Also keep in mind that no English teacher is going to grade this writing, so it doesn't matter if there are incomplete thoughts, grammar mistakes, or no clear structure to the writing. English teachers can also use this strategy by encouraging students to write in journals where students feel free to make mistakes without the pressure of a grade. The important thing is to accept yourself as you are and don't judge yourself or your writing. Cameron (1998) explains, "we can either demand that we write well or we can settle more comfortably into writing down what seems to want to come through us – good, bad, or indifferent" (p. 11). Another key component of writing narratives is to trust the writing process of what Romano (1987) refers to as "percolating, drafting, revising, editing, and publication" (p. 55).

Percolating: Thinking about ideas to possibly put on paper. Goldberg (2000) discusses the value of trusting first impressions as "our ideas and intentions can mask and cover up a story; there is a life force that will declare itself if you let it. Get out of the way" (p. 42). The truest impression of what a person thinks is usually the first impression before the writer has time to second guess thoughts and question the words.

Drafting: Capturing a vision on paper, and continuing to follow initial ideas. Writing helps the writer sort through emotions and discover insights. Often people remember something more when they write it down instead of trying to memorize the information. Goldberg (1990) describes this as, "we are going to write down what we think. Right or wrong doesn't matter. We are standing up and saying who we are" (p. 139). Hence, writing benefits the writer.

Revising: Reframing ideas to allow for new perspective. Goldberg (1986) elaborates, "so while we are busy writing, all the burning life we are eager to express should come out of a place of peace" (p. 167). Writing creates peace; the writer releases worry and stress onto the page. Rereading the words provides the opportunity to gain a new perspective.

Editing: Cleaning up a piece of writing in preparation to share with an audience. Goldberg (2013) advises writers, "you have to find the entry into what you know inside, the way to bring it out so people will listen" (p. 26). While some writing is for the writer's eyes only, sharing writing with a trusted audience brings additional healing benefits if the writer needs to share.

Publishing: Trusting someone else enough to share the written words. As Goldberg (2007) states, "it's your call, when you write. Trust the urge inside you to lead you to the right choice" (p. 165). If we trust our words, writing will lead us where we need to go.

USING CURRICULUM TO CAPTURE ONGOING STORIES

Our stories evolve as we evolve. The curriculum influences teacher's decisions, but teachers also need to adapt the curriculum to meet the needs of their students. Connelly and Clandinin (1988) write, "teachers often tell stories about the ways they have learned from their curricular milieus" (p. 210). The stories of people's lives remain ongoing, and the addition of new narratives, such as life during a pandemic, can change a story. Connelly and Clandinin elaborate, "narrative is the study of how humans make meaning of experience by endlessly telling and retelling stories about themselves that both reconfigure the past and create purpose in the future" (p. 24). Teachers can demonstrate leadership to change the curriculum, thus changing students' lives for the better, especially during difficult times.

WELLNESS RESOURCES

To help you put the theories in this chapter into practice, here are some additional wellness resources. Sandberg (2013) writes, "we cannot change what we are unaware of, and once we are aware, we cannot help but change" (p. 156). I include the following resources which helped my students and me during the pandemic, and I plan to continue implementing after the pandemic ends. I use this section to discuss strategies which provide inspiration, as well as share teaching methods which illustrate innovation both in the era of online learning and when teachers across the country and around the world return to their classrooms. Feel free to take these ideas and incorporate them into your life in whatever ways work best for you.

BIBLIOTHERAPY: READING AS HEALING

Bibliotherapy is defined by the Association of Hospital and Institution Libraries (1966) as "the use of selected reading materials as therapeutic adjuvants in medicine and psychiatry; also guidance in the solution of personal problems through directed reading" (*AHIL Quarterly*, Summer 1966, p. 18.)

People who are experiencing emotional pain may need the help of a psychologist to discuss issues that may be creating barriers to healing. However, most people can receive benefits from finding books they relate to and that inspire them. As an English teacher, I discuss the healing value of writing when students write in their journals at the beginning of each class, but literature also offers opportunities to escape or know that others share our experiences.

Even though it is a fictional story, the novel *Station Eleven* earned a place in the news cycle because it features a pandemic which destroys most of society. I remain optimistic that the real world will not end up like the dystopian fictional world where people no longer have electricity or transportation except for walking. Author Emily St. John Mandel (2014) describes a scene where a character named Clark escapes catching the highly contagious virus as, "Clark woke at four a.m. the next morning and took a taxi to the airport. These were the hours of near misses, the hours of miracles, visible as such only in hindsight over the following days. The flu was already seeping through the city" (p. 223). Rereading the passage during pandemic times feels like reading a news article instead of a novel. I like the empowering response of the characters who survive the pandemic to create art and surround themselves with the beauty they have. The novel ends with hope that the future will bring better days.

No one wants to feel like they are alone in their experiences, and books can provide hope for people if they do not know anyone personally who has experienced similar pain. Granted, reading a book is not a substitute for having a conversation with a medical professional or receiving a hug from a supportive friend; nevertheless, books make us feel that someone else has lived our experience.

During the pandemic, families cope with illness due to the coronavirus and may need inspirational stories of healing. Even if someone hasn't contacted the virus, all of us experienced a disruption in life and could benefit from inspirational stories.

Numerous nonfiction books feature true inspirational stories of people coping with health issues. Actor Michael J. Fox (2009) describes his optimism after being diagnosed with Parkinson's as, "for everything this disease has taken, something with greater value has been given – sometimes just a marker that points me in a new direction that I might not otherwise have traveled. So, sure, it may be one step forward and two steps back, but after a time with Parkinson's, I've learned that what is important is making that one step count; always looking up" (p. 6). Fox's words in his book *Always Looking Up* provide hope to anyone experiencing chronic pain while simultaneously illustrating the value of keeping a positive attitude during medical treatments.

Readers looking for additional inspiration can find advice in the words of Randy Pausch (2008), who stood on a stage in a college lecture hall with a pancreatic cancer diagnosis and months to live in *The Last Lecture*, and told his students to follow their childhood dreams. Pausch discussed his own personal legacy and wrote, "if I was able to tell my story with the passion I felt, my lecture might help others find a path to fulfilling their own dreams" (p. 10). After Randy's death, his wife Jai (2012) wrote a book called *Dream New Dreams* that encouraged people who endured loss to pick up a broken piece of an old dream and dream a new dream.

Teacher David Menasche (2013) discovered that illness necessitated early retirement from teaching, so he contacted his former students to see if he made a difference in their lives. He learned his class assignment and life lesson asking students to create a priority list of what really mattered to them resonated long after the final classroom bell rang. His book, *The Priority List* reminds us that while pain may be part of life, it shouldn't define our lives. Menasche asked his students to write a list of their priorities and "they were revealing themselves to their peers and trusting their classmates not to judge them – but that simple assignment gave the students flashes of insight into themselves, and it helped them to identify and empathize with each other. What had begun as an exercise in literature had evolved into a life lesson" (p. 71). In writing priority lists, students not only expressed their goals and values, but also learned how their priorities influenced their actions.

Anyone questioning faith during a difficult illness can turn to the books *Proof of Heaven* (2012) by Dr. Eben Alexander and *To Heaven and Back* (2012) by Dr. Mary C. Neal. Dr. Alexander, a neurosurgeon, and Dr. Neal, an orthopedic surgeon, both questioned if the science of medicine could coexist with spirituality until they each had a near death experience.

For fiction books, the following passage from *Just like Heaven* by Marc Levy (2000) sounds like it could come from a medical journal when you read the words, "after his reading, he spent evenings emailing eminent professors of medicine and researchers describing his dilemma, pretending he was working on a novel. Some of them answered. They all agreed – the situation he described was medically impossible" (pp. 89-90). But the words aren't from a medical journal; they are from a fiction story about a man named Arthur who is trying frantically to help his love Lauren while she is in the hospital. Or for a reminder of the power of love and faith, in *A Walk to Remember* by Nicholas Sparks (1999), teenager Landon sits by the bedside of his girlfriend Jamie and reads the Bible with her while she shares her hope for a miracle as she battles cancer. Don't want to read a book? The movie version of the novel, especially the scene when Jamie confesses her disease and Landon tells her he isn't going anywhere while the ballad *Someday We'll Know* plays in the background is just as powerful for finding courage during difficult times.

ROBIN AND JEN'S CD: MUSIC AS HEALING

While journal writing helps some people organize their thoughts, other people may prefer a different method of motivation other than writing. Singer Amy Grant (2007) shares, "my passion has always been the connecting power of music, connecting us to each other, to ourselves, and to the love of God" (p. 210). My cousin Robin's passion for music inspired both of us to create a mix CD to listen to while completing physical therapy exercises in 2014. Robin's insights inspired me to think of new genres of healing.

Note: This list represents a small sample of the numerous songs that have inspired us over the years. The songs are older because I wanted to include the playlist we designed in 2014. It serves as a representation for you to create your own music mix to listen to if you need to feel inspired.

Warm Up Songs (high tempo music)

1. *Firework* by Katy Perry
2. *Wow* by Kylie Minogue
3. *Oh What a Night* by Four Seasons
4. *Losing My Ground* by Fergie
5. *Whenever* by *The Black Eyed Peas*
6. *Gold* by Britt Nicole

Cool Down Songs (low tempo music)

7. *This Train Don't Stop There Anymore* by Elton John
8. *Back to December* by Taylor Swift
9. *Have You Never Been Mellow* by Olivia Newton-John
10. *There You'll Be* by Faith Hill
11. *Sail On* by Lionel Richie and Tim McGraw
12. *Takes a Little Time* by Amy Grant

CREATING YOUR MULTIGENRE HEALING PROJECT

You can use the following ideas as inspiration to create your own multigenre healing project.

1. How do you best express what you are feeling, both physically and emotionally? It may be building a model of a boat, comparing your experiences to your favorite actor or athlete, writing a poem, playing a song you wrote on the piano, or drawing a picture. It may be different on different days. Just remember that multigenre projects are a form of creative expression that do not hurt yourself or anyone else. You may want to share your feelings by throwing rocks at your neighbor's window, but that creates more problems than it solves.
2. If you need help getting started, writers Julia Cameron, Georgia Heard, and Natalie Goldberg suggest thinking of a word as a prompt and reacting to it. Start with something neutral or humorous. For example, I'm looking out a window right now. I could write about the beautiful red flowers that bloom every year in May around my birthday. I could take a picture of the flowers. I could listen to music while I look at the flowers. The word window led me to my next word, flowers. You can continue to use words like these as inspiration or you can try more serious words, such as pain. Stop the activity if you feel physical or emotional pain.

3. If you complete more than one multigenre project, look for patterns. Do these patterns tell you anything? For example, if I spend a lot of time looking out windows to describe what I see, does it mean I am avoiding something by spending too much time looking out windows and not enough time working? Other people can also help you find patterns.
4. Make a list of things you love, including people, pets, activities, television shows, music, movies, sports, and other things that bring you joy and make you smile. Spend ten minutes a day with the people and things on that list.
5. Create a pain journal and share it with your doctor or physical therapist. Refer to Jen's as an example.

HEART MAPS

When you look at heart pictures, you might think of love, Valentine's Day, and happiness. Or you might think of health or a trip to the doctor. Too often in life we worry about things, which can lead to stress on our bodies. Ever feel your heart race when you are nervous about something? One way to stress less and smile more is to spend time with people and things you love by creating a heart map.

During the routine of a busy schedule, one method people can use to remind themselves of people and things they value is to create a heart map. Heart maps help people remember not to make work their lives. Heart maps originally started as a writing strategy; teachers use them in classrooms when students can't think of a writing topic. What is important to you? Look in your heart map!

Writing teachers such as Georgia Heard discuss the value of falling in love with life and the sense of peace it can bring. Heard (2016) describes heart maps as, "heart mapping is a metaphor for what all writers know: to write is to delve into what matters to us, to keep our feelings alive, to be vulnerable, to tell the truth, to question, and to speak what many people only keep inside" (p. 1). I love drawing heart maps and creating artistic representations of my thoughts, feelings, ideas, hopes, and dreams; I also love seeing my journal writing and my formal writing that you now read as a written representation of my heart. How do you know what will make you happy? According to Heard (1995), "with the map you've already made in your heart. That's where the real home is: inside" (p. 2).

Heart maps can be a simple sketch or an intricate work of art. Heard (1999) instructs her students, "Today, I'd like you to make a map of all the important things that are in your heart, all the things that really matter to you. You can put: people and places that you care about; moments and memories that have stayed with you; things you love to do, anything that has stayed in your heart because you care a lot about it" (pp. 108-109). To create a heart map, draw a heart on a sheet of paper. In the heart, write the names of beloved people, places, and things. The important thing is to make the items in the heart map as much a part of life as possible. Heard (1999) instructs, "if it's something that you really care about then it belongs in your heart map. Only you can decide what should be in your heart map" (p. 109). In heart maps, the common thread is that the designer loves each item in it. Heard (1995) writes, "the seemingly random observations I make or the subjects I choose to write about are like the branches of a tree whose roots reach down to the depths of myself and reveal my obsessions" (pp. 69-70). Heart maps provide a vision of what the designer values.

Here's how to create your own heart map:

Table 1. Jen's Neck Pain Journal

Date	Pain Level 1=Low, 10=High	Observations
Wed 3/28 morning	Left Side = 2, Right Side =2	Feeling great after physical therapy and want to continue trend. Ask tech guy at work if I can prop computer monitor on books so I am looking up, not down. He loves idea and it makes my neck feel better.
Afternoon	Left Side =4, Right Side = 4, also dizzy	Pick up podium in classroom and move it. Pick up large box of books in classroom and move it. Have done both dozens of times in my life before neck pain. Apparently my neck isn't ready for furniture moving. Students happily move furniture.
Afternoon	Left Side = 3, Right Side =3	Students present text modernizations that are purposefully funny. Romeo and Juliet's families have a dance battle instead of a sword fight. Dorothy and her friends get lost at the mall instead of in Oz. I laugh so much I almost cry and somehow that helps neck.
Evening	Left Side = 4, Right Side = 3, also dizzy	Not sure how I feel about the guy I am going out with this weekend, but my neck doesn't like him. It's tightening up while I'm making plans for a date. Maybe my neck is trying to tell me something.
Night	Left Side = 3, Right Side = 3	9:30pm + home from work late + still need to do second set of exercises = Neck Exercise Disco Dance Party!! Turn on Kylie Minogue CD for motivation and actually have to remind myself to slow down the exercises.
Thurs 3/29/12 morning	Left Side = 1, Right Side = 3	Second set of exercises in less than 12 hours. Left side is tight but not in much pain. Think I'm still dreaming. Glad I'm not.
Afternoon	Left Side = 1, Right Side = 2	Take lunch break to play on the swings by the campus residence halls. Heaven.
Afternoon	Left Side = 2, Right Side =4, also dizzy	Playing baseball game in class for semester review and throwing ball around. I'm not getting enough sleep and all I had to eat before teaching was an energy bar. And I wonder why I'm feeling dizzy?!
Night	Left Side =0 (gone), Right Side =3	Another late night on campus. Time to turn on the Kylie CD for Neck Exercise Disco Dance Party Part II! The left side of my neck is tight, but there is no pain. Amazing. Forgot what that feels like. The right side still hurts but not as bad.
Summary	Left side is tight with occasional pain but mostly gone. Need to get over final hurdle with right side pain.	I needed to laugh more! Writing this has been entertaining, insightful, and enlightening. Hope you enjoyed it!

- Draw a heart on a sheet of paper. The artistic quality doesn't matter. What is important is that you leave enough blank space to write words inside the heart.
- Inside the heart, write down the names of people, places, and things you love. No one has to see this except you. Remember it's not always the big things in life but the small things that can cause you to smile. A walk in the park when it is sunny outside. Spending time with my family. A great book. That's part of my list. What makes you happy?

- Look at your list. How much of your day is spent with the people, places, and things in your heart map? If you are not spending part of your day with people, places, and things you love, how can you arrange your schedule so you can do this?
- No one has to see this heart map except for you, but you may want to use your heart map as a reality check. You may love things that are not healthy for you, and it's also fine to enjoy some things in moderation or occasionally, such as spending a Saturday watching reruns of a favorite television show or eating your favorite dessert. The key is balance.
- Don't have enough hours in the day for things you love? Try to rearrange your schedule to spend more time with the people and things in your heart map.
- Below is an example of a heart map I created.

Figure 1. Heart map designed by the author

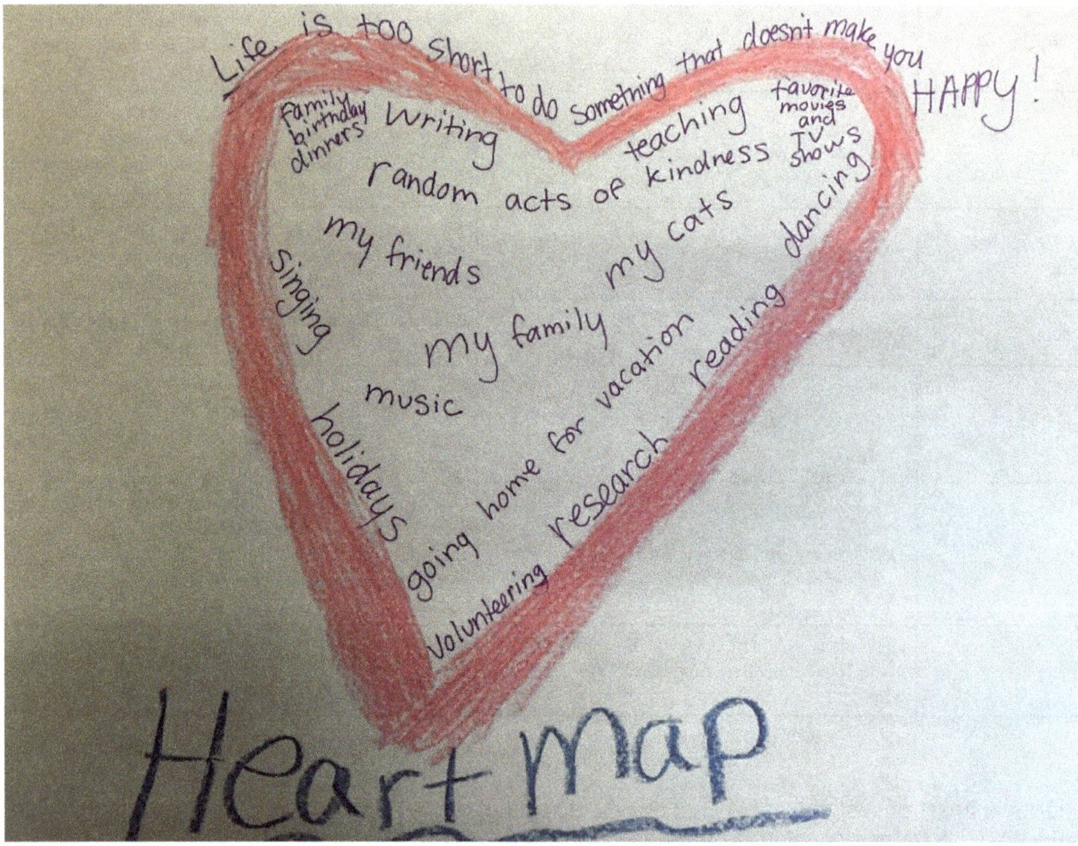

525,600 MINUTES OF WHAT BRINGS YOU ENERGY

In the song *Seasons of Love*, a year is measured in 525,600 minutes. Everyone has an equal amount of time in a year. How do you use it? Teacher Donald Graves discusses four types of activities. Graves (2001) states, "I know that you already have a sense of what takes energy, gives it, and is a waste of time. What you need now are the specifics from your own life in order to chart a different course from the one you know. Awareness that grows out of the specifics of your own situation produces energy" (p. 11). What do you do that gives you energy? What do you do that takes away energy? What do you do that is neutral? What do you do that wastes energy? Time to take a look at how you spend your time. A person can complete a variety of activities to identify what gives energy and what takes it away, such as a list of daily activities, a pie chart as a graphic organizer balance wheel of how time is spent, or writing about whatever is on his or her mind. Charting a new course can mean something as simple as minor adjustments to daily habits. If reading a favorite magazine brings energy but waiting in line takes away energy, read the favorite magazine while waiting in line. Other times, charting a new course means needing to make major life changes.

- Write out your schedule, or choose a computer program or the calendar feature on your phone that will do it for you.
- Hour by hour, list how you spend your time during a day. Be honest with yourself. No one has to see this except for you. Now look at how your energy level feels with each activity.
- Which activities give you energy? For example, I love spending time with loved ones, teaching, and making a difference in the world. List yours.
- Which activities take away energy? For example, I hate waiting in long lines, cleaning, and running boring errands. Some activities, such as a long walk, may take away physical energy but bring you emotional energy.
- Which activities are neutral? I consider driving and eating in this category, although driving may take away energy if I'm driving in a thunderstorm and eating may give energy if I am having a meal with a group of friends.
- Which activities waste energy? I have to play computer solitaire until I win. After ten or eleven games, this wastes both time and energy.
- Now that you have categorized the activities, how many of each do you have in your day? Are you spending too much time doing activities that take away energy and not enough time doing activities that give energy?
- If the answer to the above question is yes, consider pairing activities that take away energy with ones that bring you energy. For example, I might read a magazine (something that gives me energy) while sitting in the waiting room during a car oil change (something that takes away energy).
- Can you eliminate activities that take away energy or waste energy from your schedule? In other words, if you said no to someone or something, how bad would the consequences be? If you can't make the dessert for the party, the odds are someone else will do it. Probably not a big deal.
- You should notice some connections between the activities that bring you energy and the ones in your heart map. More energy = the feeling of more hours in a day.

10-10-10

Suzy Welch designed a strategy called 10-10-10. Welch (2009) explains that to reclaim her life, she needed "to start making my decisions differently – proactively – by deliberately considering their consequences in the immediate present, near term, and distant future. In ten minutes….ten months….and ten years" (p. 9). What will be important to you ten minutes from now, ten months from now, and ten years from now? Dooley (2019) shares how she uses the process as, "make sure the big and small decisions you make are good for both Present You and Future You" (p. 158). Answer these questions in your own life. Sometimes what seems like a big deal now may not be a big deal later.

Here's an example of how I used this recently:

Issue: I have numerous emails to answer but also want to meet my family for dinner. I picture how the results of my decision might look in the short term, midterm, and long term future.

Life 10 minutes from now: I really need to answer these emails so I can start work tomorrow without having to worry about them, but I also don't want to disappoint my family.

Life 10 months from now: I won't remember the content of those emails, but I will remember dinner with my family and smile when I look at the pictures of that event.

Life 10 years from now: I love my job, but I love my family more. I don't want to be a person who was so distracted by work at the expense of family relationships. So I'm going to put aside the emails and focus on being in the moment with people I love.

So if an issue is bothering you…. How will you feel about it in the immediate, distant, and really distant future?

IMPORTANT/URGENT

Stephen Covey designed a matrix of urgent vs. important. Covey, Merrill, and Merrill (1994) explain, "clearly, we deal with both factors – urgency and importance – in our lives. But in our day-to-day decision making, one of these factors tends to dominate. The problem comes when we operate primarily from a paradigm of urgency rather than a paradigm of importance" (p. 39). If something is both urgent and important (the bills need to be paid), people usually do it. If something is not urgent and not important (reading junk mail), people rarely do it. The middle categories can get confusing. Some things that seem urgent aren't that important. For example, the phone rings during a family dinner, you grab it, and it is a telemarketer. Don't take time away from family dinner (not urgent but important) to deal with the telemarketer (urgent but not important). Pipher (2006), advises, "don't let the urgent crowd out the important" (p. 91). Too often, the urgent email eclipsed the important activity that required more of my attention. Cameron (1998) reminds people that "each day, each life, is a series of choices, and as we use the lens of writing to view our lives, we see our choices" (p. 94). Sometimes the best way to delineate between the urgent and important in life is to write about choices.

Here's an example of how I used this recently:

I'm working on lesson plans for class (urgent, important). Emails appear in my inbox (urgent, not important). I also want to have dinner with my family (not urgent, important). I wonder if I will have time to watch my favorite television show (not urgent, not important). I make my decisions based on my values and priorities of what is important. I finish the lesson plans and remind myself they do not have to be perfect, enjoy dinner with my family, save the emails for later, and will watch the television show if I have time.

Don't let urgent demands eclipse what is truly important in life.

LIVING A WELLNESS NARRATIVE

As a teacher, curriculum design enables me to think of the larger goals, themes, and objectives for my lesson plans before, during, and after the pandemic. I agree with Johnson (1998) who writes, "When you walk into that classroom, know why you're there and what you want your students to learn; then relax and have some fun" (p. 359). This year, more than ever, I relied on strong leadership and innovative teaching to provide my students with teachable moments and to make learning fun during the pandemic. Beck (2021) describes teaching that connects with students' souls as, "some soul teachers are actual schoolteachers, like the Robin Williams character in *Dead Poets Society*, whose wacky methods open his pupils' hearts and souls along with their minds" (p. 44). I enjoy showing my students the clip of the movie where John Keating, played by Robin Williams, encourages his students to rip out pages of a textbook that contain outdated ideas. During the pandemic, I needed to rip out old ideas that could not work anymore based on the current circumstances. The need to change challenged me to think critically and creatively about the curriculum. While students may indeed view some of my teaching methods as unusual, I see the strategies as helping students not just intellectually, but also emotionally during a difficult time.

ACKNOWLEDGMENT

The preceding chapter contains excerpts from the following previous IGI publications:

Bird, J.L. (2020). Narratives of teaching methods. In *Using narrative writing to enhance healing* (pp. 185-237). Hershey, PA: Information Science Reference.

Bird, J.L. (2020). Narratives of patient care. In *Using narrative writing to enhance healing* (pp. 157-184). Hershey, PA: Information Science Reference.

Bird, J.L., & Wanner, E.T. (2020). Narratives of writing as healing. In *Using narrative writing to enhance healing* (pp. 295-338). Hershey, PA: Information Science Reference.

Bird, J.L., Wanner, E.T., Urenda, R., & Perry, R. (2015). Multigenre medicine. In *Innovative collaborative practice and reflection in patient education* (pp. 1-19). Hershey, PA: Information Science Reference.

REFERENCES

Adams, W., & Ferguson, S. (2010). Whenever [Recorded by The Black Eyed Peas]. On The beginning [CD]. Santa Monica, CA: Interscope Records.

Alexander, E. (2012). *Proof of Heaven*. Simon and Schuster.

Alexander, G., Brisebois, D. A., & Holland, D. (2002). Someday we'll know [Recorded by Mandy Moore and Jonathan Foreman]. On A walk to remember [CD]. New York, NY: Epic/Sony.

Association of Hospital and Institution Libraries. (1966, Summer). Bibliotherapy with children's books – reading children's books. AHIL Quarterly, 18.

Barbieri, M. (1995). *Sounds from the heart*. Heinemann.

Beck, M. (2001). *Finding your own North Star*. Three Rivers Press.

Beck, M. (2012). *Finding your way in a wild new world*. Free Press.

Beck, M. (2021). *The way of integrity*. The Open Field.

Brown, B. (2012). *Daring greatly*. Gotham Books.

Brown, B. (2015). *Rising strong*. Spiegel & Grau.

Brown, B. (2018). *Dare to lead*. Random House.

Cameron, J. (1998). *The right to write*. Tarcher/Putnam.

Clandinin, D. J., & Connelly, F. M. (2000). *Narrative inquiry*. Jossey-Bass.

Cleary, L. M. (1991). *From the other side of the desk*. Heinemann.

Connelly, F. M., & Clandinin, D. J. (1988). *Teachers as curriculum planners*. Teachers College.

Covey, S. R., Merrill, A. R., & Merrill, R. R. (1994). *First things first*. Free Press.

DiNovi, D. (Producer), & Shankman, A. (Director). (2002). *A walk to remember* [motion picture]. United States: Warner Brothers Pictures.

Dooley, J. L. (2019). *Own your everyday*. Waterbrook.

Enayati, A. (2015). *Seeking serenity*. New American Library.

Fallon, A. (2020). *The power of writing it down*. Zondervan.

Farrar, J. (1975). Have you never been mellow [Recorded by Olivia Newton-John]. On Have you never been mellow [CD]. Universal City, CA: MCA.

Ferguson, S., Sandstrom, R., Ridel, S., & Boldt, R. (2006). Losing my ground [Recorded by Fergie]. On The dutchess [CD]. Santa Monica, CA: A&M Records.

Fox, M. J. (2009). *Always looking up*. Hyperion.

Gaudio, B., & Parker, J. (1995) December 1963 (oh what a night) remix [Recorded by the Four Seasons]. On Oh what a night [CD]. Nashville, TN: Curb Records.

Goldberg, N. (1986). *Writing down the bones*. Shambhala.

Goldberg, N. (1990). *Wild mind*. Bantam.

Goldberg, N. (2000). *Thunder and lightning*. Bantam.

Goldberg, N. (2007). *Old friend from far away*. Free Press.

Goldberg, N. (2013). *The true secret of writing*. Atria.

Grant, A. (2007). *Mosaic*. Doubleday.

Grant, A., & Kirkpatrick, W. (1997). Takes a little time [Recorded by Amy Grant]. On Behind the eyes [CD]. Hollywood, CA: A&M Records.

Graves, D. (2001). *The energy to teach*. Heinemann.

Gruwell, E., & the Freedom Writers. (1999). The Freedom Writers diary. New York, NY: Broadway.

Gruwell, E., & the Freedom Writers. (2009). The Freedom Writers diary (2nd ed.). New York, NY: Broadway.

Gruwell, E., & the Freedom Writers. (2019). The Freedom Writers diary (3rd ed.). New York, NY: Broadway.

Heard, G. (1995). *Writing toward home*. Heinemann.

Heard, G. (1999). *Awakening the heart*. Heinemann.

Heard, G. (2016). *Heart maps*. Heinemann.

Heifetz, R. A. (1994). *Leadership without easy answers*. The Belnap Press of Harvard University Press.

John, E., & Taupin, B. (2001). This train don't stop there anymore [Recorded by Elton John]. On Songs from the west coast. New York, NY: Universal.

Johnson, L. (1998). *Two parts textbook, one part love*. Hyperion.

Johnson, L. (2005). *Teaching outside the box*. Jossey-Bass.

Kearns, J. (1997). *Where to begin: A guide to teaching secondary English*. Heinemann.

Lamott, A. (1994). *Bird by bird*. Anchor Books.

Larson, J. (2005). Seasons of love [Recorded by the cast of Rent]. On Rent: Original motion picture soundtrack [CD]. Burbank, CA: Warner Brothers Records.

Levy, M. (2000). Just like Heaven. New York, NY: Pocket Books. (Originally published as If only it were true).

Mandel, E. S. J. (2014). *Station Eleven*. Alfred A. Knopf.

Menasche, D. (2013). *The priority list*. Touchstone.

Minogue, K., Poole, K., & Kurstin, G. (2008). Wow [Recorded by Kylie Minogue]. On X [CD]. Hollywood, CA: EMI.

Murray, D. M. (1996). *Crafting a life*. Heinemann.

Neal, M. C. (2012). *To Heaven and back*. WaterBrook Press.

Nicole, B., Muckala, D., & Cates, J. (2012). Gold [Recorded by Britt Nicole]. On Gold [CD]. Brentwood, TN: Capitol.

Pausch, E. J. (2012). *Dream new dreams*. Crown Archtype.

Pausch, R., & Zaslow, J. (2008). *The last lecture*. Hyperion.

Perry, K., Eriksen, M., Hermansen, T., Wilhelm, S., & Dean, E. (2010). Firework [Recorded by Katy Perry]. On Teenage dream [CD]. New York, NY: Capitol.

Pipher, M. (2006). *Writing to change the world.* Riverhead.

Richie, L. (2012). Sail on [Recorded by Lionel Richie and Tim McGraw]. On Tuskegee [CD]. Nashville, TN: Mercury.

Romano, T. (1987). *Clearing the way.* Heinemann.

Romano, T. (1995). *Writing with passion.* Heinemann.

Romano, T. (2000). *Blending genre, altering style.* Heinemann.

Romano, T. (2004). *Crafting authentic voice.* Heinemann.

Romano, T. (2008). *Zigzag.* Heinemann.

Romano, T. (2013). *Fearless writing.* Heinemann.

Sandberg, S. (2013). *Lean in.* Alfred A. Knopf.

Sparks, N. (1999). *A walk to remember.* Warner.

Starratt, R. J. (1993). *The drama of leadership.* The Falmer Press.

Swift, T. (2010). Back to December [Recorded by Taylor Swift]. On Speak now [CD]. Nashville, TN: Big Machine Records.

Tindle, H. (2013). *Up: how positive outlook can transform our health and aging.* Hudson Street Press.

Tovani, C. (2011). *So what do they really know?* Stenhouse.

Wade, C. (2018). *Heart talk.* Atria.

Warren, D. (2001). There you'll be [Recorded by Faith Hill]. On Pearl Harbor [CD]. Burbank, CA: Hollywood Records/Warner Brothers.

Weir, P. (Director). (1989). *Dead Poets Society* [motion picture] United States: Touchstone Pictures.

Welch, S. (2009). 10-10-10. New York, NY: Scribner.

KEY TERMS AND DEFINITIONS

Artistic and Technical Writing: Artistic writing focuses on the writer's tone of word choice, also known as voice, while technical writing focuses on the writer's specificity of word choice. English teachers design rubrics that incorporate both artistic and technical writing.

Heart Maps: Writing teacher Georgia Heard believes in the value of heart maps, which ask writers to draw a heart and inside the heart write things that the writer loves.

Journal Writing: The process of a person responding to prompts and writing about his or her thoughts and feelings. While journal writing is typically associated with writing classrooms, writing teachers including Julia Cameron and Natalie Goldberg advocate that journal writing can be done by anyone, anywhere.

Multigenre Healing Project: This different perspective on multigenre projects connects the fields of education and medicine.

Multigenre Writing: Introduced to the field of education by Tom Romano, multigenre writing consists of creative writing in multiple genres and the writer's analysis of the genres.

Narrative Inquiry: Described in depth by F. Michael Connelly and D. Jean Clandinin, narrative inquiry is a qualitative interpretative form of research that focuses on the telling, retelling, and sharing of stories.

Neck Pain Journal: Jen created a journal of what she was doing when her neck felt pain.

Urgent vs. Important: Mary Pipher, Don Graves, and Stephen Covey all discuss the type of choices people make of how they spend their time and the resulting increased or decreased energy experienced.

Writing as Healing: James Pennebaker is a leader in the field which explores the health benefits of writing. Numerous studies have been conducted by researchers investigating the influence of writing on physical and emotional health.

Writing Process: Composing an essay using percolating, drafting, revising, editing, and publication.

Writing Voice: Voice in writing describes how a writer uses word choice and tone to reflect the unique personality of the writer. Just like each person has a unique speaking voice, each writer has a unique writing voice.

Chapter 5
Reflections of Teaching Narratives

ABSTRACT

This narrative describes the experiences of a high school English teacher who uses innovative teaching methods to adapt to online teaching during the recent pandemic. Students relied on writing to reflect on their emotional health and found comfort in relating to works of literature. The creative projects and motivational strategies discussed can apply to anyone looking to cope with difficult times, find more motivation to achieve a goal, or practice self-compassion when confronted with unexpected events.

TRANSFORMATIVE TEACHING

Like my colleagues across the country and around the world, I found my teaching career transformed by the closure of schools and the move to online teaching in the era of the coronavirus. The online teaching experience called for renovation and exploration. This narrative represents my reflection on my past teaching methods and how I used creativity and innovation to promote future success for my students.

TEACHING AND TECHNOLOGY

Change takes courage. Most people live their lives never leaving their comfort zones. Johnson (2005) observes, "teaching superbly is like running a marathon by yourself in the dark. Few people even notice what you're doing, and those who notice don't pay much attention – but their oblivion doesn't slow you down. You still enjoy the thrill and satisfaction of finishing the race, and you are definitely a winner" (p. 5). But education doesn't have to be each teacher alone in a classroom, especially with technology that makes collaboration only an email away. Teachers tend to stay in their own classrooms; every once in a while they might venture down the hall to have a conversation with a colleague, but then they lock themselves back in the world behind their classroom doors. Connelly and Clandinin (1988) believe that teachers "come to know their own practices from their work with colleagues" (p. 209). New ideas occur

DOI: 10.4018/978-1-7998-9051-5.ch005

when people venture outside their own practices and share their thoughts with others. Romano (2004) believes, "our own voices can take on strength and energy through other voices" (p. 96). My morning conversations with colleagues energized me and helped save my sanity as I prepared to put on my mask each morning during the pandemic and teach behind plexiglass.

I began my high school English teaching career in a school with a tremendous amount of energy, but not a significant amount of resources. My classroom contained a chalkboard, an old television and VCR, and an overhead projector. I made the best of it. When the overhead projector, named Elmo for the company that manufactured it, broke, I placed colorful leis on it with the note "Elmo is on vacation." For presentations, I used video clips from old VHS tapes. I wrote notes on transparencies (once Elmo started functioning again) and washed them in the restroom sink to reuse. I waited (sometimes patiently, sometimes not) for one of the four computers in the faculty workroom when I needed to send emails to parents. I returned to the same restroom sink and filled a bucket with water to scrub the chalkboard. But the lack of technology did not interfere with learning. Students loved taking out their journals and putting pen to paper to record their thoughts. This was only about ten years ago.

It frustrates me to think of inequity in school classrooms. The school where I currently teach gives every student and teacher a laptop. Technology enables us to continue teaching during a pandemic, when some students choose to learn at home with online learning, while others attend class in person. I feel grateful to erase the whiteboard in my classroom because I no longer have to clean chalkboards. I also feel grateful because the lack of technology in my first classroom prepared me to become a creative teacher; creativity helps immensely when teaching during a pandemic.

WRITING WITH TECHNOLOGY

When several students in my classes said they could not remember the last time they received a handwritten letter, I designed a class activity where everyone took out a sheet of paper and wrote a note to a friend or family member. Students shared with me stories of reconnecting with family members they hadn't seen since before the pandemic. Some things, like handwritten letters, never go out of style.

Nevertheless, when I compose my own writing for chapters such as this one, I rarely handwrite anything first. Instead, I love the feeling of my fingers flying across the keyboard and seeing words appear on the screen. As Goldberg (1986) observes, "sometimes, instead of writing in a notebook, you might want to directly type out your thoughts. Writing is physical and is affected by the equipment you use" (p. 6). And a flash drive with writing is easier to carry than a pile of notebooks. Goldberg continues, there is a time and place for both because "I have found that when I am writing something emotional, I must write it the first time directly with hand on paper. Handwriting is more connected to the movement of the heart. Yet, when I tell stories, I go straight to the typewriter" (pp. 6-7). Regardless of whether students use pen and paper or their laptop computers, I want them to write.

Revision becomes easier with a typed draft, since deleting a word makes it disappear without any of the crossed out words or erasing required of handwritten drafts. Kearns (1997) describes, "word-processing programs can help our students be better writers by encouraging students to write before they compose – to brainstorm, plan, select, focus, draft, revise, and publish." (p. 114). She elaborates, "computers can also reduce writing apprehension. For some students, writing becomes easier to manipulate and motivation becomes higher" (p. 114). Some students see a finished handwritten draft as a work of art not to be disturbed; conversely, technology enables them to save multiple drafts of an essay with a quick click of a computer mouse. Heard (1995) writes, "there are times when revision isn't necessary. These are the rare moments when what I write the first time is exactly what I want" (pp. 121-122). When I write a piece right with the first draft it is a special occasion. In fact, the words you are reading represent the fourth draft of this sentence. My computer made the magic of revision possible within a few seconds. While I will never lose my admiration for a powerful handwritten composition, technology provides methods of making writing easier and more fun for students. Technology also makes life easier for teachers. During the pandemic, I don't need to touch papers because students download and upload all documents electronically.

MULTIGENRE PROJECTS

Students do not always need to respond to a work of literature using writing. Artwork and song lyrics provide additional outlets for creative expression. Rief (1999) observes, "by watching my students and collecting their work over the years, I've learned how vision and voice matter to them. Their reader's-writer's journals are filled with sketches, drawings, and photographs; they are filled with poems and song lyrics" (p. 32). Students effectively demonstrate their comprehension of a text using multiple genres including original paintings and drawings as well as song lyrics and musical performances.

One of my favorite projects is the multigenre project, where students view a text through multiple genres and multiple lenses. In describing multigenre writing, Romano (2013) explains, "multigenre places students in a situation that demands narrative thinking. It's risky. Readers might not 'get' the writer's intentions. Writers must work hard on the writing. They must craft it" (p. 22). Multigenre writing encourages writers to look beyond traditional expository writing when discussing research. A narrative thread connects the genres of a project and focuses on a central theme. For example, if a student completes a multigenre project about a novel, the narrative thread is that each project illuminates a different aspect of the text. Romano elaborates, "instead of producing expository papers, students are writing in many genres. Although each piece is self-contained, making a point of its own, taken together, all the writing creates a unified whole" (p. 2). Technology adds a new dimension to multigenre projects, as students now design digital collages, blogs from a character's perspective, and movies starring their friends and family to recreate scenes from the novel. Students then include a short section of end notes to explain why they designed the projects they did. Clandinin and Connelly (2000) remind me that "the teacher is part of the curriculum and therefore part of the establishment of the goals in the first place and part of the ensuing achievement" (p. 29). In my classroom, I observe students learning more if they have fun in the process, so my goals which lead to student achievement incorporate both creativity and critical thinking.

Multigenre projects served as a staple in my classroom since my first year of teaching, but students appreciate creative projects more during the pandemic era because creativity provides a fun outlet during times of stress. Multigenre projects are not limited to this list, since some students use technology to create additional innovative ideas, and I also offer students the opportunity to propose their own projects that they imagine. Multigenre projects can include the following:

Project #1: Vocabulary Project

- A board game featuring words from the novel
- A poem featuring words from the novel

Project #2: Interactive Reading Project

- A magazine collage symbolizing parts of the novel
- A mix CD containing songs that represent the characters
- Artwork depicting a scene from the novel
- An invitation, menu, or other art project related to the novel
- A news article describing an event in the novel

Project #3: Writing Project

- A "missing scene," such as a conversation between two characters that could have taken place but didn't actually happen in the novel
- A prequel or sequel
- Rewriting an existing scene from another character's point of view
- Pretending you are a minor character and explaining your connection to the main character
- A journal entry from a character's perspective
- An advice column helping a character solve a problem.

COMPARING BOOKS AND MOVIES

My passion for using video clips that relate to the texts discussed in class has not changed even after transitioning from using a VCR to using a DVD player. And some video clips don't even need a DVD player. When enrolled in an eLearning class, I learned that YouTube videos can be embedded into the online Blackboard site for courses. I was ecstatic! No more taking class time to cue a clip! Gaughan (1997) believes, "as teachers, we can help students become more visually literate by making them aware of how they read films" (p. 137). I also ask students to complete a book vs.movie chart to discuss the similarities and differences between the two texts. Students enjoy comparing and contrasting the book vs. movie versions of a text and debating why the changes may have occurred. Some book to movie changes are significant, such as the Nicholas Sparks novel *Dear John*, where the movie ends in a completely different way from the book. Other changes are more subtle, such as in the Randall Wallace novel *Pearl Harbor*, where in the book Rafe gives Evelyn a rose and in the movie he gives her a paper crane. Students use Venn Diagrams (showing the degree of overlap between concepts) to describe similarities and differences between the book and the movie.

By watching video clips, instead of only discussing a concept, students can experience it. Gaughan (2001) argues, "but teaching strategies are not enough. Long-term, sustained thinking requires immersion" (p. 137). I believe in the learn by doing approach, and if I can immerse students in learning while making connections to things that already interest them, the sparks of knowledge fly. Numerous students admit that the movies provide a visual of the characters which assists in comprehension of the text. I frequently model strategies before asking students to complete assignments. Johnson (1998) recommends, "even when I have a cooperative class, I do every assignment with my students. Working with them keeps me on track and makes them feel important" (p. 193). Therefore, when students studied explicit (stated) and implicit (implied) themes in a music video, I demonstrated the media literacy analysis using Katy Perry's song and video *The One That Got Away*. I dissected the song lyrics, highlighting literary terms such as similes (comparison using like or as) and metaphors (comparison not using like or as) and an example of Deus ex machina (God from the machine, a literary device where a character is unexpectedly rescued from an impossible situation) when Katy laments that all the money in the world can't buy a time machine to undo a decision she regrets. After analyzing the lyrics (explicit text), students watched the video (implict text) to see Katy Perry's visual interpretation of the song. Students gasped when an unexpected twist happened in the video that they never could have predicted from the lyrics. Literature came alive that day with an assist from technology. I also give students the opportunity to choose (school appropriate) music videos and analyze them.

Another powerful strategy involves building a theme unit containing texts with similar themes. One of my favorites is pairing Jennifer E. Smith's young adult novel *The Statistical Probability of Love at First Sight* with the movie *Serendipity*. The book is about a teenager named Hadley who gets separated from Oliver, a guy she just meets and likes, in an airport before they can exchange phone numbers. The same thing happens to the characters of John and Sara in the movie, when they get separated from each other in a crowded hotel before they can exchange phone numbers. I introduce the theme unit by playing Kylie Minogue's song *Love at First Sight* and conclude by asking students to write advice to the characters of Hadley and Oliver who were separated from the person they believed to be their soul mate. Interestingly, most students gave the advice to move on because there was nothing that could be done, thus illustrating real life students are much more practical than their fictional counterparts in the novel. As Brooks (1998) observes, "it is important for the English teacher to develop a useful, practical method for helping teenagers evaluate the products of mass media" (p. 21). Because media plays a significant role in the lives of my students, I find value in using this technology to enhance reading comprehension for my students.

MODERNIZING CLASSIC LITERATURE

Sometimes students struggle to relate to texts written a couple hundred years ago, even though the texts have literary value. Maxwell, Meiser, and McKnight (2011) write, "traditional literature has long served as a window to understand humanity. In an era where technology develops at a mind-boggling pace, our students must learn how to decipher messages that they receive daily. These messages transmit powerful ideas about our society and humanity. Being able to use and create these messages and texts is another means for powerful personal expression" (p. 255). Traditional literature, frequently called classic literature, can coexist with rapidly developing technology. In this way, teachers modernize classic texts and make them more relevant to students' lives. One method used to modernize classics is to ask students to imagine text message conversations between characters. I always smile when reading the scene in Jane Austen's novel *Pride and Prejudice*, where the characters of Elizabeth and Mr. Darcy realize they have feelings for each other. Austen (1813) describes the scene as "Elizabeth feeling all the more than common awkwardness and anxiety of his situation, now forced herself to speak; and immediately, though not very fluently, gave him to understand, that her sentiments had undergone so material a change, since to the period to which he alluded, as to make her receive with gratitude and pleasure, his present assurances" (p. 346). After reading this, students usually comment that the passage is too wordy. I show students the corresponding clip of the scene from the movie and ask them to imagine that the story took place in 2020 instead of 1813. If the story took place in modern times, Elizabeth and Darcy would most likely exchange text messages with each other. So what would that text message conversation look like? I ask them to write it. Students live in the world of texting, so laughter, creativity, and comprehension ensue.

Students also live in a world of music, so designing a mix CD for a work of literature becomes another modernization of a classic novel project enhanced by technology. Students enjoy building playlists of songs they feel symbolize the characters and themes in a text, even if the songs aren't in the story or aren't even of the era in which the novel takes place. They further analyze each song by creating a main idea wheel. Johns and Lenski (2010) instruct, "draw a wheel with spokes on the chalkboard and tell students that the center of the wheel represents the main idea and the spokes represent the supporting details" (p. 438). I use various songs from the television show *Glee* about a high school choir to create main idea wheels, putting the song title in the center and details from the lyrics on the spokes. Other times, like in the next example, I prefer to make connections using narratives instead of graphic organizers. The following is a playlist I designed for F. Scott Fitzgerald's *The Great Gatsby* with connections between the song list and the scenes from the novel:

Song: *A Public Affair* by Jessica Simpson

Passage from *The Great Gatsby:* "Sometimes they came and went without having met Gatsby at all, came for the party with a simplicity of heart that was its own ticket of admission" (p. 45).

Connections: The song lyric about the party never stopping highlights the fact that Gatsby's parties never seemed to stop. One party ended, only to have another begin. Like the tabloids gossip about modern celebrities, people gossiped about Gatsby's parties and turned a private event into a public affair.

Song: *Don't Lie* by The Black Eyed Peas

Passage from The Great Gatsby: "It made no difference to me. Dishonesty in a woman is a thing you never blame deeply – I was casually sorry, and then I forgot" (p. 63).

Connections: Jordan lied enough that she often didn't know who she was, but it didn't matter to Nick because he loved her. Nick believes lying is wrong, although his relationship with Jordan causes him to rationalize her behavior. Jordan's lies, however, eventually create tension between her and Nick.

Song: *Love Will Wait* by Wild Orchid

Passage from The Great Gatsby: "I went in – after making every possible noise in the kitchen short of pushing over the stove – but I don't believe they heard a sound. They were sitting at either end of the couch looking at each other as if some question had been asked or was in the air, and every vestige of embarrassment was gone" (p. 94).

Connections: Nick sees Daisy and Gatsby together and in that moment, without knowing what happens later in the novel, their love has appeared to wait for the time when they have the opportunity to be reunited after the passage of years. According to the song, if a love is true, it will wait, which is why Gatsby believes he and Daisy are meant to be together.

Song: He'll Never Be...(What I Used to Be to You) by 98 Degrees

Passage from *The Great Gatsby:* "He wanted nothing less of Daisy than that she should go to Tom and say: 'I never loved you'" (p. 116).

Connections: Even though Daisy is with Tom, Gatsby believes he loves Daisy more than Tom ever can or will. In Gatsby's mind, Tom can never be what Gatsby was to Daisy. Even when Daisy expresses the desire to return to Tom after the car accident, Gatsby truly believes that Daisy will return to him because he doesn't believe that Daisy really loves Tom.

Song: *Losing My Ground* by Fergie

Passage from *The Great Gatsby:* "And as I sat there, brooding on the old unknown world, I thought of Gatsby's wonder when he first picked out the green light at the end of Daisy's dock" (p. 189).

Connections: Nick ponders the events of his life in New York and asks himself the questions of what he should do next and where he should go. His life for the previous months has been a whirlwind of chaos; Nick feels he has lost himself and needs time to reflect about his life and his identity, since so much of it has been entangled with Gatsby's.

While modernizing classic texts helps students comprehend literature, the activities do not take the place of meaningful class discussion. I want students to compare the literature they read to other texts, themselves, and the world around them. Asking how a literary character would deal with the pandemic enables students to relate to the text as well as demonstrate both critical and creative thinking. And if students think a novel no longer relates to their lives, that novel needs additional literary analysis and perhaps retirement from the curriculum.

VALUING FEEDBACK

While nothing can take the place of field experiences in classrooms, when I taught college students who prepared to become teachers I wanted to provide students with as many experiences as possible that simulate what they will encounter when they go to their field experiences. I shared with students my own stories of teaching mistakes and my recovery from them. Providing feedback helps students think both critically and creatively about their own classroom decisions. Towell (2010) believes, "teachers should provide frequent feedback, giving their students the motivation and support needed for improvement" (p. 113). Feedback does not take much time when it is a comment shared during a class discussion. However, when students turn in writing assignments, teachers find themselves with a seemingly overwhelming amount of comments to write on papers or type into a computer program.

To save teachers from neck pain caused by hunching over a pile of papers or hand cramps from writing numerous comments, technology can help in the form of audio comments. When I was a college student, one of my professors asked each student for a blank cassette tape. The following week, each of us received our tape returned with recorded comments about our papers. At first it felt weird to play the tape and hear my professor's voice, but it became easy to listen to the tape with my paper in front of me and revise based on the suggestions. Instead of using an old cassette tape recorder, my version of technology involves looking at student writing while speaking comments into the microphone app on my iPhone. I then email the audio file directly to the student. All comments are limited to the student's writing so there are no concerns if students decide to play the comments for a larger audience. Students also love the instant feedback of audio comments.

Other apps for smart phones enhance reading comprehension. I love the *Talking Tom* app, part of the *Talking Friends* series, where students can read aloud and hear their words repeated back to them in the voice of a cartoon cat. According to Daniels and Zemelman (2004), "listening to, as well as making taped recordings connects students to the printed word with the human voice that gives it life in every subject" (p. 236). And students are more likely to smile with a cartoon animal reading their words back to them instead of a cassette player.

READING AND RESEARCH

Technology can give new life to existing reading strategies. According to Routman (2003), "partner reading, shared reading, listening to tapes (when students can keep up), Readers Theatre, and reading series books are all great ways to help students gain fluency" (p. 128). In addition to listening to audio recordings using apps, technology offers different perspectives for series books. Some students express frustration when they don't like the ending of a book series. Using the technology of fanfiction, students can write new scenes and alternate endings for existing stories. Alvermann, Gillis, and Phelps (2013) define, "fanfiction – a term for stories that fans of an original work write by using the settings, characters, and plot from the original to imagine and create different situations that sometimes include curious mixes across genres and media" (p. 79). An internet search (another example of how technology can find resources in seconds) revealed a long list of fanfiction websites for two popular book series, *The Hunger Games*, *Catching Fire*, and *Mockingjay* by Suzanne Collins and *Divergent*, *Insurgent*, *Allegiant*, and *Four* by Veronica Roth. Students can also use fiction writing to rewrite an ending they don't like or imagine a scene from the perspective of a different character.

Since technology can find resources in seconds and since students walk into the classroom attached to their smart phones, I use the opportunity to design internet inquiries for research. Vacca, Vacca, and Mraz (2014) describe, "the Internet inquiry engages students in research using information sources on the Internet" (p. 52). In class, my students choose one of four *Newsweek* articles by author Anna Quindlen. After reading the article, students share what they learn with each other. I then ask them to pull out their smart phones and conduct a short internet inquiry about the topics presented in the articles including standardized tests, journal writing, censorship of literature, and teacher salaries. The resources they find allow for new insights and provide more depth to the discussion.

LESSONS LEARNED

I believe that the best teachers never stop learning. Graves (2001) believes, "it is essential that teachers have the same freedom to create. The energy-filled teachers are continually creating new materials, investigating new approaches, or revamping the ways they use time" (p. 137). Learning about new resources simultaneously placed me out of my comfort zone and enhanced my creativity as a teacher. Graves writes, "teaching is an emotional roller coaster" (p. 1). On this emotional roller coaster, I have faith and trust the process. The most important thing as a teacher is to meet the needs of students, regardless of the format in which strategies are implemented.

Education is a journey. Romano (1987) describes his classroom as, "most students will risk saying more among their peers than with me. And, of course, the students can learn from each other in this close contact" (p. 70). The key becomes active learning. Walk into any teacher's classroom and notice that students learn more if they can participate in an activity instead of only talking about the strategy. Johnson (1998) advocates, "unsuccessful students are rarely good goal setters. They blame their failure on other people, circumstances or luck. One of the most valuable lessons you can teach your students is how to set realistic goals, make a list of steps to move them forward, evaluate their progress, revise goals when necessary, and to set a new, higher goal, once a goal has been reached" (p. 137). Work = progress. You need to actively do something to get somewhere. Teaching in the pandemic era, when students need to keep socially distant from each other without close contact, I found ways to engage students in learning through discussions such as Socratic Seminars and games with the technology resource Kahoot, where students could interact with each other by clicking a computer mouse button.

During the pandemic, I discovered my teaching methods needed additional reinvention. I ask a discussion question and ask all students to respond, alternating between students in the classroom and students learning online so everyone hears each other's voices and feels more connected to each other. I use the messaging function in the online Teams platform the school uses so students will share their comments about the literature they read in an academic group chat (which of course I participate in and monitor). I choose literary works which offer a theme of hope and connect the narratives to teaching methods designed to motivate students to continue sharing their opinions. I discovered I could apply the strategies I learned as a health coach to teaching by practicing active listening and asking open-ended questions. I tell my students I love teaching literature because literature is about life stories. In the following sections, I describe my teaching methods that work both in school classrooms for students and the classroom of life for anyone who becomes a patient during the pandemic and anyone who desires to change behavior and reinvent life after the pandemic.

RICE

My writing, teaching, and research reflect my philosophy of RICE (Reflection, Innovation, Collaboration, Evaluation). Educators need to reflect on their practice. They also need to use innovation to develop a lesson plan. Collaboration becomes essential for learning to take place. And finally, educators need to evaluate the needs of their students or patients.

For teachers, the process is RICE, because like all teachers I need to reflect on each class I teach before planning the next one. However, physical therapists and other clinicians need to complete the evaluation step first with patients so their process is ERIC. When we first started working together, my physical therapist colleague, Dr. Eric Wanner, found it interesting that his work was the same as his name. We discovered English professors and physical therapists can learn from each other's fields of expertise.

MICE

When people align their goals with their vision and values, they become more likely to enact change in their lives. Change begins with four components: motivation, importance, confidence, and expression. I use the acronym MICE to refer to these components. By using both conversational methods such as motivational interviewing and writing strategies such as expressive writing, both teachers and health coaches can help people identify the stories they are telling themselves. Rankin (2015a) argues, "it's not life's stressors per se that make us sick and miserable. It's the stories we make up about these events, which translate into negative beliefs that activate chronic repetitive stress responses, shorten our life expectancy, and lead us into despair" (pp. 37-38). Conversely, Rankin (2015b) believes, "when the mind heals from loneliness, anxiety, fear, depression, resentment, anger, and negative beliefs about health and life, at least a percentage of the time, the health of the body follows suit" (p. 204). As far as implications for your life, you do not have to be a patient to practice the components of MICE which will help you the next time you set a goal that requires sustained behavior change.

PART I: MOTIVATION

Motivation manifests as two types, extrinsic and intrinsic. What inspires you to do something? External or internal factors? Does a student write a research paper to earn a specific grade or for the love of the topic? Does a patient complete exercises to earn a compliment from a physical therapist or for a personal desire to heal? One of the foundations of health coaching is the field of motivational interviewing.

Caldwell, Gray, and Wolever (2013) explain, "while some professionals are actually using the terms health coaching and MI synonymously, this analysis suggests there are overlapping but also distinct elements to health coaching" (p. 55). Despite the slight delineation, the essence of both motivational interviewing and health coaching is in the conversation. Miller and Rollnick (2013) clarify, "motivational interviewing is a collaborative conversation style for strengthening a person's own motivation and commitment to change" (p. 12). Strengthening motivation and commitment to change is important in all areas of a person's life. As Rollnick, Miller, and Butler (2008) explain, "MI works by activating patients' own motivation for change and adherence to treatment" (p. 5). From this perspective of collaboration, a patient sees the health care provider as a partner, not an authority figure giving orders. Miller and Rollnick (2002) elaborate, "we define motivational interviewing as a client-centered, directive method for enhancing intrinsic motivation to change by exploring and resolving ambivalence" (p. 25). Or as Tindle (2013) addresses patients, "You know what you want to do. The big question is, how do you get there? MI helps answer that question. It's a tool that helps the road open up before you. MI shows you how to see the path and gives you a starting push in the right direction" (pp. 117-118). Grant (2021) believes, "motivational interviewing requires a genuine desire to help people reach their goals" (p. 155). This statement describes my role as a teacher: I want to help my students reach their goals, but I can't accomplish their goals for them. I can, however, help motivate my students to succeed.

Motivation is frequently connected to the sense of purpose a person has in life. Pink (2009) asks the question, "as you contemplate your purpose, begin with the big question: What's your sentence?" (p. 155). In other words, at the end of your life, if you could only have one sentence on your memorial stating what you accomplished in life, what would that sentence be? My sentence would be: Helped others find their voices and use writing to heal both physically and emotionally while simultaneously living a strong life filled with family and faith.

Other researchers argue that moving beyond extrinsic motivation to intrinsic motivation can make people happier. Enayati (2015) believes, "this reason to be happy – this essential "why" – is why we must be resolute in our quest to move beyond extrinsic motivations" (p. 135). Since extrinsic motivation involves doing something to either please someone else (getting a compliment from a teacher when turning in an essay) or avoiding pain from someone else (getting a lecture from that same teacher when not turning in that essay) we can experience stress. Carter (2015) believes, "we also need intrinsic motivation, or passion – and the space to pursue our passions" (p. 183). This intrinsic motivation means finding the things that bring joy in life and provide both passion and purpose, such as signing up for a dance class for the pure joy of it or completing an essay for the love of learning regardless of what the teacher thinks.

Pursuing passions can lead to improved health. As Carter (2015) explains, "when we are happy, we are more creative and motivated, more productive and skilled socially because blood flows freely to our pre-frontal cortex, allowing us to make better decisions than we would if we relied on the more primitive, instinctive regions of our brain that are activated when we are under stress" (p. 20). So while there are times in life where we may need extrinsic motivation from others to help us get through a situation, it also becomes essential to find the internal motivation that drives us to succeed and makes us happy. Milkman (2021) elaborates, "research has proven time and time again that rather than relying on willpower to resist temptation, we're better off figuring out how to make good behaviors more gratifying in the short-term. Big payoffs far down the road just aren't enough to keep us motivated" (p. 58). You know yourself better than anyone else, and what you need to do to stay motivated.

Finding purpose and self-motivation can lead to growth. Dweck (2006) describes students with the growth mindset as "even if they thought the textbook was boring or the instructor was a stiff, they didn't let their motivation evaporate. That just made it all the more important to motivate themselves" (p. 61). The goal of learning eclipsed the potential barriers of a boring textbook or a passionless instructor. Johnson (1998) advises teachers, "you can harness the power of words to motivate and inspire your students by displaying inspirational quotations in your classroom where students will see them every day. Some teachers ask their students to discuss the quotations or write responses to them in their journals. Others let them speak for themselves. Whether you discuss them or not, your students will read them and think about them – although they may never admit that they do" (p. 141). The power of words is not limited to classrooms with desks. The power of words can be used with patients, clients, students, friends, family, colleagues, and everyone else we encounter.

By sharing words and stories, we support each other. We rely on our own intrinsic motivation but know where to find positive extrinsic motivation when needed. Sandberg (2013) states, "sharing emotions builds deeper relationships. Motivation comes from working on things we care about. It also comes from working with people we care about" (p. 88). Extrinsic motivation and intrinsic motivation can coexist beautifully in supportive environments where people care about each other and encourage each other to achieve positive change.

PART II: IMPORTANCE

Are we willing to change? The answer to that question is how important change is to a person. Miller and Rollnick (2002) explain, "one factor is the extent to which the person wants, desires, or wills change. We tend to talk about this dimension as the perceived importance of a particular change" (p. 10). We all know there are things we probably should do. But the importance of each thing to us determines if we make a change.

Connected to importance is another word that starts with I, intuition. People often have an intuitive sense of what is truly important to them. Individuals who have a strong sense of intuition can appear to others as having a psychic sixth sense of what to do and when to do it. While intuition is unique to each person and highly individualized, a significant amount of theory exists to explain the practice of intuition. Dimitrius (1998) provides the description, "what we call intuition is nearly always the surfacing of a submerged memory, a barely noticed event, or some combination of the two" (p. 216). Perhaps we have experienced something similar in the past, so we have a feeling of how we want to act in the present, even if we can't explain the feeling. Or maybe we notice something out of the corner of the eye that we know is significant information before the brain has the opportunity to process it. Dimitrius advises, "since your intuition depends on the quality and quantity of your information, your first step is clear: Improve the database" (p. 218). The more experiences people have, the more they are able to synthesize the experiences and file the information away in the database to help in the future. Starratt (1993) states, "professionals develop intuitions of what works over years of experience" (p. 39). What seems like magic or everything falling into place is a result of a person collecting experiences and calling up those experiences when they are most needed to appear in a moment of intuitive insight.

As an FBI security expert, DeBecker (1997) tells people that intuition helps keep them safe and always provides helpful information. He explains, "intuition is always learning, and though it may occasionally send a signal that turns out to be less than urgent, everything it communicates to you is meaningful" (p. 70). So if something catches our attention, it is important to pay attention to it, because our intuition is trying to communicate something to us. DeBecker provides the valuable advice, "listen to your intuition" (p. 74).

Deep inside, we know the answers for what we truly feel is important in our lives. The key is to stop and listen. Baty (2003) concurs, "you hear it time and time again: Listen to your gut instinct, or intuition. Fact is, it works" (p. 3). Why does it work? Baty answers, "intuition just means acknowledging what you already know inside" (p. 4). If we ask ourselves the questions and trust our intuitive insights, we frequently get the answers right. DeBecker (1997) emphasizes the importance of listening without judgement because, "when free of judgment, we inherently respect the intuition of others" (p. 25). In medicine, it's always best to consult a medical professional if you have an intuitive sense something is wrong with your health. But if in your personal life, if you sense someone sinister behind you, listen to your intuition and keep yourself safe.

While security experts focus on the value of intuition to keep you safe, intuition can also help you assess what is important to achieve your goals in life. Beck (2001) believes, "your intuition has a more refined understanding of your right life than any other part of your consciousness" (p. 221). If we are asked to do something we don't find important, intuition helps delineate whether we need to do that thing anyway to reach a goal or achieve a dream, or whether we think that thing is unimportant because it has no benefit. Beck describes this feeling as, "the more you listen to your intuition, the more it will change your life; and the more bravely you set forth into the territory of change, the more you'll come to rely on it" (p. 239). You are more likely to achieve success if you listen to your intuition and follow the path that makes you happy instead of listening to anyone who doubts your insight. If you do experience doubt, opportunities exist to make a fresh start. Milkman (2021) explains, "so, if you're hoping to make a positive change in your life but are pessimistic about your chances, perhaps because you've failed before and worry another attempt is likely to turn out similarly, my advice is to look for fresh start opportunities. Is there an upcoming date that could represent a clean break with the past? It could be a birthday, the start of summer, or even just a Monday" (p. 35). By listening to our intuition, we become aware of what we find important and what we value.

PART III: CONFIDENCE

Do we feel we have the ability to change? The answer to that question is how confident a person feels about making a change. Miller and Rollnick (2002) explain, "sometimes a person feels willing but not able to change" (p. 11). We may feel that making a change is important, but we don't have the confidence we can make the change.

Connected to confidence is another word that starts with C, compassion. Compassion for others, and specifically the self-compassion we must have with ourselves when things don't go as planned. Often people can be their own worst critics, and when something doesn't happen the way we want it to happen, it becomes easy to give up and focus on self-blame instead of searching for methods to overcome the obstacles and other pathways to achieve the goal. Germer (2009) defines, "self-compassion is simply giving the same kindness to ourselves that we would give to others" (pp. 33-34). Since we cannot change the past, all we can do is move forward and show ourselves the same kindness that we demonstrate for others. Neff (2011) believes something meaningful can happen from a less than perfect experience and states, "by giving ourselves unconditional kindness and comfort while embracing the human experience, difficult as it is, we avoid destructive patterns of fear, negativity, and isolation. At the same time, self-compassion fosters positive mind-states such as happiness and optimism" (pp. 12-13). No one is immune from negative events, both the minor annoyances of daily life as well as the major life changing catastrophes, but keeping a positive attitude and demonstrating the kindness to ourselves that we would demonstrate to others can diminish the severity of an event's impact.

If a person practices self-compassion and sees that the hard times in life can be obstacles to overcome rather than insurmountable barriers, he or she can get creative in problem solving and build confidence in the process as each problem is solved. Germer (2009) explains the value of practicing self-compassion because, "research on self-compassion is demonstrating that it softens the impact of negative events in our lives. Self-compassionate people are more likely to recognize when their efforts turn out badly and to take responsibility for their part" (p. 98). Neff (2011) adds, "by giving ourselves unconditional kindness and comfort while embracing the human experience, difficult as it is, we avoid destructive patterns of fear, negativity, and isolation. At the same time, self-compassion fosters positive mind-states such as happiness and optimism. The nurturing quality of self-compassion allows us to flourish, to appreciate the beauty and richness of life, even in hard times. When we soothe our agitated minds with self-compassion, we're better able to notice what's right as well as what's wrong, so that we can orient ourselves toward that which gives us joy" (pp. 12-13). Self-compassion is not the same thing as self-confidence, but self-compassion can contribute to self-confidence. Once someone achieves or overcomes something, it becomes possible to draw on that memory of confidence to know something similar that was achieved in the past can be achieved in the future.

People face fear and lack of confidence when encountering a new situation. Cameron (2002) calls these moments creative U-turns; just like a car may need to make a U-turn when going the wrong direction on the road, people may have to make U-turns when going the wrong direction in life. Cameron encourages, "have compassion. Creative U-turns are always born from fear – fear of success or fear of failure. It doesn't really matter which. The net result is the same" (p. 157). Whatever caused the U-turn, it led to the discovery of a new way to overcome an obstacle along with the confidence of finding a solution to a problem.

When we demonstrate compassion for others and ourselves, we find a support system of people to walk with us on our journey. Brown (2012) believes, "self-compassion is key because when we're able to be gentle with ourselves in the midst of shame, we're more likely to reach out, connect, and experience empathy" (p. 75). When people accept us and our stories, we experience the confidence that we are okay as we are and that we do not need to be anyone other than ourselves. Our confidence decreases when we feel shame at what we have done or how we have acted. By finding the courage to share our stories and be compassionate with ourselves, we own our story and while we cannot rewrite what has already happened, we can find the confidence to pick up a pen and write a new ending. Brown (2012) describes this story sharing process as, "whether we're on the purging end or the receiving end of this experience, self-compassion is critical. We have to give ourselves a break when we share too much too soon, and we have to practice self-kindness when we feel like we weren't able to hold space for someone who hit us with the floodlight" (p. 161). When we find the right person with whom to share our story, we have the confidence that we will not be judged and that our words will be heard.

By demonstrating compassion, people earn the right to hear our stories. Goldberg (2013) advises writers, "always have tremendous kindness for yourself. You'll get a lot more writing done" (p. 21). The same advice applies to all parts of life; demonstrating self-compassion means a lot less time thinking about regrets and a lot more time getting things accomplished. Milkman (2021) elaborates, "this turns out to be a good summary of one of the most influential discoveries psychologists have made in the past fifty years – that how we think about something affects how it is" (p. 156). A change in perspective can lead to a change in reality.

PART IV: EXPRESSION

Are we ready to change? The answer to that question is the expression of where change falls on a person's priority list. Miller and Rollnick (2002) explain, "One can be willing and able to change, but not ready to do so" (p. 11). We may feel making a change is important and we may have the confidence to make the change, but we are not ready to take action.

Expression is articulating a plan for what is needed to be done in order to enact change. It means stating one's goals and making a commitment to the accountability of achieving them. It is one thing to say you will do something, but another thing to actually do it. Expression, however, allows for the exploration of possibilities. It puts experiences into words. This is often best done in writing. Goldberg (2016) believes, "you don't have to change a thing. Writing doesn't ask you to be any different from who you are right now" (p. 161). When writing, you are who you are. Looking at a piece of paper and seeing a plan for achieving goals in writing is a method of making the plan seem like a series of concrete steps to focus on and be accountable for instead of a series of ideas swirling around in one's head. Like a camera lens focusing on a subject, everything suddenly zooms into possibility. Seeing the words on the page allows an issue to become present and eliminate the maybe someday attitude people have when thinking of specific steps needed to transform a dream into reality.

People can experience success when speaking their goals or drawing pictures of them; however, expressive writing possesses power. Romano (2000) provides a description of expressive writing as, "we use expressive writing when we are trying to explain or render something for the first time, when we're seeking to recover information, make connections, generate ideas. Expressive writing is exploratory and new and focused on meaning" (p. 137). By capturing our words on paper, we not only share our story of what happened to us, but also explore what we want to happen next. Pennebaker and Evans (2014) explain, "expressive writing (EW) – can positively affect people's sleeping habits, work efficiency, and their connection to others. Indeed, when we put traumatic experiences into words, we tend to be less concerned with the emotional events that have been weighing us down" (pp. 3-4). Brown (2015) concurs that Pennebaker's work with writing as healing is "some of the most important and fascinating research I've seen on the power of expressive writing in the healing process" (p. 87). While Pennebaker and Evans have studied the positive effects of people writing about traumatic experiences, writing does not always have to be negative and people always have the power to rewrite their narratives. According to Goldberg (1986) "we must continue to open and trust in our own voice and process" (p. 12). She provides the encouragement, "understanding this process cultivates patience and produces less anxiety" (p. 15). Revision is always possible; the first few pages of a draft might not end up being used, but may provide an idea that can later be implemented.

Similar strategies apply when designing a plan for achieving a goal. The initial plan may not end up being used, but leads to exploration of an idea that can later be implemented. Exploration of the initial draft may lead the writer to discover that he or she believes a version of the story that is not entirely true. Brown (2015) advises that when writing, "don't hold back. There is no rising strong without a true accounting of the stories we're making up" (p. 92). And when we hold ourselves accountable for the stories we're making up that we may emotionally believe to be true but that factually may not be true, we do become emotionally strong so we can become physically strong in our health as well. Fallon (2020) believes, "writing in which you name the facts, thoughts, and feelings becomes a diagnostic tool you can use any time to get at the root of what's really going on with you, see clearly the stories you've been telling yourself, unwind the complicated emotions swirling beneath the surface, and carve a brand-new path forward" (p. 100-101). Naming facts, thoughts, and feelings can help sort through complex emotions as well as provide insight into life.

Writing also allows the writer to turn negative emotions into positive ones. As Cameron (1998) observes, "we are so skilled in the art of negative imagination, we are so adroit at the art of writing out of anxiety, what might our writing and our world look like if we allowed ourselves to inhabit our positive imagination?" (pp. 125-126). And what might our world look like if we reframed a negative attitude into a positive one and realized there is more than one road that can lead to our destination?

TEACHERS AS REFLECTIVE PRACTITIONERS

Since the beginning of my teaching career, taking the time to reflect on my experiences provides me with clarity and enhances the quality of my teaching. Connelly and Clandinin (1988) explain, "teaching provides little opportunity for reflection. 'Doing things' is such a significant part of our daily pressures that we have little occasion to sit back and ask ourselves 'what am I doing?' We move forward but we find it hard to think back" (p. 33). When critiquing a lesson, I might think it could have been better, although students experiencing that lesson love it. In teaching and in life, I learn from my experiences and try not to be too critical of myself. Psychologist Grant (2021) argues, "I believe that good teachers introduce new thoughts, but great teachers introduce new ways of thinking" (p. 203). I know I introduced my students to new ways of thinking during this pandemic.

I also needed to find the strength to stay strong for my students. Gruwell (2007) writes, "writing in my diary was one of the ways I found strength. I thought if my students saw that everyone has a story – even their teacher – maybe the writing process could be cathartic for them too" (p. 148). She became a writing role model for her students, just as I am for my students, and because she shared her story with them it "seemed to intensify my desire for my students to write what needed to be written" (p. 148). During the pandemic and the resulting unusual school year, my students and I used our journals to maintain our strength and resilience.

Sometimes people can mentally beat themselves up and relieve a story, thinking what could have, should have, or would have been different if only another outcome occurred. Once again, writing can help. Conner (2008) believes, "writing can't change the story, but it can change how you think about it. It can change how you feel about it. It can change what it means to you" (p. 122). Writing about an experience helps people see it from a new perspective with the benefit of reflecting on the learning experience. Handler (2013) states, "you've started to accept that your story is part of you" (p. 225). Some call it intuition, others call it purpose, but writers trust the writing to process the past, accept the present, and lead them where they need to go in the future.

Stories will unfold on the page and words can lead to needed answers. Not only can words lead to the answers we need, but words can also help people heal both physically and emotionally. As Goldberg (2007) writes, "let your mind first believe you are dedicated, that you sincerely want the truth, are willing to take what comes through. Keep moving the pen. Keep practicing" (p. 4). Romano (2013) believes, "we can gain strength through giving words to the pain, through crafting language around it" (p. 176).

I found strength by writing through both physical and emotional pain in my life; as a teacher, I want to help my students find strength through writing their stories.

Thanks to the magic of editing and revision, writers can rearrange words into different combinations, but the original intent of the writing, the heart of the piece, often appears in the initial draft. Zimmermann (2002) believes, "writing about the same thing repeatedly from slightly different angles is a healthy part of the process. You create new dimensions. You gain distance and clarity" (p. 27). If writers wrestle too much with words, the message they really want to say gets lost along the way. Brown (2018) believes, "writing slows the winds and calms the seas" (p. 263). The calm after the storm often results in clarity and peace.

Someday soon, the storm of the pandemic will pass, hopefully leaving behind moments of calm and clarity. During the pandemic, my student Writing and Reading Center tutors and I inspired the school community by practicing kindness and helping others. On a memorable day in May, tables placed throughout the school displayed green mental health awareness ribbons for students to take and remind them they belong to a community willing to help them. By the end of the school day, I noticed students with ribbons on their shirts, shoes, computers, or backpacks. Bernstein (2014) believes, "therefore, we must learn to dissolve all boundaries with love by taking responsibility for our own energy. In doing so, we'll raise the energy around us" (pp. 4-5). The positive energy shared by one act of kindness can have a positive ripple effect that leads to larger transformation. Even if an act of kindness only affects one person, it is still worth doing. Every day in the classroom, our actions as teachers influence the lives of our students.

ACKNOWLEDGMENT

The preceding chapter contains excerpts from the following previous IGI publications:

Bird, J.L. (2020). Narratives of teaching methods. In *Using narrative writing to enhance healing* (pp. 185-237). Hershey, PA: Information Science Reference.

Brown, S., Bird, J.L., Musgrove, A., & Powers, J. (2016). The digital journey: integrating technology into teaching and learning. In V.C.X. Wang (Ed.), *Handbook of research on learning outcomes and opportunities in the digital age* (pp. 612-643). Hershey, PA: Information Science Reference.

Bird, J.L., Wanner, E.T., Urenda, R., & Perry, R. (2015). Multigenre medicine. In J.L. Bird (Ed.), *Innovative collaborative practice and reflection in patient education* (pp. 1-19). Hershey, PA: Information Science Reference.

REFERENCES

Abrams, P., Levy, R., & Fields, S. (Producers), & Chelsom, P. (Director). (2001). *Serendipity* [motion picture]. United States: Miramax Pictures.

Adams, W., Gomez, J., Pineda, A., Ferguson, S., Peters, C., Peters, D., & Walters, R. (2005). Don't lie [Recorded by The Black Eyed Peas]. On Monkey business [CD]. Santa Monica, CA: Interscope Records.

Alvermann, D. E., Gillis, V. R., & Phelps, S. F. (2013). *Content area reading and literacy* (7th ed.). Pearson.

Austen, J. (2005). *Pride and prejudice*. Penguin. (Original work published 1813) doi:10.5117/9781904633013

Baty, K. (2003). *A girl's gotta do what a girl's gotta do*. Rodale.

Beck, M. (2001). *Finding your own North Star*. Three Rivers Press.

Bernstein, G. (2014). *Miracles now*. Hay House.

Bowen, M., Godfrey, W., & Kavanaugh, R. (Producers), & Hallstrom, L. (Director). (2010). *Dear John* [motion picture]. United States: Sony Pictures.

Brooks, J. (1998). Teenagers evaluating modern media. *English Journal, 87*(1), 21–24. doi:10.2307/822014

Brown, B. (2012). *Daring greatly*. Gotham Books.

Brown, B. (2015). *Rising strong*. Spiegel & Grau.

Brown, B. (2018). *Dare to lead*. Random House.

Bruckheimer, J. (Producer), & Bay, M. (Director). (2001). *Pearl Harbor* [motion picture]. United States: Touchstone Pictures.

Caldwell, K., Gray, J., & Wolever, R. Q. (2013). The process of patient empowerment in integrative health coaching: How does it happen? *Global Advances in Health and Medicine: Improving Healthcare Outcomes Worldwide, 2*(3), 48–57. doi:10.7453/gahmj.2013.026 PMID:24416672

Cameron, J. (1998). *The right to write*. Tarcher/Putnam.

Cameron, J. (2002). *The artist's way* (2nd ed.). Tarcher/Putnam.

Carter, C. (2015). *The sweet spot*. Ballantine.

Clandinin, D. J., & Connelly, F. M. (2000). *Narrative inquiry*. Jossey-Bass.

Collins, S. (2008). *The hunger games*. Scholastic.

Collins, S. (2009). *Catching fire*. Scholastic.

Collins, S. (2010). *Mockingjay*. Scholastic.

Connelly, F. M., & Clandinin, D. J. (1988). *Teachers as curriculum planners*. Teachers College.

Conner, J. (2008). *Writing down your soul*. Conari.

Daniels, H., & Zemelman, S. (2004). *Subject matters*. Heinemann.

DeBecker, G. (1997). *The gift of fear*. Little, Brown and Company.

Dimitrius, J. (1998). *Reading people*. Ballantine.

Dweck, C. (2006). *Mindset*. Ballantine.

Enayati, A. (2015). *Seeking serenity*. New American Library.

Fallon, A. (2020). *The power of writing it down*. Zondervan.

Ferguson, S., Ridel, S., Sandstrom, R., & Boldt, R. (2006). Losing my ground [Recorded by Fergie]. On The dutchess [CD]. Santa Monica, CA: A&M Records.

Fitzgerald, F. S. (1925). *The great Gatsby*. Scribner.

Gaughan, J. (1997). *Cultural reflections*. Heinemann.

Gaughan, J. (2001). *Reinventing English*. Heinemann.

Germer, C. K. (2009). *The Mindful path to self-compassion*. The Guilford Press.

Goldberg, N. (1986). *Writing down the bones*. Shambhala.

Goldberg, N. (2007). *Old friend from far away*. Free Press.

Goldberg, N. (2013). *The true secret of writing*. Atria.

Goldberg, N. (2016). *The great spring*. Shambhala.

Grant, A. (2021). *Think again*. Viking.

Graves, D. (2001). *The energy to teach*. Heinemann.

Gruwell, E. (2007). *Teach with your heart*.

Gruwell, E.Freedom Writers. (1999). *The Freedom Writers diary*.

Handler, J. (2013). *Braving the fire*. St. Martin's Griffin.

Hayward, D., & Chasin, L. (Producers), & Wright, J. (Director). (2005). *Pride and prejudice* [motion picture]. United States: Focus Features.

Heard, G. (1995). *Writing toward home*. Heinemann.

Johns, J. L., & Lenski, S. D. (2010). *Improving reading* (5th ed.). KendallHunt.

Johnson, L. (1998). *Two parts textbook, one part love*. Hyperion.

Johnson, L. (2005). *Teaching outside the box*. Jossey-Bass.

Kearns, J. (1997). *Where to begin: a guide to teaching secondary English*. Heinemann.

Magness, C., Ridel, S., Sandstrom, R., & Ferguson, S. (1996). Love will wait [Recorded by Wild Orchid]. On Wild orchid [CD]. Hollywood, CA: RCA.

Maxwell, R. J., Meiser, M. J., & McKnight, K. S. (2011). *Teaching English in middle and secondary schools* (5th ed.). Pearson.

Milkman, K. (2021). *How to change*. Portfolio/Penguin.

Miller, W. R., & Rollnick, S. (2002). *Motivational interviewing* (2nd ed.). The Guilford Press.

Miller, W. R., & Rollnick, S. (2013). *Motivational interviewing* (3rd ed.). The Guilford Press.

Minogue, K., Stannard, R., Gallagher, J., Howes, A., & Harrington, M. (2001). Love at first sight [Recorded by Kylie Minogue]. On Fever [CD]. Hollywood, CA: EMI Records.

Murphy, R., Falchuk, B., & Brennan, I. (2009-2015). *Glee* [Television series]. Beverly Hills, CA: 20th Century Fox.

Neff, K. (2011). *Self compassion: The proven power of being kind to yourself.* HarperCollins.

Outfit 7 Limited. (2010). *Talking Tom* [Mobile Application Software]. Retrieved from http://itunes.apple.com

Pennebaker, J. W., & Evans, J. F. (2014). *Expressive writing: words that heal.* Idyll Arbor.

Perry, K., Gottwald, L., & Martin, M. (2010). The one that got away [Recorded by Katy Perry]. On Teenage dream [CD]. New York, NY: Capitol.

Pink, D. (2009). *Drive.* Riverhead Books.

Quindlen, A. (2005, November 28). The wages of teaching. *Newsweek, 146*, 100.

Quindlen, A. (2006, February 20). None of the above. None. *Newsweek, 147*, 78.

Quindlen, A. (2007, January 22). Write for your life. *Newsweek, 149*, 74.

Quindlen, A. (2008, July 21). Write and wrong. *Newsweek, 152*, 68.

Rankin, L. (2015a). *The fear cure.* Hay House.

Rankin, L. (2015b). *The anatomy of a calling.* Rodale.

Rief, L. (1999). *Vision and voice.* Heinemann.

Rogers, E., Sturken, C., & Timmons, J. (2000). He'll never be (what I used to be to you) [Recorded by 98 Degrees]. On Revelation [CD]. New York, NY: Universal.

Rollnick, S., Miller, W. R., & Butler, C. C. (2008). *Motivational interviewing in health care: helping patients change behavior.* The Guilford Press.

Romano, T. (1987). *Clearing the way.* Heinemann.

Romano, T. (2000). *Blending genre, altering style.* Heinemann.

Romano, T. (2004). *Crafting authentic voice.* Heinemann.

Romano, T. (2013). *Fearless writing.* Heinemann.

Roth, V. (2011). *Divergent.* Katherine Tegen Books.

Roth, V. (2012). *Insurgent.* Katherine Tegen Books.

Roth, V. (2013). *Allegiant.* Katherine Tegen Books.

Roth, V. (2014). *Four.* Katherine Tegen Books.

Routman, R. (2003). *Reading essentials.* Heinemann.

Sandberg, S. (2013). *Lean in.* Alfred A. Knopf.

Simpson, J., Austin, J., Kurstin, G., Watters, S., Biancaniello, L., Mendez, L., Ashford, N., & Simpson, V. (2006). A public affair [Recorded by Jessica Simpson]. On A public affair [CD]. New York, NY: Sony.

Smith, J. E. (2012). *The statistical probability of love at first sight*. Little, Brown, and Company.

Sparks, N. (2006). *Dear John*. Grand Central Publishing.

Starratt, R. J. (1993). *The drama of leadership*. The Falmer Press.

Tindle, H. (2013). *Up: how positive outlook can transform our health and aging*. Hudson Street Press.

Towell, J. L. (2010). *Hooked on books*. KendallHunt.

Vacca, R. T., Vacca, J. L., & Mraz, M. (2014). *Content area reading* (11th ed.). Pearson.

Wallace, R. (2001). *Pearl Harbor*. Hyperion.

Zimmermann, S. (2002). *Writing to heal the soul*. Three Rivers Press.

KEY TERMS AND DEFINITIONS

Interdisciplinary Collaboration: This describes the teamwork that occurs when colleagues from different disciplines work together in order to learn about each other's field of expertise. As a result of interdisciplinary collaboration, opportunities are created that may not have been discovered if the collaboration had not taken place.

Journal Writing: The process of a person responding to prompts and writing about his or her thoughts and feelings. While journal writing is typically associated with writing classrooms, writing teachers including Julia Cameron and Natalie Goldberg advocate that journal writing can be done by anyone, anywhere.

Motivational Interviewing: A method of using reflective statements and open ended questions to enhance intrinsic motivation for change.

Multigenre Writing: Introduced to the field of education by Tom Romano, multigenre writing consists of creative writing in multiple genres and the writer's analysis of the genres.

Story Sharing: By sharing a story with a supportive audience, either in conversation or in writing, it frees the storyteller of unneeded physical and emotional stress caused by holding the story inside and worrying about it. Brene Brown explains that it helps people to share stories instead of numbing pain with unhealthy choices.

Writing as Healing: James Pennebaker is a leader in the field which explores the health benefits of writing. Numerous studies have been conducted by researchers investigating the influence of writing on physical and emotional health.

Chapter 6
Reflections of Emotional Truth Narratives

ABSTRACT

This narrative provides fictional examples based on factual experiences of patients who worked with a health coach and the story of a grieving daughter who experienced her mother's death. Factual truth focuses on facts, while emotional truth focuses on the emotions associated with a memory. Sometimes when life brings difficulties, discussing the emotional truth of events through the writing process can provide a coping mechanism for emotional trauma and insight of a path forward leading to better days.

BEYOND TRADITIONAL HORIZONS OF WRITING

As the character of Nick memorably reflects in the novel *The Great Gatsby* (Fitzgerald, 1925), "so we beat on, boats against the current, borne back ceaselessly into the past" (p. 180). While memories of stories often pull us back into the past, they don't define our future. Expanding the horizons of how writing becomes implemented leads to innovation. Differences exist between happening truth (the factual truth of events people experience) and story truth (the emotional truth of how each person interprets the events). When I explain this concept to my students, I tell them to look at the clock. The exact time is a factual, verifiable truth. We count the desks in the room to learn another factual truth. Then I tell my students when they leave the classroom, if a friend or family member asks them what they learned in English class, each student will share a slightly different story, and each story represents the individual emotional truth of the person who shares it. I tell myself the emotional truth of an event and sincerely believe it, but a photograph of that event shows I wore a different sweater than I remembered. Details may be different than I remember, although my experience remains a true story.

DOI: 10.4018/978-1-7998-9051-5.ch006

USING EMOTIONAL TRUTH TO PROCESS GRIEF

My mom died when she was too young to die and when I was too young to lose her. Almost eighteen years later, I still look for meaning in the narrative. Edelman (2020) explains the reason for this as, "organizing disordered thoughts into a coherent, manageable account is what helps us make sense of a crisis and fit it into a larger system of personal meaning" (p. 142). I used writing, specifically fiction writing, to cope with my grief in the immediate aftermath of losing my mom. One week, in the midst of the pandemic, I reminded my students to tell their parents they loved them. My mom and I knew we loved each other, but I didn't know the last conversation we had would be the last time we ever spoke. Edelman elaborates, "a sudden loss offers no opportunity for a logical progression of cause-and-effect relationships that lead to an inevitable conclusion" (p. 175). If I want to spiral into a dark mood, I can relive every moment of that horrible afternoon and wonder if anything could have been different. I'm a writer; I want the narrative to make sense. Because it doesn't, I wrote a different, redemption narrative. I became determined to make my mom's senseless death have meaning by using my loss to help others. According to Edelman, "finding a balance between acknowledging the gravity of a distressing event and creating a narrative that includes redemption scenes appears key toward achieving hope, sustenance, and positive long term adjustment after a trauma or loss" (p. 251). Maybe I tried to find too much meaning in a tragedy, because my mom would have been happy with any decision I made which made me happy. Nevertheless, my journey of discovery helped students in my classroom while simultaneously helping me feel better, so I have no regrets.

During pandemic times, I use my past experiences with grief to help me with my present reality. Soukup (2019) believes, "struggle and pain and adversity aren't fun, but they do make us better. It's where we learn how to be stronger and wiser and humbler and more patient and empathetic" (p. 158). I agree that adversity isn't fun, but what are the options? Give up on life or move forward in life? Sometimes it feels easier to not try. After my mom died, whenever I found myself in those moments of darkness for more than a day or two, I knew to get help from my doctor or therapist. If you are reading these words and feel despair, contact a medical professional. There are people willing to help and your life is too valuable. There is hope, and there is light in future life. My life story would have been different had I not lived through this loss, but my narrative became part of who I am. I honor my life story, just like Hale (2018) honors her narrative when writing, "it was time to let it be. To let it all be. Not to let it all go, necessarily, but to let it be" (p. 143).

MEMORIES OF MARILYN

Winter in Kettering, Ohio was more brutal than usual this year. Marilyn Kepler Bird looked out the window of the hospital at the blizzard. She had been a patient in the hospital for some minor medical tests and felt ready to go home. However, no one was going home in this storm.

Things seemed serious. The hospital employees who had been snowed in at the hospital were on the front lines of dealing with any medical crisis. The doctors and nurses on call were snowed in at their homes and could not travel to the hospital to provide relief. In this era before cell phones, patients couldn't send a quick text home to let loved ones know they were okay. The landline looming on the desk at the nurses' station provided the only lifeline to the outside world. The phone started ringing. No nurses stayed at the station; they needed to be dispatched to various parts of the hospital to help patients.

A trained hospital volunteer, Marilyn picked up the phone and reassured the frantic caller his loved one was okay. Marilyn put her hands on her hips, and her green eyes surveyed the chaos around her as she flipped her brown hair over her shoulders. Time to get to work.

During that blizzard week, Marilyn worked more volunteer hours than some of the paid hospital staff. To her, reassuring patients was not a job, but a calling. They needed her, and she was there. Trained as a high school social studies teacher, Marilyn liked teaching but loved health care. She counseled hospital patients scared by their internal medical conditions as well as the external blizzard. Before the medical field had a name for the role she played, she used the skills of listening and inquiry implemented by health coaches.

END NOTES FOR "MEMORIES OF MARILYN"

The previous scene you just read was a work of fiction based on fact. That scene happened before I was born, so of course I did not witness my mom Marilyn helping patients. I heard the story from her when I was a kid, and as I was getting ready to begin my health coach training I discovered an article my dad wrote about my mom's heroism. Finding that article served as an affirmation that I was on the right path in my life.

Writing about emotional truth helps heal people. I first explored multigenre writing as healing when I wrote my doctoral dissertation and used a fictional character to share factual information. I created a character named Jenna Kepler, who was a thinly disguised variation of me, and sent her into horrific circumstances worse than my reality in order to process some of the events in my life. I used emotional truth to capture the essence of an issue while freeing myself from being obligated to remember every single factual detail. Writing Jenna Kepler's story helped me heal. That's the real truth.

When writing fiction, Jenna the character said things Jenny the author couldn't because I was hurting too much. As DeSalvo (1999) explains, "if the emotional aftermath of our trauma is similar to O'Brien's, we, too, can use semifictional alter ego to tell our stories, to help us feel" (p. 167). After a crisis, fiction can help us find our way back to a new reality as we skate the fine line between fact and fiction. O'Brien (1990) describes this experience as, "I'm skimming across the surface of my own history, moving fast, riding the melt beneath the blades, doing loops and spins, and when I take a high leap into the dark and come down thirty years later, I realize it is as Tim trying to save Timmy's life with a story" (p. 246). Goldberg (2000) describes her reaction to reading O'Brien's words as, "tears sprang to my eyes. I, too, have attempted many times to keep my childhood safe, warding off death with a story" (p. 131). I agree with this sentiment. By writing a story about my mom's experiences volunteering in a hospital, for a few moments she is alive again and I get to spend a little more time with her.

One of my former professors, Tom Poetter (2013) describes the feeling of freedom in teaching as, "I was allowed to teach instead of sentenced to follow someone else's script" (p. 102). I felt grateful he applied the same philosophy to writing and gave me the opportunity to tell my story when he advised my doctoral dissertation. My dissertation committee encouraged me to write about my experiences as a method for helping me heal emotionally, but I couldn't write about my mom without crying. So I turned to fiction and created my character Jenna Kepler. Beck (2001) describes, "narrative therapy teaches people to literally rewrite their life stories, so that they tell themselves the happy truth, instead of the miserable truth" (p. 96). I used writing as a form of therapy to discuss my feelings while hiding behind my fictional character. But Jenna wasn't really a fictional character. Her first name was close to mine and her last name was my mom's maiden name. While I made up details about Jenna's life, I couldn't run from the emotional truth of my experiences. I could rewrite the fiction story and give it a happy ending, but I couldn't change how the story ended in real life.

My doctoral dissertation featured a narrative inquiry approach discussing how stories help people heal emotionally. I never imagined writing could also help people heal physically until years later when I completed research at a physical therapy clinic and continued research at a hospital.

FACT AND FICTION

I present a longer merger of fact and fiction, where you will read fictionalized narratives of a health coach's factual experiences. The fictional stories have their foundation in factual truth. Health coaches adhere to a code of ethics and must honor confidentiality to provide patients with a safe place to share their stories. Creating that safe space includes not sharing any real patient stories in a publication. To protect confidentiality, no real names of patients are used in the following narrative. All patients described are composites of several patients, and no patient described is based on the experiences of a single real person to add an additional layer of confidentiality. Furthermore, additional details have also been fictionalized so there is no possibility of a single patient being identified.

Think of the patients in this narrative as fictional characters. While their stories were inspired by real patients, the important thing for you as a reader is to experience what the health coach felt when learning the patient narratives, and all the emotions are true. All of the patients received total knee arthroplasty (TKA) surgery and spoke to the health coach while in a hospital inpatient orthopedic setting. In addition to speaking with a health coach, the patients all received treatments from a physical therapist and an occupational therapist, as well as hospital care from nurses and physicians. The narrative is told in the first person "I" from my perspective as a health coach who is also an English teacher and Stephen Minister. End notes follow the narrative and elaborate on the concepts discussed. In the original version of this narrative, I named the patients after literary characters. Upon rereading and reflecting, that decision proved too distracting, so in the revision I named the patients in the memory of my four grandparents and two uncles. After the fictional narrative, I explain in my end notes section an additional rationale for my writing decisions.

These narratives took place before the pandemic and as I reread them, they seem like they took place in a different world. During the pandemic I and other volunteers stayed away from the hospital, and I watched on the news as the corridors I once walked filled with patients fighting for their lives from the virus. In the following narratives, the patients recovering in the orthopedic wing of the hospital of course do not experience the same recovery process as patients with the coronavirus, but the orthopedic patient stories provide a glimpse into how different people feel about healing.

PATIENT NARRATIVES

I sling my lanyard with my ID badge around my neck and pick up the list of patients I am scheduled to visit today, as I look forward to another day of health coaching and helping people. A gift card I received from my family enabled me to afford a stack of composition books for hospital patients. Every patient did not receive a journal due to the fact that some patients experienced surgical complications that made neither coaching nor writing possible for them. When patients in the hospital received a journal, there was a note on it that read as follows:

This is your journal!
Use it to…

1. Write questions for your medical team.
2. Write a list of your goals.
3. Freewrite about anything on your mind.
4. Draw pictures.
5. Annotate medical advice so you remember.

I refer to my first patient of the day as William. On the one hand, this William loves being surrounded by the constant visitors to his room; on the other hand, he is tired and in pain. Overall, William feels at peace with his life and very optimistic. He is telling jokes with the physical therapist and occupational therapist who are in the room when I arrive and I notice his great sense of humor. I appreciate the support for health coaching from all the members of the medical team. The physical therapist and occupational therapist tell William they think it would be good for him to talk to me before they leave to help another patient.

"What are you looking forward to the most when you go home?" I ask. Questions like this motivate patients to envision their lives after the hospital.

"Outdoors. My bike. My boat. My dog. Being pain free when going on a drive." He smiles and describes a beautiful scene of going for a drive, which I hope comes true for him after he leaves the hospital.

"Sometimes it's the little things we miss most." I try to add meaning while reflecting one of his statements. William changes the direction of the conversation.

"I'm happy, but exhausted. I love all my visitors, but they won't leave." He leans back against his pillows, signaling he would like to rest. Health coaching conversations in the hospital are usually short, since patients are on medication and need their rest between physical and occupational therapy treatment sessions. I have learned to make the most of the short time I have. We talk about ideas of how he could get some rest without being rude to his guests. As a health coach in a hospital, I have to accept that patients are in my life for only the duration of their short hospital stays; therefore, I do not have the opportunity to know the next chapters they write in their stories.

I then stop by to check on the writing of my second patient of the day. I call her Martha, and she is quiet and reluctant to talk about her feelings. I'm hoping that the composition notebook I gave her will encourage her to write what she is feeling. Martha was excited to write in her journal. I knock on the door and push it open. A nurse is in the room with Martha.

"These notebooks are a great idea," Martha says. The nurse smiles. Typically patients open up more when I am the only person in the room with them, but Martha keeps on talking. "I have no pain today."

"That's great news." I look at the journal buried under a book, a food tray, and other items on the table next to her and know she won't be reading her writing to me. That's okay; I've learned from the college students I teach and a large amount of research that it is the act of writing that helps people, regardless of whether or not the writing is shared. Writing in a journal gives patients such as Martha the opportunity to explore their thoughts on paper without worrying about staying awake to talk to a visitor in their hospital rooms.

"I need some rest," Martha says, but she is smiling and seems happy as she says it. "I'm excited to write more."

"Writing can help you remember things," I tell her. "Sometimes you think of your best questions after your medical team leaves the room." I notice the nurse nod in agreement while I mentally reprimand myself, because I've just lapsed into teaching, and health coaches are supposed to listen, not teach.

"Very true," Martha picks up on my thread of conversation anyway. "Oh. I'm starting to feel some pain now." That's my cue to leave as the nurse takes over Martha's care. I wonder how much she can focus on her future goals while she is in pain. Even if she's not sharing her feelings with me verbally, at least she is writing them in her journal. The nurse stops me before I go into the next patient's room and tells me the journals are a great idea.

My third patient of the day I refer to as Steven. His wife hovers over him like a bird that doesn't know where to land. "This machine is making too much noise," she remarks as she reaches for one of the machines.

"Let me get a nurse," I quickly tell her, not knowing much about the machine in question but suspecting that unplugging it would be bad. After the situation is resolved, I evaluate my options. The purpose of health coaching is to have individual conversations with people; family members, as well meaning as they are, can easily redirect a conversation.

"Will I ever leave this hospital?" Steven asks. I can still encourage him on his healing journey and talk to his wife about practicing self-care so she can better take care of him once he returns home from the hospital. I switch from a coaching role to that of motivational speaker and notice that Steven's wife has been writing in the journal. I am reminded that the hospital patients are receiving care from all the medical professionals, but who is taking care of the caregivers?

"I gave her the journal," Steven explains.

"That's fine." I look at his wife, wondering if she needs coaching more than her husband the hospital patient.

"Take care of yourself so you can better take care of him," I tell her.

"I will," she promises, but she is already reaching for her husband's pillows. This wasn't a coaching session, but hopefully I helped both of them. All I can do is my best, I tell myself. The good news about seeing patients one right after another is that I can't dwell too much on one conversation. I need to practice mindfulness and focus on each patient in the moment, not think about the ones I spoke to earlier or the ones I am going to speak to later.

"Get out of my room! Go away!" That is my introduction to my fourth patient of the day, who I name Mary Ann. The mystery I need to solve immediately is why Mary Ann has never met me, yet doesn't like me. "I can't watch my favorite singer in peace!" Mary Ann yells, and slumps against the pillow angrily. I glance at the television screen and see a singer typically more popular with the college students I teach than members of Mary Ann's older generation, and remind myself of the advice I tell my college students when I teach a reading diagnosis class. Interest + Area of Need = Effective Assessment. I assess I am not going to have an effective coaching session at this moment in time, especially when I see Mary Ann is not alone in the room. Her daughter is there with her.

"She's in pain. Please leave," Mary Ann's daughter orders. Concern of family members is understandable; anytime my grandma had surgery, my mom insisted on staying in the hospital room with her even after visiting hours.

"I'll be back," I tell Mary Ann, leaving her to her concert. A physical therapist and occupational therapist who heard the exchange with Mary Ann smile at me encouragingly. Don't let it get to you, I tell myself. As I walk past the patient admitting desk, the kind receptionist who I see multiple times a day asks me how much I've walked today. Thanks to my iPhone app, I already know that by the end of the day I will walk six miles and climb ten flights of stairs. I'm grateful a colleague advised me to wear comfortable shoes as I go to the cafeteria for a free cup of coffee I won't finish because it takes too long to drink and I want to return to my patients. I stop by the documentation room, greet the physical therapists and occupational therapists who are there, and quickly write my notes for the patients I have seen so far. The team is listening to a mix CD I made during a team development workshop, and I realize I am not just helping patients while I am here, but also my colleagues. By the time I don't finish my coffee and do finish my notes, Mary Ann's television concert has ended and I try talking to her again.

One of the physical therapists is in the room helping Mary Ann and suggests we work together. While the physical therapist teaches Mary Ann exercises, I ask her to visualize her ideal health. Her focus remains in the present, not in the future. She visualizes a peaceful scene while completing the exercises the physical therapist gives her. While health coaching encourages the setting of long term goals in timeframes of three to six months in the future, Mary Ann can only visualize one moment to the next. For her, that is what she needs. She mentions her love of antiques. My dad has been known to keep things for years and now has an impressive collection of antiques. I found the opening I needed to get her to trust me and talk. Once the physical therapist leaves, Mary Ann glares at me.

"I'm glad my daughter left. A three day hospital stay means a three day vacation from family. Where are my glasses? Have you seen my toothbrush?" Confusion has taken over her. The ethics of doing what is best for a patient overrule any additional coaching, so it's time for me to leave and let her sleep.

My fifth patient of the day wants to talk about Shakespeare instead of his health goals. I refer to him as Harold.

"Have you read this book?" Harold asks, holding up a popular contemporary novel.

"I have," I confirm. "My students like it too."

"You're a professor!" Harold claps his hands. "I always believe reading and writing have value. What's your favorite Shakespeare play? If I tell you a quote from a Shakespeare play, can you identify it? My son in high school needs to learn more quotes and appreciate the value of reading!" He is not doing it intentionally, but he is trying to distract me. This could easily turn into a conversation about literature, which I love, but that would put the focus on me and not on Harold.

"How would you compare your journey to the journey of a literary character?" I ask. While, as health coaches, we do self-manage our own thoughts and feelings, we are only human and sometimes patients learn parts of our stories. And just as English teachers discuss poems in the literature we teach, health coaches often use metaphors to reflect part of the stories they hear. In Harold's case, he compared himself to various characters in a Shakespeare play. He was on a quest just like they were, and his quest was to heal from his surgery. By the time I leave, I'm pleased with the session, and happy Harold now sees himself as the hero of his life story, just like his favorite Shakespeare characters.

"Please pray with me," instructs my sixth patient of the day, a happy and peaceful woman I refer to as Bobbie, and I soon learn of her strength. I find my dual roles as Stephen Minister and health coach emerging as I hold her hand and pray. Often when people pray, they don't know the words to say and that's okay. Word choice doesn't matter as much as the intent of the message; the same can be said for writing. I have learned to trust my heart with both prayer and writing and try not to overthink the words of my prayer. "That was beautiful," Bobbie wipes away a tear.

"How are you feeling?" I ask, knowing that one of the physical therapists told me she experienced complications during her surgery.

"What happens when we die?" Bobbie asks. I pause before answering. While she had complications during her surgery, they were not life threatening, but sometimes medical experiences cause patients to reflect on their lives.

"What do you think happens when we die?" I turn her question back to her, using another health coaching strategy of exploring what the patients feel instead of asking as experts answering all their questions. Both health coaches and Stephen Ministers guide others to find their own answers. Unlike teaching, we don't direct others what to do. In both of my roles, reflective listening and being present for another person becomes essential. I believe Heaven is a beautiful place with peace and love and happiness, where I will be reunited with everyone in my family who died, but I don't want to tell her what to believe if she has a different opinion. Bobbie starts telling me about a book she read where the author had a near death experience.

"I'm scared," she admits.

"It's okay to feel that way," I assure her. "What are you looking forward to the most when you go home?" I ask, bringing my day full circle by asking my last patient of the day the same question I asked the first.

"Watching football. Eating chocolate. Can we pray again?" Bobbie reaches for my hand. While we are praying, her doctor arrives. He bows his head and remains silent as I finish the prayer.

"Spirituality has value. It helps patients," the doctor remarks. Since patients have limited time with their doctors, I always leave the room when a doctor arrives. I never want patients to miss a moment of discussing their medical care. Bobbie's story will become another one to which I will never know the sequel. Spirituality is one of the dimensions of health explored by health coaches and it was the one that Bobbie wanted to discuss the most during my coaching session with her.

Before I conclude my day at the hospital, I leave the orthopedic wing of the hospital where I visited my six patients because I am asked to visit an oncology patient coping with a cancer diagnosis. I try to offer some comfort to a shocked patient immediately after the cancer treatment didn't work and there are no more medical options. For this patient, there is no setting of long term goals but reflecting on the question: What do you need to do to feel at peace with the time you have left? Health coaches don't usually make visits to the emergency room, but I am asked to sit with a patient's family until they receive an update on their loved one's condition from someone on the medical team. Mixed with the tragedy of sad diagnoses are the triumphs, as I walk through the hospital hallways and witness a physical therapist and occupational therapist help a patient walk again against the odds. The best moments are the ones talking to patients, learning their narratives, and know that for a short moment in time, my life story intersected with theirs and I hopefully helped make a difference in their lives by being there.

END NOTES FOR "PATIENT NARRATIVES"

These notes focus primarily on the role of using health coaching with physical therapy patients since that is the setting where I worked as a health coach, but health coaching can also be used with cardiac patients, oncology patients, or even healthy patients who desire lifestyle changes.

Some health coaches have medical backgrounds; for example, many health coaches are nurses. But other health coaches bring our own unique knowledge to the field and offer different perspectives. My area of expertise is writing, so I am able to use that skill to help patients.

Regardless of background, all health coaches need to receive specific training in order to practice. The goal of using journaling as a health coach is to provide patients with another way to think about their progress. Germer (2009) discusses the value of journals and writes, "journaling is an opportunity to monitor habit change, to troubleshoot, and, most important, to notice new ways you might be responding to problems in your life" (p. 241). Journals may be used for recording narratives, tracking pain, setting goals, and celebrating the small victories in life. Neff (2011) believes in the power of gratitude journals and states, "after a relatively short time, keeping a gratitude journal can make a substantial contribution to your level of happiness" (p. 279). Writing in journals contributes to the positive outlook that helps people heal. Writing reminds patients to take their recovery process during physical therapy one day and one step at a time, because small steps can lead to big changes.

Journal writing provides accountability for achieving goals. Lea Michele (2015) explains, "this might be a way for you to hold yourself accountable for achieving everything you want. Keeping a journal and asking yourself hard questions about what you really want to get out of your life is the best way, in my experience, to actually help you achieve your dreams" (p. 11). Displaying the list of goals in a prominent place is another way of remaining accountable and providing inspiration during the healing journey.

Using the theory of writing can benefit the practice of medicine. In addition to helping clinicians learn their patients' stories, writing empowers patients to take control of their own stories. Statistics and objective data serve as a cornerstone of medical practice. Wheelan (2013) argues, "statistics is more important than ever before because we have more meaningful opportunities to make use of data" (p. 255). Nevertheless, statistics do not capture a patient's entire story. Fallon (2020) explains, "the research is clear: writing can help us manage negative emotional states, process our lives, and even heal from trauma. One of the reasons writing does this, I believe, is because it invites us, and even requires us, to look at our pain in a new way and for a long time. It requires contemplation" (p. 154). Writing about pain does not replace a medical treatment plan, but it does help patients manage the complex emotions associated with pain by providing a safe space for contemplation and reflection.

While Romano (1987) is describing a writing conference in an English classroom instead of a health coaching session, the same goal of establishing a safe environment applies to both a student in an English classroom and a patient in a health coaching session because, "once a comfortable, reassuring atmosphere is established, the conference proceeds. How it proceeds depends upon many things: where the student is in the writing process, what her attitude is toward the work, what problem is foremost in her mind at the moment, how far she has moved or been nudged in previous conferences. The teacher must listen and take cues from the student" (p. 87). The same description applies to health coaching, as the health coach must listen and take cues from the patient before proceeding with the conversation.

Health coaching is not therapy but shares similarities with solution-oriented brief therapy (SBT) in psychology. As Weiner-Davis (1995) describes, "the secret to its brevity is that, instead of taking a long introspective journey into the past, SBT helps people to envision a positive future and to identify fail-safe strategies for getting there" (p. 18). In her practice, she found that people often know what they need to do but need someone to ask them the right questions to help them get there. The difference is that psychologists use narratives to help patients understand the past, whereas health coaches use narratives to help patients set goals for the future.

Health coaches help patients make sense of their lives in the present. Clandinin and Connelly (2000) believe, "narrative inquiry, from this point of view, is one of trying to make sense of life as lived" (p. 78). As people make sense of life, they live, tell, retell, and relive their stories. Clandinin and Connelly elaborate, "living, telling, retelling, and reliving mark the qualities of a life" (p. 187). Narrative inquiry shares similarities with narrative therapy and narrative medicine. In narrative therapy, Madigan (2011) draws a parallel between narratives used in literature and narratives told in therapy settings by stating, "if there was to be any interest and/or consistency between narrative therapy theory, practice, and research, the task of any research would be akin to that of the literary critic, insofar as cultural behavior can be treated only as a text that requires interpretation" (p. 140). English teachers encourage students to interpret the texts they read. Similarly, medical practitioners can help patients interpret the stories they tell themselves. The only difference is that the endings of classic works of literature will never change. People's lives, however, are not a book that has already been written; their lives contain unwritten pages waiting to be filled with new stories.

Most caregivers find joy and purpose in helping others. As Carter (2015) describes it, "it's the person. It isn't about the prestige or even the helping nature of our work. It's about the meaning we personally find in it and express through it, and the effort and commitment we give to it" (p. 241). While the patient must be the one to do the work of recovery, it becomes comforting to be surrounded by members of the medical team who will remain a supportive presence. Brown (2015) writes, "when we decide to own our stories and live our truth, we bring our light to the darkness" (p. 75). By living our truth, we write a narrative of health and wellness.

END NOTES FOR HEALTH COACHING

Health coaching is still new to the field of medicine; consequently, research studying the benefits of health coaching is only emerging as of this writing. According to Caldwell, Grey, and Wolever (2013), "the major tenets of the health coaching process are patient-centeredness and patient-control focused around patient-originated health goals that guide the work within a supportive coaching partnership" (p. 48). The health coach works with the patient to explore the patient's attitude about change. What are the factors causing the patient to not be motivated to take care of his or her health, not think the treatment plan is important, not feel confidence in completing the treatment plan, or not feel ready to express why changing is not a priority? The health coach does not tell the patient what to do, but asks open ended questions while the patient finds his or her own answers. Defined by Smith, Lake, Simmons, Perlman, Wroth, and Wolever (2013) as "through techniques sourced from humanistic and positive psychology, solution-focused and mindfulness-based therapies, and leadership coaching, Integrative Health Coaching (IHC) provides a mechanism to empower patients through various stages of learning and change" (p. 66). The health coach partners with the physical therapist and any other member of the patient's medical team to not only help the patient comply with goals set by the medical team, but also any personal goals the patient may have which align with the treatment goals.

END NOTES FOR STEPHEN MINISTRY

Helping people through their experiences is a role of not only health coaches, but also Stephen Ministers. Haugk (2000) provides the definition as, "Stephen Ministers are lay Christians carefully recruited, selected, trained, commissioned, and supervised for lay caring ministry" (p. 17). Both roles are similar yet different. Health coaches use the same skills as Stephen Ministers of reflective listening, maintaining boundaries, encouraging people to express their feelings, asking open ended questions to lead to solutions, and providing a supportive presence. However, they differ in that health coaches encourage people to set goals to improve their health while Stephen Ministers provide prayers. Prayers provide comfort to patients as they heal. Alexander (2012) demonstrates belief in the science of medicine because "I'm still a scientist. I'm still a doctor, and as such I have two essential duties: to honor truth and to help heal" (p. 171). Alexander (2014), however, also argues, "the fact is, science and faith, the two ways of knowing the world that have defined our culture, are much, much more entwined than we tend to think they are" (p. 63). While patients need all the advantages of modern medicine, if saying a prayer or writing in a journal helps a patient feel better, such techniques effectively supplement their medical treatment.

Helldorfer and Moss (2007) believe, "in health care, we have a distinct mission to relieve suffering and restore hope" (p. 213). Helping a patient with the awareness that just because pain exists now doesn't mean it will exist in the future can provide a patient with hope and courage to rewrite an existing narrative. Adams (1990) describes the writing as healing process as journal therapy and explains, "when you move your negative emotions out of your body through exercise or writing, they aren't lurking around to cause tension or disease via tight muscles, stiff necks, headaches, ulcers, or heart attacks" (p. 39). She continues, "if there is one inviolate rule of journal writing, it is that there are simply no rules. Writing naturally means that you do what works for you and that you don't worry about what you're not doing in the journal" (p. 42). Therefore, writing has the potential to help relieve both emotional pain and physical pain.

Obviously, if a patient experiences pain, no amount of journal writing will take the place of a treatment plan prescribed by a medical practitioner. However, writing can be used in conjunction with the treatment plan to enhance patient healing. Zimmermann (2002) believes, "by giving voice to fears, anger, and despair, by letting go of old dreams and hopes, our self-healing powers come into play" (p. 18). Writing helps us figure out our concerns so we will help our own healing process; we then share our concerns with medical professionals so they can use the information to design a treatment plan that will best help us continue to heal.

CREATIVE WRITING AS HEALING

Research exists that supports using creative writing as a healing device. Pennebaker (1997) explains, "the mind torments itself by thinking about unresolved and confusing issues. One reason that writing about traumas can be so beneficial is that it is a powerful tool to discover meaning. Writing promotes self-understanding" (p. 93). But if reporting the facts of a trauma causes too much emotional pain for the writer, it may help for the writer to write about the event using creative writing. As Pennebaker and Evans (2014) believe, "you can't help but wonder where personal narrative ends and fiction begins. Does writing fictionalized stories improve health as much as exploring your own experiences? Possibly" (p. 94). Lepore, Greenberg, Bruno, and Smyth (2002) discuss a study by Greenberg and her colleagues where study participants were asked to write about personal traumas, imaginary traumas, or nonemotional events and learned, "both real and imaginary trauma groups visited the student health center for illness less often at 1-month follow up relative to controls" (p. 106). In the original study, Greenberg, Wortman, and Stone (1996) reflect that "writing about a hypothetical trauma could also facilitate development of a more resilient version of self" (p. 600). In other words, we save our lives with stories.

And we can save other lives too.

NARRATIVE MEDICINE

Since it values narratives, narrative medicine provides the foundation for presenting a patient's story using a multigenre format. Rasminsky (2012) tells the story of Dr. Rita Charon, "the founding director of the Program in Narrative Medicine at Columbia University, where future MDs participate in writing workshops and examine texts by authors" (p. 88). Charon uses information about writing and literature typically found in an English teacher's classroom to inform her practice because she "realized that the clues she needed weren't confined to lab results and diagnostic scans. They were hidden in her patients' habits, fears, beliefs, family circumstances, even their insurance battles" (p. 88). Writing provides subjective qualitative information often missing in quantitative objective measures. Now when talking to patients, "she sits with her hands in her lap – no notes, no typing – and lets the patient tell her story" (p. 88). Narrative medicine presents an integrative approach to medicine that focuses on the patient's story.

Patients benefit from focusing on what Duke Integrative Medicine (2010) calls the Wheel of Health. By asking patients to reflect on movement, exercise and rest; nutrition; personal and professional development, physical environment; relationships and communication; spirituality; mind-body connection; and mindful awareness, "the Wheel of Health represents a comprehensive perspective of well-being and it addresses all the resources available to you to optimize your health" (pp. 5-6). Integrative medicine provides patients with the opportunity to take ownership of their health, frequently by partnering with a health coach, and set wellness goals to achieve. Charon (2006) discusses narrative medicine and argues, "by virtue of being trained in the style appropriate to the genre of the chart, doctors learn to suppress their own authorial voice, their own I" (p. 142). Narrative medicine encourages medical practitioners to see each patient as living a story, not as only a name on a chart and a list of notes. Health coaches listen more than they talk, which opens the door for patients to reflect on their narratives and think how minor differences, like a change in routine for the day, will lead to major behavior change.

NARRATIVE INQUIRY

Life takes unexpected directions. After we live our stories, we decide whether or not to share them. Too often, people don't share their stories because sharing takes courage, trust, and vulnerability. Sharing stories, however, can help the author process and comprehend them. Clandinin and Connelly (2000) explain, "therefore, difficult as it may be to tell a story, the more difficult but important task is the retelling of stories that allow for growth and change" (p. 71). You may tell a story to someone as soon as that story happens and have one perspective. Years later, you may retell that same story to a different person and gain additional insight about how you changed between sharing sessions. Narrative inquiry, the discipline of research that encourages researchers to share stories, is described by Clandinin and Connelly (2000) as, "we imagine, therefore, that in the construction of narratives of experience, there is a reflexive relationship between living a life story, telling a life story, retelling a life story, and reliving a life story" (p. 71). In retelling a story, you relive the moments once experienced and see them from a new perspective. It helps us see where our lives are heading and opens our eyes to things we may want to adjust or keep the same.

Our stories evolve as we evolve. Clandinin and Connelly (2000) continue, "narrative inquiry carries more of a sense of continual reformulation of an inquiry than it does a sense of problem definition and solution" (p. 124). We live our stories, tell our stories, and in the reliving and retelling of our stories we often find new answers and think of new questions. Whether it is in a classroom, a clinic, or in life, we take the theories we learn and transform them in to practical strategies. Connelly and Clandinin (1988) believe, "we may think of our own education through curriculum situations in terms of theory and practice" (p. 89). In the field of narrative inquiry, a research project may end, but the stories of the participants continue.

Stories of people's lives remain ongoing, and the addition of new narratives can change a story. Cameron (1998) believes, "valuing our experience is not narcissism. It is not endless self-involvement. It is, rather, the act of paying active witness to ourselves and to our world" (p. 50). By writing, we witness our experiences as we retell them and thus relive them. Reliving an experience, especially in writing, offers the benefit of reflection. We learn from our past experiences so we can move forward. We learn from an experience, but gain more insight from reflecting on the experience.

MULTIGENRE WRITING

Narrative inquiry theory supports the practice of multigenre writing. Tom Romano, one of my former professors at Miami University in Oxford, Ohio, inspired his students to use multigenre writing. Multigenre writing provides authors the opportunity to share their narratives using creative and unique perspectives. The practice of multigenre writing originated in the field of English Education, where Romano (2008) provides the definition as, "instead of producing one long expository paper, students wrote about their topics in many genres. Although each piece was self-contained, making a point of its own, taken together, all the writing created a unified whole. I called the assignment a multigenre research paper" (p. 180). Multigenre writing helps writers surprise the reader and let creativity shine through traditional reporting of research. Romano (2004) elaborates, "it isn't simply one expository or narrative monolog. In multigenre papers, writers put together information from many perspectives, angles, and voices" (p. 34). Of course, as with all research papers, all the facts reported in a multigenre paper must be accurate. The most important thing with multigenre writing, however, becomes for the author to use the research to tell a compelling story.

Multigenre perspectives present two sides of a story as researchers live their narratives through creative genres and then step back to report on the research, much like a journalist reporting the news. Journalist Anna Quindlen (2004) describes this perspective as, "it's a strange job, covering and commenting on the news. Life washes over us as it does all our fellows, and yet we see it in a completely different way than they do" (p. xxi). In multigenre writing, means narratives become the driving force. As Romano (2013) explains, "while expository forms like clear explanations, succinct position statements, and tight arguments surely have a place in multigenre papers, genres of narrative thinking carry the cognitive load" (p. 20). Multigenre writing opens up additional dimensions for research by giving the author of a multigenre paper the opportunity to present findings using innovative formats such as artwork, creative writing, and fictionalized interpretations of stories.

For example, in the practice of both health coaching and Stephen Ministry, specific accounts of patient conversations cannot be repeated in order to protect confidentiality. Consequently, sometimes the best method to present facts is by using fiction. The essence of the story remains true, but details have been changed to maintain confidentiality for participants. Romano (2000) advises teachers, "whether your students are doing secondary research and writing multigenre papers out of that or whether they are exploring aspects of their lives, urge them to use the techniques of fiction" (p. 72). Fictionalized experiences protect details confidential to people involved in the narrative while retaining the emotional truth of a story. It becomes possible for readers to feel what the author felt without needing to know names or identifying details of other participants in the story. Romano (1995) believes, "by creating fictional dreams peopled with fully realized characters driven by tension amid enough detail of setting to create atmosphere, students can create truths that show what they know" (p. 8). Fiction frees the writer of having to remember factual details, or in this case, allows for the reader to gain a better comprehension of health coaching without the author compromising confidential information unable to be shared in a publication. The goal becomes to tell a captivating story while simultaneously honoring the lives of the patients who made the story possible.

Planning a successful multigenre paper is similar to a teacher planning a lesson or a city planner planning a city. Harper (1996) writes, "monitoring implementation is the only way to know if a plan is becoming effective" (p. 196). She's writing about city planning, but multigenre writers also need to monitor if the implementation of ideas is effective. Throughout my life, I have heard my dad use the terms survey, analysis, plan, implementation, and feedback to describe the city planning process. Whether working with a city or a multigenre paper, careful planning is required. So I became a planner, just like my dad; I just plan lessons and writing pieces instead of cities.

EMOTIONAL TRUTH

While writers quote factual truth, the emotional truth will always be told from the perspective of each individual writer. Examples of emotional truth include a clinician fictionalizing part of a patient's story to change identifying details or a teacher not remembering the exact clothes worn during a class but remembering perfectly the emotional resonance of the lesson taught that day.

Here is a good description of emotional truth from an author with the same last name but no relation to my research teammate Eric. Wanner (1994) says, "stories may claim to be factual truth at one end of the spectrum or metaphoric truth at the other, with all shadings in between. A story's 'truth' depends more upon its coherence than upon its faithfulness to actual events" (p. 18). So I maintain my responsibility to my readers by informing them that not every detail may be true, but the message of the piece becomes its emotional resonance. As Handler (2013) states, "what's emotionally true for you may not have the ring of truth for others who were present in the same situation" (p. 63). This is because "emotional truth isn't always provable truth" (p. 155). If the emotional truth of the story resonates with you, do the details really matter? For example, a medical practitioner can share the essence of a patient's story to provide life lessons for readers while simultaneously changing personal details to protect the patient's confidentiality. That enables the reader to comprehend the emotional truth of the experience regardless of the modification of specific details of the story. Goldberg (2007) explains, "you can develop the right compass to reach emotional truths inside your own life without having to fabricate your experience. Your life is good – or bad – enough. Your suffering is real" (p. 111). Emotional truth does not ignore facts, but focuses primarily on feelings.

Most fiction has some foundation in factual experiences. For example, a conversation as presented by the author is based on subjective memory and not objective facts, and therefore may not be presented in this book as exactly as it originally occurred. However, the emotional resonance of the conversation is true. As fiction writer Cleaver (2002) writes, "when you deepen the connection to your character, you deepen your connection to yourself" (p. 85). In research methods such as narrative inquiry, the lines between fact and fiction often become blurred. Clandinin and Connelly (2000) elaborate, "when pressed, what seemed like fact appears more and more as memory reconstruction, either ours or participants'. Are these reconstructions best thought of as fiction? (p. 179). As Romano (2000) says when teaching multigenre writing, " I encourage students not just to report fact in a multitude of genres but also to fictionalize what they cannot know in order to create what could or should have happened" (p. 68). Fiction, as well as other creative writing, gives writers the opportunity to present the emotional truth of a story while experiencing freedom from details either too trivial or painful to remember.

One notable example of an author reconstructing fact as fiction is *The Things They Carried*, where O'Brien (1990) writes, "I'm forty-three years old, true, and I'm a writer now, and a long time ago I walked through Quang Ngai Province as a foot soldier. Almost everything else is invented. But it's not a game. It's a form" (p. 179). As Goldberg (2000) writes when discussing *The Things They Carried*, "as I read I knew the book was all true, but he's also saying what is truth?" (p. 129). DeSalvo (1999) provides another insight about the book by stating, "but he says too, that to tell truthfully what happened to him as a foot soldier in Quang Ngai Province in Vietnam, he has had to resort to invention" (p. 165). The important thing about all stories that use fiction or other forms of creative writing to present facts is that the reader comprehends the emotional truth of the story.

Clandinin and Connelly (2000) observe, "in narrative inquiry, the distinction between fact and fiction is muddled" (p. 179). Sometimes when remembering a story in preparation for retelling it, details blur together. Lamott (1994) believes, "a writer paradoxically seeks the truth and tells lies every step of the way. It's a lie if you make something up. But you make it up in the name of the truth, and then you give your heart to expressing it clearly" (p. 52). Sometimes the emotional truth of a story resonates more than the happening truth when the emotions the writer felt mean more than specifics such as the name of a street or the color of a sweater. In *The Things They Carried*, O'Brien (1990) needed a method to provide the emotional truth of his war experiences in Vietnam while freeing himself of specific details; he explains, "I want you to feel what I felt. I want you to know why story-truth is truer sometimes than happening truth" (p. 179). The story-truth of fiction helps a writer focus on an experience without feeling confined by specific details that exist in happening-truth life. In fact, fiction helps writers focus on the facts. Goldberg (2000) describes her perspective on *The Things They Carried* and elaborates, "so O'Brien walks out into the land of fiction and looks back and tells the story from that perspective. Maybe then he can get a handle on it. Sometimes the more fictional a writer becomes, the closer he actually gets to dead center. Fiction lets us unhinge from facts and unleashes the soul of a thing" (p. 129). DeSalvo (1999) concurs that *The Things They Carried* "brilliantly solves many problems inherent in writing about extreme trauma. In the novel he writes what is, ostensibly, a memoir. But then he tells the reader the only way to tell the truth about his life is to make it up, to use "story-truth." He does this, in part, he says, because all memory is fictive" (p. 165). She continues, "we can write, not to express feelings we don't have, but to discover what we might have felt if we hadn't been terrified. This is best done, O'Brien believes, when we strive for 'story truth' rather than literal truth, when we describe semifictional stand-ins for ourselves" (p. 166). Or as O'Brien (1990) states, "what stories can do, I guess, is make things present" (p. 180). Sometimes the happening-truth feels too painful for a writer to explore in writing, so the only way for the writer to share the experience becomes to use story-truth and share the soul of the story without reliving the trauma during the retelling of events.

I experienced the converging of story-truth and happening-truth during the writing of my doctoral dissertation. With the story-truth of fiction, I felt free to focus on the emotional truth of experiences without feeling confined by specific details that existed in my happening-truth life. While fiction writing helped me heal from emotional pain, I had to leave story-truth behind and share the happening-truth of my life in order to help me heal from physical pain. In my neck pain journal, I needed to be specific in order to help my physical therapist help me heal. I needed to be honest and share my story. When using writing to heal from emotional pain, the form, such as fiction, poetry. or personal essay, doesn't matter as much as the processing of emotional truth. Conversely, when using writing to heal from physical pain, the essential thing is telling the specific truth of events as they happen and sharing them with a medical professional who can help.

When focusing on finding the emotional truth of a narrative, I followed the advice of Files (2016) who suggests, "when it's emotional truth you seek, trust memory's details to find it" (p. 79). Brown (2015) concurs, "stay in the story until you touch every part of it" (p. 92). This process of trusting my memories until I touched every part of the story meant reconnecting with my mom and knowing I honor her whenever I write about research or help a student or patient.

EMOTIONAL TRUTH MEMORIES

I sometimes find myself waking up in the middle of the night having pandemic teaching dreams, where I am stuck in a plexiglass box and can't find my mask or lesson plans. I don't remember all the details of that particular nightmare, but I do remember the emotional truth of the experience, which led me to better manage my stress.

Writing captures moments in time and provides perspective as history unfolds. Journalist Anna Quindlen (2004) describes the perspective of her personal feelings about an event needing to coexist with her role as a reporter to objectively tell the facts of a story. When she and another bystander witnessed the scene after September 11, she relates, "I took a notebook from my bag and wrote down what he said and how it looked and how I felt" (p. xxv). Just like Quindlen captured her experiences of September 11 for readers in her role as a journalist, we can use our words to capture moments from the pandemic so we never forget how we remained strong and survived. As Goldberg (2000) explains, "I believe that this is a primary commitment a writer makes to her writing, an essential commitment she makes to her reader: a willingness to be open to encounter, to experience – and to the suffering this may bring" (p. 86). When my cousins' children, who are too young to fully comprehend the pandemic, are older, I want them to read my stories of how our family suffered but survived, how we stayed connected and stayed resilient, how we learned lessons about ourselves and each other. I want them to read my narrative and feel the emotional truth of my experiences.

ACKNOWLEDGMENT

The preceding chapter contains excerpts from the following previous IGI publications:

Bird, J.L. (2020). Narratives of emotional truth. In *Using narrative writing to enhance healing* (pp. 101-128). Hershey, PA: Information Science Reference.

Bird, J.L., Wanner, E.T., Urenda, R., & Perry, R. (2015). Multigenre medicine. In *Innovative collaborative practice and reflection in patient education* (pp. 1-19). Hershey, PA: Information Science Reference.

REFERENCES

Adams, K. (1990). *Journal to the Self.* Warner Books.

Alexander, E. (2012). *Proof of Heaven.* Simon and Schuster.

Alexander, E. (2014). *The map of Heaven.* Simon and Schuster.

Beck, M. (2001). *Finding your own North Star.* Three Rivers Press.

Brown, B. (2015). *Rising strong.* Spiegel & Grau.

Caldwell, K., Gray, J., & Wolever, R. Q. (2013). The process of patient empowerment in integrative health coaching: How does it happen? *Global Advances in Health and Medicine: Improving Healthcare Outcomes Worldwide, 2*(3), 48–57. doi:10.7453/gahmj.2013.026 PMID:24416672

Cameron, J. (1998). *The right to write.* Tarcher/Putnam.

Carter, C. (2015). *The sweet spot.* Ballantine.

Charon, R. (2006). *Narrative medicine: honoring the stories of illness.* Oxford University Press.

Clandinin, D. J., & Connelly, F. M. (2000). *Narrative inquiry.* Jossey-Bass.

Cleaver, J. (2002). *Immediate fiction.* St. Martin's Press.

Connelly, F. M., & Clandinin, D. J. (1988). *Teachers as curriculum planners.* Teachers College.

DeSalvo, L. (1999). *Writing as a way of healing.* Beacon Press.

Duke Integrative Medicine Staff. (2010). *Personalized health plan manual.* Duke Integrative Medicine.

Edelman, H. (2020). *The AfterGrief.* Random House.

Fallon, A. (2020). *The power of writing it down.* Zondervan.

Files, M. (2016). *Writing what you know.* Allworth.

Fitzgerald, F. S. (1925). *The great Gatsby.* Scribner.

Germer, C. K. (2009). *The Mindful path to self-compassion.* The Guilford Press.

Goldberg, N. (2000). *Thunder and lightning.* Bantam.

Goldberg, N. (2007). *Old friend from far away.* Free Press.

Greenberg, M. A., Wortman, C. B., & Stone, A. A. (1996). Emotional expression and physical health: Revising traumatic memories or fostering self-regulation. *Journal of Personality and Social Psychology, 71*(3), 588–602. doi:10.1037/0022-3514.71.3.588 PMID:8831163

Hale, M. (2018). *You are enough.* FaithWords.

Handler, J. (2013). *Braving the fire.* St. Martin's Griffin.

Harper, A. N. (1996). Tooling up for effective planning. In B. W. McClendon & A. J. Catanese (Eds.), *Planners on planning* (pp. 190–198). Jossey-Bass.

Haugk, K. C. (2000). *When and how to use mental health resources*. Stephen Ministries.

Helldorfer, M., & Moss, T. (2007). *Healing with heart*. Moss Communications.

Lamott, A. (1994). *Bird by bird*. Anchor Books.

Lepore, S. J., Greenberg, M. A., Bruno, M., & Smyth, J. M. (2002). Expressive writing and health: self-regulation of emotion-related experience, physiology, and behavior. In S. J. Lepore & J. M. Smyth (Eds.), *The writing cure* (pp. 99–117). American Psychological Association.

Madigan, S. (2011). *Narrative therapy*. American Psychological Association.

Michele, L. (2015). *You first: journal your way to your best life*. Crown Archetype.

Neff, K. (2011). *Self compassion: The proven power of being kind to yourself*. HarperCollins.

O'Brien, T. (1990). *The things they carried*. Broadway Books.

Pennebaker, J. W. (1997). *Opening up: the healing power of expressing emotions*. The Guilford Press.

Pennebaker, J. W., & Evans, J. F. (2014). *Expressive writing: words that heal*. Idyll Arbor.

Poetter, T. S. (2013). Stemming the tide. *Kappa Delta Pi Record*, *49*(3), 100–104. doi:10.1080/00228958.2013.819195

Quindlen, A. (2004). *Loud and clear*. Ballantine.

Rasminsky, A. (2012). The story doc. *Oprah*, *13*(7), 88.

Romano, T. (1987). *Clearing the way*. Heinemann.

Romano, T. (1995). *Writing with passion*. Heinemann.

Romano, T. (2000). *Blending genre, altering style*. Heinemann.

Romano, T. (2004). *Crafting authentic voice*. Heinemann.

Romano, T. (2008). *Zigzag*. Heinemann.

Romano, T. (2013). *Fearless writing*. Heinemann.

Smith, L. L., Lake, N. H., Simmons, L. A., Perlman, A., Wroth, S., & Wolever, R. Q. (2013). Integrative health coach training: A model for shifting the paradigm toward patient-centricity and meeting new national prevention goals. *Global Advances in Health and Medicine: Improving Healthcare Outcomes Worldwide*, *2*(3), 66–74. doi:10.7453/gahmj.2013.034 PMID:24416674

Soukup, R. (2019). *Do it scared*. Zondervan.

Wanner, S. Y. (1994). *On with the story*. Heinemann.

Weiner-Davis, M. (1995). *Fire your shrink*. Simon & Schuster.

Wheelan, C. (2013). *Naked statistics*. W.W. Norton.

Zimmermann, S. (2002). *Writing to heal the soul*. Three Rivers Press.

KEY TERMS AND DEFINITIONS

Expressive Writing: Writing that is exploratory and focuses on meaning and first impressions.

Journal Writing: The process of a person responding to prompts and writing about his or her thoughts and feelings. While journal writing is typically associated with writing classrooms, writing teachers including Julia Cameron and Natalie Goldberg advocate that journal writing can be done by anyone, anywhere. Students in an English classroom, patients in a physical therapy clinic, and readers of this chapter in their living rooms can pick up pen, paper, and just write.

Multigenre Writing: Discussed in the field of education by Tom Romano, a multigenre paper consists of two parts: creative writing in multiple genres and the writer's analysis of the genres.

Narrative Inquiry: Discussed in the field of research by F. Michael Connelly and D. Jean Clandinin, narrative inquiry is a qualitative interpretative form of research that focuses on the telling, retelling, and sharing of stories. Researchers who complete narrative inquiries interpret stories and search for common threads to find patterns. They are encouraged to tell their research stories in first person as they look back to find meaning in past stories and look forward to set future goals.

Narrative Medicine: The field of medicine, used by programs such as the one Rita Charon founded at Columbia University, which encourages medical practitioners to use theories from the fields of literature and composition to enhance comprehension of the stories patients share.

Story-Truth and Happening-Truth: Happening-truth is an objective factual account of events which occurred. Story-truth, sometimes referred to as emotional truth, is a subjective reflection of a person's thoughts and feelings about the same event when retelling that story. Writers such as Tim O'Brien, Natalie Goldberg, and Anne Lamott believe in the power of emotional truth that enables writers to switch back and forth from objective observations to subjective emotions when sharing a story.

Writing Voice: Voice in writing describes how a writer uses word choice and tone to compose a journal entry or other written composition that reflects the personality of the writer. Just like each person has a unique speaking voice, each writer has a unique writing voice.

Chapter 7
Reflections of Curriculum Narratives

ABSTRACT

This narrative represents the foundation for the PAGES program and shares examples from physical therapy patients, high school students, and people coping with life changes during the recent pandemic. PAGES serves as an acronym for practice patience, accept the present, gather information, encourage, and self-care. The strategies can apply to a variety of settings, and anyone wishing to implement change may use all parts of the acronym collectively or choose useful individual components of the advice.

DESIGNING PAGES

PAGES, the program described in this narrative, happened because of a large foundation of writing. Rarely does any single piece of writing happen in isolation. Program development and new learning opportunities occur because of the outcomes of previous writing and research. Often different pieces of writing fit together like puzzle pieces to form a larger picture. Heard (1995) confirms, "the obstacles I face – lack of time, too many projects at once – as well as the obstacles all writers face – rejection, criticism, doubts and insecurities, unfinished poems and stories – are impossible to avoid and can be valuable teachers" (pp. 38-39). Writers consistently overcome obstacles to develop new ideas. I, as an English teacher and health coach, completed extensive writing and research with Eric Wanner, a physical therapist and research consultant, which provided a foundation upon which to scaffold this new idea. Family involvement becomes the heart and soul of PAGES. While physical therapists, health coaches, and other medical professionals can offer support to a hospital patient, when the patient goes home from the hospital, the relay baton of care gets passed to the family member caregiver. Similarly, while teachers, academic advisors, and other education professionals can offer support to a student, when the student goes home from the school, the relay baton of care gets passed to the family member caregiver. Recently, when dealing with life during a pandemic, people may use the foundation of PAGES to take care of themselves and others.

DOI: 10.4018/978-1-7998-9051-5.ch007

This narrative provides a foundation for the PAGES program. While the program was originally designed for the families of hospital patients, the same strategy was later adapted to help the families of high school students. It may also be adapted to other fields that you as the reader view appropriate. PAGES is an acronym that serves as a reminder for families of hospital patients to reflect on what they need to do to help their loved ones recover after surgery. It also serves as a reminder for families of students to reflect on what they need to do to help their loved ones achieve success in school. The designers used expertise in health coaching, curriculum design, teaching, writing, and research in a physical therapy clinic to create the PAGES program with the intent it will make a difference to people who apply the strategy to their lives.

THE PAGES FAMILY COACHING PROGRAM

Helping patients turn new pages and write new chapters in their healing journeys

To help your loved one who is a patient:

Practice patience: Healing is a journey. No one can wave a magic wand and provide an immediate cure. Celebrate progress, no matter how small.

Accept the present: Feelings of guilt, anger, and frustration are normal, but are not helpful when coaching. No matter what happened in the past, this is where you are now. Worrying about the future only causes additional stress. Try your best to remain in the present moment. Consider writing in a journal to sort through your feelings.

Gather information: The medical professionals such as doctors, physical therapists, occupational therapists, nurses, and speech therapists are here to help you. Ask questions, and listen to their instructions. Consider bringing a notebook with you to write down information so you don't have to remember it.

Encourage: During the healing journey, patients need cheerleaders. You are a source of hope and light during this process and a little support can make a large difference.

Self-Care: In order to take care of your loved one, take care of yourself too. You can better help someone else when your own needs, such as hunger and sleep, are met too.

PAGES CURRICULUM

In 2015, I completed a health coaching internship at a hospital, where I served as a member of the inpatient physical therapy team and helped patients with the emotional side of healing. When we both worked at the hospital, Eric and I designed a family coaching program called PAGES. Due to the changing needs of programs at the hospital, the program never reached the implementation stage. In a serendipitous moment, I joined the advisory committee at the high school where I teach with the goal of designing mentoring strategies to enhance the lives of high school students. The PAGES program, which incorporates strategies from a variety of relationship based leadership curricula, can easily adapt to fit the needs of high school students.

Practice patience: As high school students continue their journeys through life, they need supportive adults as role models. Often, the most significant goals cannot happen overnight. Empower students by celebrating progress, no matter how small. Students have numerous people giving them advice, so active listening proves valuable in a role as advisor.

Accept the present: Try to remain in the present moment. It becomes easy for both teachers and students to think of the myriad of tasks to accomplish in a day, but advisory time provides a break for students from past mistakes and future worries. Journal writing also helps students sort through their feelings.

Gather information: Ask open ended questions, and listen to student answers. As an advisor, use reflective statements to acknowledge student feelings. If students need additional assistance, refer them to the appropriate resource such as college counseling or the school psychologist.

Encourage: During the high school journey, students need support. As an advisor, you provide a source of hope, which makes a difference.

Self-Care: In order to take care of your students, take care of yourself too. You can better help someone else when your own needs, such as hunger and sleep, are met.

PAGES THROUGH A PANDEMIC LENS

Practice patience: Even during feelings of pandemic fatigue, know that this era in time won't last forever. It will take time for places to open, people to receive vaccines, and for the virus to be controlled.

Accept the present: We are where we are. Whatever each individual circumstance may be, accept what is beyond control and what can be controlled. Focus on things that can be controlled, such as mindset and perspective.

Gather information: Numerous news resources exist for information. Find a reputable source and learn from it. Take periodic breaks from the news to avoid information overload, or search for stories of people helping others.

Encourage: Reach out to people and connect with them. It is possible for people to become lonely and isolated during the pandemic, and a phone call to check that someone is okay makes a difference.

Self-Care: Make sure to find moments for self-care. Dealing with the constant reminders of wearing masks, social distancing, washing hands, and cleaning can be exhausting, so find time for healthy moments of comfort.

FOUNDATION FOR PAGES

Skills such as being in the present moment, practicing active listening, asking open ended questions, and using reflective statements to acknowledge the feelings of others appear in several training programs. Kenneth Haugk (2000) and the team at Stephen Ministries designed a program to prepare lay caregivers to assist ministers in helping members of a congregation who experience losses. For people looking to improve or maintain health, the team at Duke University Integrative Medicine (2010) designed a health coaching program. To promote care of self and others, the team at Creative Health Care Management (2003) designed a relationship based care model for showing compassion in the workplace. The PAGES program combines elements from all of these programs, as well as the theory and practice of curriculum design in schools, to meet the needs of high school students.

Some educators may feel concern that advisory represents time away from classes. However, teacher Graves (2001) argues, "curriculum is the sum total of the content of human experience from the time we arise until we go to bed in the evening" (p. 47). Hence, curriculum does not only represent the lesson plans and textbooks teachers use in their classrooms; curriculum also represents life and lived experiences. Johnson (1998) explains, "life is magnified and feelings are intensified for children" (p. 173). Advisory represents a place where students can discuss topics with an adult mentor, or write about feelings in a journal to process emotions on the page. English professor Romano (2000) describes the value of students writing in journals and elaborates, "when we write expressively in a journal, we imprint ideas, information, and experience deeply within us. We live topics by re-creating them with words on paper, by pulling images and dialog from the flow of our lives" (p. 138). When students explore their thoughts and feelings in writing or through conversation, it becomes important for both teachers and students to remember that, while teachers may serve as mentors and advisors, teachers cannot play the role of counselor. Brown (2018) explains, "if struggle is being down in a hole, empathy is not jumping into the hole with someone who is struggling and taking on their emotions, or owning their struggle as yours to fix. If their issues become yours, now you have two people stuck in a hole. Not helpful. Boundaries are important here" (p. 142). If teachers see signs of depression, anxiety, or any other emotional distress in students, the teacher should refer the student to the school psychologist.

With an advisory curriculum, it becomes essential to give students a voice in their learning experiences. Beane (1997) believes, "since curriculum integration is tied to the larger concept of democratic education, the matter of student participation in planning their own experiences must eventually become a crucial aspect of the design" (p. 9). Therefore, even though teachers may develop a plan for advisory, student experiences should play a role in an advisory session. Connelly and Clandinin (1988) advise teachers to use reflection when learning student narratives because, "it is their curriculum, their personal practical knowledge and narratives of experience that fall within your guidance" (p. 197). In order for students to feel comfortable sharing their stories, teachers need to provide a safe space for such conversations. Brown (2018) advises teachers, "we must be guardians of a space that allows students to breathe and be curious and explore the world and be who they are without suffocation. They deserve one place where they can rumble with vulnerability and their hearts can exhale" (p. 13). Small advisory groups provide such a place for students. Sandberg and Grant (2017) describe the launch of "Lean In Circles, small groups of peers who meet regularly to support and encourage one another" (p. 134). Like a Lean In Circle for adults, a high school advisory represents a place where peers encourage and support each other.

Moments of connection become essential during the pandemic. Students often struggle with questions similar to those asked by Williams (2019) such as, "do you want to get to the end of your life and question whether you've really lived? Or worse, regret not going for your dreams?" (p. 12). Finding the answers to questions about future goals and purpose can be difficult during times when there isn't a pandemic, but a virus that restricts college tours to online visits and eliminates or changes rituals including graduation and prom causes additional stress. A time during the school day such as advisory where students talk to a trusted adult about issues and concerns in their lives becomes a brief moment of calm during a chaotic time.

PAGES, the acronym for this program, symbolizes the idea of turning new pages in life. The skills of practicing patience, accepting the present, gathering information, encouragement, and self-care provide the foundations of a supportive learning community. Through a regular advisory meeting, advisors help students turn the pages of their own life stories and write new chapters of success.

TURNING PAGES FOR NEW POSSIBILITIES

This idea for the PAGES program occurred once I began working as a health coach at a hospital. During my time at the hospital I worked with staff members who wanted to make health adjustments to their lives. Since the foundation for PAGES exists in curriculum development, which usually takes place in a school, it became easy to modify the strategy from a group classroom environment in a hospital to a classroom environment in a school. Regardless of whether a hospital patient experiences recovery from a surgical procedure or a high school student experiences a difficult day at school, family support provides a foundation for success. Havrilesky (2018) describes how people create change as, "we are called to plant these seeds in our world: to dare to tell every living soul that they already matter, that their seemingly mundane lives are a slowly unfolding mystery, that their small choices and acts of generosity are vitally important" (p. 217). Lee (2018) provides a similar description of change as, "the lesson of renewal is that from small seeds big things grow" (p. 298). She continues, "it's not far-fetched to believe that from the seeds of our own joy, a whole world can be reborn" (p. 298). Every person needs to know that he or she matters to other people; therefore, a support network provides the necessary environment to demonstrate care and community. Support networks become even more critical during the pandemic era, when it becomes easy for people to feel isolated when having to quarantine.

CREATING A CARING CURRICULUM

If energy is put into the curriculum design and lesson plans, the energy will be reflected in the teacher as the lesson is taught and the students will subsequently benefit from it. Graves (2001) states, "the energy of the curriculum lies in the making, learning, and planning of what is ahead" (p. 49). Sometimes, however, the curriculum is not explicitly stated but implicitly implied. This is called the hidden curriculum. As Connelly and Clandinin (1988) define, "generally speaking, people think of the hidden curriculum as falling in the area of attitudes and values" (p. 154). The hidden curriculum encompasses everything from the posters hanging on the walls to the smiles on the instructors' faces. Patients also bring their own hidden curriculum to their treatment sessions. A patient may not want to complete exercises as part of a treatment plan, but may want to achieve the goal of being pain free for a vacation. Health coaches build bridges to link the information in the patient's mind to illuminate the fact that doing the exercises will lead to a pain free vacation. Health coaches enlist the support of family members to offer additional encouragement during the healing journey.

Similarly, students bring their own hidden curriculum to a classroom. A student may not want to complete an assignment as part of a lesson plan, but may want to achieve the goal of earning a high grade in the class. Advisors for a student play more of a coaching role than a teaching role; therefore, advisors build bridges to link the information in the student's mind to illuminate the fact that studying will lead to a high grade.

Both health coaches and teacher advisors may choose to use writing as a method of managing the myriad emotions experienced in a coaching setting. Cameron (1998) believes, "every time I put my hand to the page, I am altering the energy that flows through my life" (p. 201). Whether writing encourages the venting of frustrations or the setting of goals, it brings clarity to the writer and eases anxiety. Clark (2018) explains, "both in writing and in speech, embracing a narrative of healing can be powerful in constructing a present and a future not at the mercy of the past" (p. 325). However, before writing takes place in any type of coaching setting, the coach must establish a safe environment. People often serve as their own worst critics. Neff (2011) confirms it helps "to treat ourselves with the same kindness, caring, and compassion we would show to a good friend, or even a stranger for that matter. Sadly, however, there's almost no one whom we treat as badly as ourselves" (p. 6). A safe environment creates space for members of a community to honestly speak their feelings.

Whether a person has a goal of a pain free vacation or a high grade in a class, emotions make a difference in the achievement of the goal. Medical doctor Tindle (2013) explains, "the evidence shows that people with a high degree of anger do worse healthwise" (p. 29). Medical doctor Rankin (2013) agrees that, "when you make efforts to increase your happiness, the health of the body tends to follow" (p. 142). Hope creates a desire to achieve goals, leads to increased motivation, and paves the way for a possible shorter road to achieve a goal; conversely; anger creates obstacles or adds to existing obstacles, leads to decreased motivation, and paves the way for possible longer road to achieve a goal.

Encouragement provided by supportive communities transforms the emotions of participants. Social worker Brown (2015) discovered, "in my work, I've found that moving out of powerlessness, and even despair, requires hope" (p. 202). Brown (2017) advocates turning negative emotions into positive ones because "anger is a catalyst. Holding on to it will make us exhausted and sick" (p. 67). She continues, "it's an emotion that we need to transform into something life-giving: courage, love, change, compassion, justice" (p. 68). Even if people want to transform their emotions, such a change requires trust and vulnerability. Brown (2018) explains, "trust is the stacking and layering of small moments and reciprocal vulnerability over time. Trust and vulnerability grow together, and to betray one is to destroy both" (p. 34). Change may not immediately occur, but over time a supportive community creates the environment for participants to trust each other and feel vulnerable with each other.

Turn on the news during the pandemic and witness stories of communities coming together to deliver groceries to each other, make masks for each other, design cards to send to each other, and numerous other acts of kindness which make a difference in the lives of others. From all the discouraging news about the coronavirus, moments of hope emerge. Since everyone's life has been touched in some way by the pandemic, whether it is the severe trauma of losing a loved one or the mild inconvenience of having to stay at home, people need each other and their communities for sustenance.

While the theory described in the subsequent sections focuses on hospital patients and schools, the practice of PAGES adapts to multiple learning environments. Use the examples as inspiration to fill unwritten pages in an organization's future with new ideas and possibilities.

ASSESSMENT REVELATIONS

When implementing a program, assessment occurs to ensure the program meets its goals.

When I became the Director of the Writing and Reading Center (WRC) at Oxbridge Academy, I inherited the twenty-five high school student peer tutors who worked in the WRC during their study hall. We used the book *The Longman Guide to Peer Tutoring* to inspire us to practice the strategies of non-judging, open-ended questions, presencing, reflective statements, and active listening during peer tutoring conferences. In my role as WRC Director, I reflect on how teachers assessed student assessments. Reflection led to revelations about assessment.

What if I evaluated students at the beginning of the class instead of the end?

What if I approached evaluation like a physical therapist does?

I thought about how Eric, a physical therapist, evaluates patients. I arrive at the clinic and he asks me to rate on a number scale how I am feeling (numeric evaluation) and why (narrative evaluation). For example, my pain might be a 5 (on a scale of 10) because I looked down too long when reading a book. While I do my initial stretches (warm up), he takes his exercise plan (lesson plan) and adjusts it based on the information I just told him (differentiation). I leave the clinic feeling better (what learning should be).

So here is how this could work in my classroom. Instead of exit slips, where students answer questions as they leave, I use entrance slips. Students arrive with a post-it note (ideally completed for homework, but I can have post-its by the door if they forget). Students have to tell me how they would rank their comprehension numerically and give me a reason why. Students would then have to write their responses on the board so their classmates can see. For example, after reading a scene in *The Great Gatsby*, one student might give comprehension a 3 because he did not understand why Gatsby received a strange phone call. Another student might give comprehension a 7 because she loved the romantic scene where Daisy and Gatsby were staring at the green light.

While students write in journals (warm ups), I would quickly use their numbers and narratives to modify my lesson plans to inform my teaching for the day (differentiation). For example, if I have high numbers, I can ask higher level learning questions or have a Socratic seminar where students share their opinions. If I have low numbers, I may ask students to complete a double-entry journal where they choose a confusing quote and write what they think it means. If I have numbers all over the scale, I may break students into small groups and ask them to share their thoughts with each other. Then (hopefully), students leave the classroom feeling better about the text (what learning should be).

Assessment for a program such as PAGES does not have to look identical to the previous example, but should demonstrate thought and reflection to ensure the program meets its objectives.

My students complete self-assessment of how they can help other members of the school community. During pandemic times, the writing center tutors have started a garden, designed bulletin boards with inspirational quotes, completed online programs which being peers together, and delivered thank you notes to members of the school staff. As a team we set the goal of making the Writing and Reading Center (even with all the plexiglass barriers) a welcome, comforting place for students to learn. Lee (2018) describes this concept as "specifically, it is what designers call aesthetics – the properties that define a way an object looks and feels – that give rise to the feelings of joy" (p. 7). Creating a welcoming environment illustrates the importance of comfortable community spaces, even during a time when visitors to the community space need to social distance.

PRACTICING PAGES

Throughout the pandemic, families found themselves separated from each other either due to the physical distance of geography or the emotional distance of wanting to give someone a hug but not being able to because of the lurking threat of the virus. The words of Havrilesky (2018), although written before the pandemic, still feel relevant because, "even as depression and anxiety, or else simple dissatisfaction with the state of things, are as prevalent as ever, we are urged to get over these feelings, to recover from them, to bounce back quickly, or else conceal them" (p. 8). Whatever feelings may arise during the pandemic, those feelings have value. I might feel hope, despair, anger, loss, and joy all on the same day, and that is okay.

For families seeking to stay connected to each other, for families who have experienced a loved one's illness as a coronavirus patient, and for anyone looking to build a community, here's how to practice PAGES.

GREATER HEALING GAINS THROUGH FAMILY INVOLVEMENT

Similar to how family support can lead to educational success for a child, evidence exists that family involvement leads to greater healing for patients. Ryan, Wade, Nice, Shenefelt, and Shepard (1996) discovered, "family involvement was found to be a significant aspect of a patient's rehabilitation" (p. 159). Through a series of interviews with forty physical therapists, the researchers learned, "the shift from hospital to home care increases the effect on the family unit and significantly expands the role of the physical therapist in involving the family in the rehabilitation process. Such trends in healthcare require that physical therapists have effective, time-efficient strategies for involving family members in a way that ensures the highest potential for optimal recovery of the patient" (p. 160). However, family members may have barriers in their family dynamics to work thorough while attempting to provide support for their loved one who is a physical therapy patient going through an exercise treatment plan.

Physical therapists expertly inform family members about the patient's at home treatment plan. Nevertheless, due to demands by insurance companies and the health care system for clinicians to consistently demonstrate increased productivity, a physical therapist may not be able to have a lengthy conversation with a patient's family about how the family is navigating the crisis of the patient's surgery and how everyone can move forward together as a family unit. This is where health coaches provide much needed assistance for both physical therapists and families. The authors of the family involvement research study observed, "the success with which a family adapts to crisis depends on a variety of factors from financial resources to the family's expectations and knowledge of the patient's condition" (p. 160). The role of the health coach is to help the patient, and therefore also the family members, focus on the present situation and offer strategies and resources for breaking down barriers and overcoming obstacles which help maintain forward momentum. The researchers concluded that "the physical therapist's knowledge of what the family is experiencing is crucial in guiding the family towards appropriate goal setting" (p. 175). The emerging field of health coaching did not exist when this research study was conducted, but health coaches, physical therapists, and families all work together to ensure elite results for the patient.

DESIGNING A CURRICULUM OF FAMILY INVOLVEMENT

Creating a new curriculum, whether it is at a school or a hospital, takes thought and effort. A teacher doesn't just walk into a classroom, wave a copy of *The Great Gatsby* at students, and teach without a lesson plan or a curriculum to support that lesson plan. Similarly, it helps the families of patients to know the expectations of the physical therapist for the exercise plan. As Marshall, Sears, and Schubert (2000) explain, "we believe that the essence of curriculum studies lies in the way each educator internalizes fundamental questions of what curriculum is and should be – and the attendant whys, whens, and whereas of its enactment" (p. 3). Anyone designing a new curriculum needs to ask the questions of why a lesson is being taught, when the lesson is going to be taught, and how it is going to be presented.

In one example, when family members coach patients, the why is that as the primary caregivers, a family member will have to take over supervision of the patient's home exercise plan once the patient leaves the hospital and help the patient remember to do the exercises. The when begins when the family member attends group physical therapy classes with the patient and learns instructions about the exercises from the physical therapist. And the how happens when family members offer encouragement and support to become an extra member on the team that helps motivate the patient to achieve success.

In another example, when teachers coach students, the why is that as the educator, a teacher will use a variety of instructional techniques to inspire students to learn. The when begins when the students step into the classroom and the teacher sets the tone for learning. And the how happens when the teacher offers encouragement and support to become an extra member on the team that helps motivate the students to achieve success.

To be successful, a curriculum also needs to incorporate goal setting. Beane (1997) explains, "curriculum integration centers the curriculum on life itself rather than on the mastery of fragmented information within the boundaries of subject areas. It works off a view of learning as the continuous integration of new knowledge and experience so as to deepen and broaden our understanding of ourselves and our world" (p. 18). Curriculum integration encourages democratic education and active learning, where participants have ownership of the curriculum instead of having someone else tell it to them. The goals of a curriculum often evolve from evidence based practice, such as action research. Action research occurs when a teacher develops a new idea and tries it in a classroom setting. Or as Connelly and Clandinin (1988) explain, "action research is, therefore, a deliberate way of creating new situations and of telling the story of who we are" (p. 153). If an idea is implemented and succeeds, it often becomes adapted into the curriculum. While action research has its foundation in the field of education, it can be modified for use in other fields. Part of health coaching involves encouraging people to set goals to take ownership of their healing. In this instance, the goal setting process becomes collaborative. A curriculum which provides the foundation of effective information that sets people up for success enhances the goal setting process. Just as teachers celebrate their student's successes in a classroom, physical therapists celebrate their patient's successes in a clinic. The creation of SMART (specific, measurable, action oriented, realistic, timed) goals in both settings means that learning becomes a collaborative team effort, with the successful outcome of one goal leading to the setting of a new goal. Connelly and Clandinin (1988) continue, "administering the curriculum meant the narrative living out of a personal philosophy of education" (p. 196). The best teachers combine the artistic and technical when teaching. They teach the required elements of the curriculum using methods that make the lessons come alive for students. The execution of an effective lesson resembles a beautiful figure skating or dance routine. Skaters and dancers must complete required technical elements, but also infuse their performance with artistic interpretation and passion.

Every curriculum needs a solid theoretical foundation to support the practice of teaching. The next sections highlight the dimensions of PAGES and why they are important. Teachers, family members of hospital patients, physical therapists, health coaches, other medical practitioners, other educators, and readers interested in learning something new will all benefit from the following information.

PRACTICE PATIENCE

In children's stories, a fairy godmother frequently shows up to save the day. There is a literary term for this too, called "Deus ex machina," Latin for God from a machine, meaning unexpected rescue. It appears in superhero stories too, when characters are rescued from a seemingly impossible situation. Real life doesn't work that way, and people must do the work to reach their goals. Having a positive attitude helps make everything easier. Tindle (2013) believes that if one person has a positive attitude it can influence an entire community because, "when we learn to see the interconnectedness of things in this way, we understand how a positive attitude in one person can benefit countless others, because every person who is able to look up to mental and physical health gives herself maximal opportunity to develop her unique talents. Whenever even one of us can accomplish this feat, it not only stokes the enthusiasm of the entire group but also adds to our collective resources. To this end, cultivating a healthy outlook may perhaps be society's ultimate return on investment" (p. 218). Therefore, if everyone involved in the patient's healing journey (such as doctors, nurses, physical therapists, health coaches, and family members) promotes positivity the patient will know it is okay to take the time needed to heal. Comparatively, if everyone involved in a student's educational journey (such as teachers, advisors, counselors, and family members) promotes positivity the student will know it is okay to take the time needed to learn.

Promoting positivity helps patients not only emotionally, but also physically. Rankin (2013) discusses the connection between mind and body and asks, "so what happens to the body when the mind is in a dark place? Emotional suffering might start in the mind, but it is ultimately an embodied experience. You don't just experience unhappiness in your mind. You feel it in your body, as suffering cascades through your body via the stress response" (p. 132-133). If a patient feels upset about the length of time it is taking to heal, it is possible that the emotional stress will manifest itself as additional physical symptoms.

In order to have a positive attitude, patients need to feel they are in a safe environment. It takes time and patience to establish trust. Advice given by Johnson (1998) can apply to hospitals as well as schools because, as is true with anyone being taught, "they need time to see that we sincerely care about them, have something valuable to teach them, and will not embarrass them when they make mistakes. We need time to get to know their personalities and maturity levels, as well as their intellectual abilities and academic needs. It also takes time to create an environment in our classrooms that is comfortable and secure, so students can relax and concentrate on their lessons" (p. 101). Physical therapists collaborate with health coaches and family members to establish a supportive environment for the patient during group physical therapy classes just like teachers collaborate with advisors and family members to establish a supportive environment for students.

ACCEPT THE PRESENT

When a loved one needs surgery and physical therapy, family members experience a myriad of emotions. They may feel anger at the circumstances that landed the patient in the hospital, or frustrated that the patient is not healing faster. They may feel guilty if their actions contributed to the patient's condition or helpless because they can't take away the pain. All of these feelings are normal, but do not help the patient. Therefore, it is important for family members to deal with their feelings by writing in a journal or talking to someone such as a supportive friend or professional counselor if additional help is needed. Writing in a journal helps patients heal and helps family members sort through their feelings.

Zimmermann (2002) explains, "there is now extensive research that shows writing – the simple act of putting down your deepest thoughts and feelings on paper – is one of the most powerful and effective means to ease and ultimately heal sorrow" (p. 18). Anyone visiting the English Department at a high school or college will hear discussion of research studies illustrating how writing improves emotional health. Writing helps caregivers process their emotions so they can better help their family members who are patients. Caregivers may choose to keep their writing to themselves or share it with a health coach or other professional if they need to discuss their feelings.

Health coaches help a patient see the importance of a treatment plan and increase the patient's confidence in completing the treatment plan by connecting the treatment plan to the patient's vision and values. Pipher (2006) explains, "in both therapy and writing, we want to help people see the connections between their actions and consequences of those actions" (p. 97). It remains important for family members to realize they cannot force change on their loved one. In order for a person to make a change, he or she needs to reach the conclusion that change is necessary. Pipher continues, "people do not change unless they have a powerful emotional turning. This may be thorough epiphanies, insights, or deep connecting moments between the people in the room" (p. 100). While one person cannot make another person change, showing acceptance and being a supportive presence can set the stage for powerful insights by the patient to occur. The same process occurs in classrooms. If a teacher, advisor, or family member serves as a supportive presence the safe environment creates insightful student learning moments.

Another part of the health coaching process is accountability. Health coaches work with people to set goals and make connections, but they also ask the people they are coaching to be accountable for their actions. With family members, sometimes emotions get in the way when trying to hold a loved one accountable for his or her actions. As Brown (2010) explains, "it's hard for us to understand that we can be compassionate and accepting while we hold people accountable for their behaviors" (p. 18). Sometimes when coaching a family member, emotions take over when the patient is not demonstrating accountability for complying with the treatment plan. Since health coaches have an objective distance from the patient that family members do not, health coaches remind family coaches to continue to show compassion and acceptance during the patient's healing journey.

With family relationships, dynamics get complicated. Beck (2008) elaborates, "you may be one of the lucky people whose loved ones and associates are all delighted and inspired when you set out to live your right life. More likely, though, you'll encounter some level of resistance. After all, the most common reason we stray from our best lives is that we're socialized to behave in ways that aren't right for us. Our social groups, almost by definition, tend to disapprove when we drop those behaviors" (p. 191). Regardless of what happened between family members in the past, it is important for family members to put any issues aside when coaching the patient. If the family member felt disappointed in the patient's behavior in the past, bringing those emotions into a group physical therapy class does not help the patient heal in the present moment. Change can be difficult for everyone, especially family members who did not ask for their lives to be disrupted by the patient's surgery. However, as Nick tells Gatsby in *The Great Gatsby* by Fitzgerald (1925), "you can't repeat the past" (p. 116). This quote from literature is powerful advice for families too.

In addition to family members demonstrating acceptance for the patient's current medical reality, the patient has to accept that even when the family is accepting and supportive, the patient still has to do the work to reach his or her healing goals. Beck (2001) states, " people whose families were accepting and supportive have to face the fact that familial love can't take them all the way to their right lives" (p. 70). Beck continues with the reminder, "but you will still have to do the physical therapy to get your bones and muscles to work again. The same thing is true of psychological wounds" (p. 70). No matter how many people are cheering in the audience, the patient still needs to stand on the metaphorical stage of the physical therapy clinic and perform the exercises.

GATHER INFORMATION

The more information a patient knows, the more empowered he or she feels while on the healing journey. Family members help the patient by being another person to listen to the advice and instructions given by the medical professionals treating the patient. Medical professionals such as physical therapists want the patient to succeed and will provide helpful suggestions for how to complete the treatment intervention and make lifestyle adjustments during the healing process. By continuing to be a supportive presence, family members make this gathering of information a team effort to ensure the comprehension of all information.

Sometimes when patients are in pain they have difficulty remembering important information given to them by the therapist or information they want to share with the therapist. Family members help make sure patients fully understand the important information once they get home or ask the important questions to the therapist. Knowing a patient's initial thoughts about factors causing pain can assist clinicians in developing a treatment plan. Juhan (1998) explains, "this missing link of conscious, active engagement is of enormous importance when it comes to strategies of therapeutic intervention. Some of the habits I am unconsciously perpetuating are reinforcing – sometimes even creating – my current difficulties" (p. 350). Writing illuminates such habits for both the patient and the clinician so ineffective old habits will be replaced by effective new ones. English teachers use journals and writing conferences with students to discover patterns in student writing. Family members use journals to record information stated by the clinician so it is remembered, and patients use journals to track their pain so the clinician can see patterns. By doing this, patients provide an additional dimension of information for the clinician, and family members make sure they have all information correctly written down for when the patient arrives home. Barrett (2013) writes about her own experiences with chronic pain and describes, "I started to track my experience with just pen and paper. I recorded when I felt best (and worst) and began making deliberate changes to my environment and behavior. One at a time, I assessed the factors in my life" (p. 37). Writing prompts and surveys assist patients in writing their thoughts. Nevertheless, asking a patient to write becomes only half the story. The other half involves a supportive clinician willing to read the writing.

ENCOURAGE

If patients know their loved ones will walk with them on their healing journey and be a source of comfort and support, they know they are not alone and part of a supportive community while they heal. If a patient is completing a set of exercises and looks across the room to see a health coach or family member offering words of encouragement, the patient will most likely experience increased motivation to comply with the treatment plan. By celebrating accomplishments and providing the reassurance that mistakes and setbacks are part of the healing journey, the best possible environment will be created for the patient. Likewise, when teachers give students the reassurance that mistakes are part of the learning journey, the best possible environment will be created for the student.

No one needs to be alone while on a healing journey. Helldorfer and Moss (2007) discuss the importance of a climate of care because "while our focus at work is always on our patients, we are also part of a larger community of colleagues where we care for one another, and where each person has a role to play in creating the climate" (p. 163). A climate where patients feel encouraged to achieve their goals can make a positive difference in healing.

Some communities, such as the schools children attend or the neighborhoods where families live, become permanent fixtures in people's lives. Other communities, such as the hospital community where patients spend only a few days, are temporary. Nevertheless, a supportive community of any kind, even if it is for a short amount of time, makes a lasting impact. If a patient attends a group physical therapy class to learn exercises from the physical therapist, discuss goals with the health coach, and receive encouragement from a family member, it makes the patient feel accepted. Even talking with other patients who are experiencing similar health issues creates a sense of community and belonging. Brown (2012) explains that people need to feel unconditional belonging and elaborates, "what makes that such a challenge is that most of us struggle to feel a sense of belonging – to know that we are part of something, not despite our vulnerabilities, but because of them" (p. 233). When a patient is in a hospital room after surgery, it becomes easy to feel vulnerable. A strong community that makes the patient feel part of something greater than oneself can provide encouragement for the patient. The same philosophy applies to a classroom or advisory group in a school, where a strong community provides encouragement for the student.

It becomes essential for patients to feel part of a community as they heal because loneliness leads to additional stress. Rankin (2013) discovered, "the reality is that loneliness causes stress, while loving community relaxes you. The effects of stress and relaxation don't just affect the mind; they affect the body. When you lack supportive community and feel you must handle life alone, the daily overwhelm may trigger anxiety, which the brain perceives as a threat" (p. 86). Additional stress influences the body's ability to heal, so it becomes important to counteract the stress response with the relaxation found in an encouraging community.

As part of her popular *Lean In* movement discussed in her book of the same title, Sandberg (2013) encourages people to create their own Lean In Circles to provide a network of colleagues for each other to share ideas, since "communication works best when we combine appropriateness with authenticity, finding that sweet spot where opinions are not brutally honest but delicately honest" (p. 78). A Lean In Circle can easily be created in a hospital where patients talk to each other and learn from each other. The patients' families become part of the circle by offering encouragement to each other. If one family is having a difficult day, another family who has gone through a similar experience will be there to provide support as stories are shared. Baldwin (1998) discusses the value of calling a circle because "calling a circle doesn't have to be a huge risk or lengthy experiment. We can start small, start with one evening" (p. 14). Patients sitting in a circle sharing their stories with a health coach during a group coaching session or families sitting in a circle leaning on each other and learning from each other becomes a method to lean in and start a conversation.

Advisors in a school may also call a circle for their advisory group by gathering students to sit in a circle and asking a question such as, "how did you feel about last week's assembly?" Students then respond one at a time without interrupting each other. If someone tries to interrupt, the advisor provides a reminder for that comment to wait until after each student in the circle has the opportunity to share. After each person in the circle speaks, the advisor then leads a discussion based on the comments students shared during circle time. This process reminds students that their voices and ideas matter to others, especially their advisor.

Through their encouragement of a patient going through treatment, family members become healers. Physical therapists, health coaches, and other clinicians are drawn to healing professions because of a desire to help others. Beck (2012) describes the healers as, "every now and again, though, I've met individuals who seem to embody the whole premise of the healer's archetype. These people are walking generators of peace, hope, compassion, and restoration. The things they accomplish often seem miraculous, but they themselves are universally humble, insisting that their work is simple and pragmatic" (p. xxi). Family members join the team and become a source of peace, hope, compassion, and restoration for the patient.

SELF-CARE

Most people want to help others before they help themselves. However, taking care of someone else to the point where one's own needs are neglected is not healthy. If the caregiver collapses from exhaustion, there is no one to help the patient.

Practicing self-care also applies to teachers in a classroom. With all the students to help, reports to complete, and papers to grade, it becomes easy for teachers to neglect their personal lives. Teachers need to remind themselves to practice self-care in order to best help their students.

One way to practice self-care is to engage in mindful awareness. Tindle (2013) defines, "mindfulness is simply choosing to be aware of whatever you are thinking, feeling, and sensing right now" (p. 105). Being the caregiver for a loved one might cause stress and lead to burnout. Mindfulness means providing permission to not have to do anything for anyone for awhile and just be with one's own thoughts and feelings in the present moment. Mindfulness means simply closing your eyes for a few minutes in meditation, or practicing a more formal meditation such as a Mindfulness Based Stress Reduction (MBSR) workshop or yoga class. Kabat-Zinn (2013), one of the leading experts in the field, shares the advice, "learning how to suspend all your doing and shift over to a being mode, how to make time for yourself, how to slow down and nurture calmness and self-acceptance in yourself, learning to observe what your mind is up to from moment to moment, how to watch your thoughts and how to let go of them without getting caught up and driven by them, how to make room for new ways of seeing old problems and for perceiving the interconnectedness of things – these are some of the lessons of mindfulness" (p. 6). Reading these words does not take the place of a yoga class or MBSR class taught by an experienced instructor, so consider taking classes in your community if you want more formal mindfulness training than just closing your eyes to meditate.

When experiencing stress from caregiving, relaxation time becomes essential for the caregiver to maintain his or her own health. Rankin (2013) suggests "other relaxing activities such as laughter, playing with pets, journaling, prayer, napping, yoga, getting a massage, reading, singing, playing a musical instrument, gardening, cooking, tai chi, going for a walk, taking a hot bath, and enjoying nature may also activate your parasympathetic nervous system and allow the body to return to a state of rest so it can go about the business of self-repair" (p. 153). Writing in a journal becomes another resource. Baldwin (2006) describes how journals provide a record of our lives because "each journal's contents are eclectic: reports of the day's events, recorded feelings, dreams, dialogues, fantasies, sketches, recipes, quotes from current reading material, cartoons and clippings, photographs and four-leaf clovers – whatever writers want to leave recorded in their passage through time" (p. 5). Journals provide a place to share any emotions experienced during an emotional day of caregiving. If you need additional resources for caregivers, visit websites such as Caregiver.com (2021) that have current articles, places to find support groups in your community, and other helpful information.

TEACHING LESSONS

Teachers have a positive impact whether they set up their classrooms in a school, a hospital, or another location. Brady and Vega (2009) believe, "the best way to learn is to teach" (p. 128). However, as Brady and Vega observe, "most places lack a teaching and learning culture, because no one has organized it" (p. 128). The hospital has the teaching and learning culture because it has organized group physical therapy classes for patients. Patients in the hospital receive the same powerful learning moments as students in a classroom due to the effective educators who teach them.

Gruwell (2009) describes such learning moments as "those priceless moments when students' faces lit up, their hands flew in the air, and I knew they 'got it,' validated all the sleepless nights and began to ease my self-doubt" (p. xix). All the effort becomes worth it when the teacher, whether it is a high school writing teacher demonstrating the craft of revision or a physical therapist demonstrating a series of exercises, makes a connection to the subject area in such a way that the students grasp the concept. Group physical therapy classes use modeling. As Johnson (2005) explains, "modeling is one of the most effective ways to teach new skills" (p. 169). When a patient sees the physical therapist or physical therapist assistant demonstrating exercises, the patient is more likely to remember the concept. Another effective educational component of the group physical therapy classes is using family members as assistant coaches. Johnson continues, "teachers tend to be nurturing souls. We like to help other people. But we also like to be in control, and many of us find it difficult to delegate any of our authority. Sharing your authority can provide huge dividends, however" (p. 95). Sharing authority with family members, especially since the family members will take over the supervision of the exercises when the patient returns home, makes everyone share the work and makes the patient's healing journey a team effort.

Granted, as every teacher who has ever stood in front of a group of students will share, teaching can be challenging. But with modeling by an excellent physical therapist teacher, goal setting from a health coach, and support from family members, patients will experience powerful learning moments as they heal.

HEALING THROUGH WRITING

Health coaches lead group coaching sessions and writing workshops for either patients or their family members. While a circle sharing session may look like group therapy, it is important to remember that group health coaching and writing workshops are not group therapy. Instead of focusing on past issues like group therapy, group coaching focuses on meeting the needs of people where they are in the present and finding strategies to help them move forward. Beck (2008) reminds people that it is never too late to make changes in life because, "if you feel stuck in your present life, if you feel no enthusiasm for anything, if you think you have no purpose or that you lost that purpose somewhere along the way, I guarantee you are living in a dungeon made of stories – and that none of those limiting stories are true" (p. 53). Sharing stories in a supportive environment help people feel encouraged to regain their sense of purpose.

Sometimes people experience stress when they find themselves struggling to focus on the myriad of thoughts occupying their minds. Goldberg (2000) reports, "we don't own our thoughts, even if they are filled with all our own details. They come through us, like heartbeat and breath" (p. 30). And the more thoughts come through, the more overwhelmed a person feels. Expressive writing helps control the chaos when an individual has time to reflect. Pennebaker and Evans (2014) concur, "expressive writing can force you to deal with important emotional experiences that you may have been avoiding" (p. 27). No matter the age of a person, whether teenager or senior citizen, writing helps the author articulate emotional experiences so physical and emotional healing can begin. Fallon (2020) describes of expressive writing, "this is not to say that writing is a cure-all or that we should all ditch our pharmaceutical drugs in favor of a regular writing practice. It is to say that writing – if we're open to it – can have a measurable impact on every area of our lives, including our mental and emotional health" (p. 19). And no one has to read the writing except the writer.

WRITING THE NEXT CHAPTER IN THE HEALING JOURNEY

Writing practice enhances a group coaching class led by a health coach or other medical professional. A group class provides accountability and structure for hospital patients and their families, similar to the way a school classroom provides accountability and structure for students. Students in a classroom receive advice from teachers like Rief (1992) who instruct, "we take at least thirty minutes each Monday for silent writing. I begin my writing with the students during this time" (p. 30). After attending a group physical therapy class or occupational therapy class, attending a group coaching class with writing activities becomes another part of the patient's schedule. Group coaching enables people to walk through their healing journeys together, empower patients, and provide families with the educational resources they need to assist physical therapists with exercises. Murray (1996) writes, "we forge communities when we share who we are, what we feel, what we think; and writing allows a sharing beyond the room, even beyond our lifetime" (p. 7). After participating in discussion as part of the community, patients will then be encouraged to write their goals for the next day. The written goals can be displayed in a location of the patient's hospital room and later the patient's home to provide a visual reminder of goals. Patients celebrate any successes and vent any frustrations through writing. The same writing strategies apply to students in an English classroom or advisory group. As Johnson (2005) advises her students, "say whatever you want. Then rip up the paper into tiny shreds and throw it away" (p. 263). Patients have the option of ripping up writing if it helps them vent frustrations or saving their writing as a powerful reminder of celebrating success. And know that regardless of what happened today, tomorrow is another day.

MORE CHAPTERS FOR PAGES

PAGES was chosen as an acronym for this program because it symbolizes turning a new page in life. People turn pages of a book to get to the next chapter in the story, just as people can use the PAGES program to get to the next chapter of their own life stories. Unlike a book that has already been written, life represents a series of unwritten pages for the author to narrate and experience. Clandinin and Connelly (2000) describe the study of narratives as, "we characterized narrative inquiry as a kind of fluid inquiry, a kind of inquiry that challenges accepted inquiry and representation assumptions. It is a kind of inquiry that necessitates ongoing reflection, what we have called wakefulness" (p. 184). Wakefulness and reflection echo the mention of mindfulness earlier in this narrative, when healing can occur by practicing patience, accepting the present, gathering information, encouragement and self-care.

In living this pandemic life, some families find themselves in the role of caregivers for family members recovering from the coronavirus or other illness, and also in the role of teacher for students navigating online learning. Juggling multiple demands becomes exhausting. Hollis (2020) feels, "I believe it's possible to find meaning in anything; I believe how I deal with the hard parts of my past and how I manage them in the present is me taking back ownership" (p. 24). It becomes possible to find meaning and moments of gratitude during this difficult time in our world. Even when life seems overwhelming, people take care of each other as part of a kind, compassionate community. People take ownership of the things they can control, acknowledge their feelings, and help each other. We discover our collective strength. It takes time for a pandemic to end, but we manage our mindsets while taking care of ourselves and connecting with other people. We don't know other people's stories until we have a conversation with them. We do, however, turn the PAGES to learn more.

ACKNOWLEDGMENT

The preceding chapter contains excerpts from the following previous IGI publications:

Bird, J.L. (2020). Narratives of curriculum design. In *Using narrative writing to enhance healing* (pp. 129-156). Hershey, PA: Information Science Reference.

Bird, J.L., & Wanner, E.T. (2016). Turning PAGES with health coaching and family involvement. In V.C.X. Wang (Ed.), *Handbook of research on advancing health education through technology* (pp. 213-233). Hershey, PA: Information Science Reference.

Reprinted in the IGI publication:

Bird, J.L., & Wanner, E.T. (2019). Turning PAGES with health coaching and family involvement. In *Chronic illness and long-term care: Breakthroughs in research and practice* (pp. 255-276). Hershey, PA: Information Science Reference.

REFERENCES

Baldwin, C. (1998). *Calling the circle*. Bantam.

Baldwin, C. (2006). *One to one*. Rowman and Littlefield.

Barrett, D. (2013). What is paintracking? *Pain Pathways*, *6*(1), 36–41.

Beane, J. A. (1997). *Curriculum integration*. Teachers College Press.

Beck, M. (2001). *Finding your own North Star*. Three Rivers Press.

Beck, M. (2008). *Steering by starlight*. Rodale.

Beck, M. (2012). *Finding your way in a wild new world*. Free Press.

Brady, L., & Vega, P. (2009). 5 keys to structural success. In Orthopedics and spine (pp. 107-132). Danvers, MA: HCPro.

Brown, B. (2010). *The gifts of imperfection*. Hazelden.

Brown, B. (2012). *Daring greatly*. Gotham Books.

Brown, B. (2015). *Rising strong*. Spiegel & Grau.

Brown, B. (2017). *Braving the wilderness*. Random House.

Brown, B. (2018). *Dare to lead*. Random House.

Cameron, J. (1998). *The right to write*. Tarcher/Putnam.

Caregiver.com. Inc. (2021). *Today's caregiver*. Retrieved from https://caregiver.com/

Clandinin, D. J., & Connelly, F. M. (2000). *Narrative inquiry*. Jossey-Bass.

Clark, A. H. (2018). *Hack your anxiety*. Sourcebooks, Inc.

Connelly, F. M., & Clandinin, D. J. (1988). *Teachers as curriculum planners*. Teachers College.

Creative Health Care Management Staff. (2003). *Re-igniting the spirit of caring*. Creative Health Care Management.

Duke Integrative Medicine Staff. (2010). *Personalized health plan manual*. Duke Integrative Medicine.

Fallon, A. (2020). *The power of writing it down*. Zondervan.

Fitzgerald, F. S. (1925). *The great Gatsby*. Scribner.

Gillespie, P., & Learner, N. (2008). *The Longman guide to peer tutoring* (2nd ed.). Pearson.

Goldberg, N. (2000). *Thunder and lightning*. Bantam.

Graves, D. H. (2001). *The energy to teach*. Heinemann.

Gruwell, E. (2009). Teaching hope. New York, NY: Broadway.

Havrilesky, H. (2018). *What if this were enough?* Doubleday.

Heard, G. (1995). *Writing toward home*. Heinemann.

Helldorfer, M., & Moss, T. (2007). *Healing with heart*. Moss Communications.

Hollis, R. (2020). *Didn't see that coming*. Dey St.

Johnson, L. (1998). *Two parts textbook, one part love*. Hyperion.

Johnson, L. (2005). *Teaching outside the box*. Jossey-Bass.

Juhan, D. (1998). *Job's body* (2nd ed.). Station Hill.

Kabat-Zinn, J. (2013). *Full catastrophe living* (2nd ed.). Bantam.

Lee, I. F. (2018). *Joyful*. Little, Brown Spark.

Marshall, J. D., Sears, J. T., & Schubert, W. H. (2000). *Turning points in curriculum*. Merrill/Prentice Hall.

Murray, D. (1996). *Crafting a life*. Heinemann.

Neff, K. (2011). *Self compassion: the proven power of being kind to yourself.* HarperCollins.

Pennebaker, J. W., & Evans, J. F. (2014). *Expressive writing: words that heal.* Idyll Arbor.

Pipher, M. (2006). *Writing to change the world.* Riverhead.

Rankin, L. (2013). *Mind over medicine*. Hay House.

Rief, L. (1992). *Seeking diversity*. Heinemann.

Romano, T. (2000). *Blending genre, altering style*. Heinemann.

Ryan, N. P., Wade, J. C., Nice, A., Shenefelt, H., & Shepard, K. (1996). Physical therapists' perceptions of family involvement in the rehabilitation process. *Physiotherapy Research International, 1*(3), 159–179. doi:10.1002/pri.56 PMID:9238732

Sandberg, S. (2013). *Lean in*. Alfred A. Knopf.

Sandberg, S., & Grant, A. (2017). *Option B*. Knopf.

Stephen Ministries Staff. (2000). *Stephen Ministry training manual*. Stephen Ministries.

Tindle, H. (2013). *Up: how positive outlook can transform our health and aging*. Hudson Street Press.

Williams, E. (2019). *I heart my life*. Hay House.

Zimmermann, S. (2002). *Writing to heal the soul*. Three Rivers Press.

KEY TERMS AND DEFINITIONS

Accept the Present: Feelings of guilt, anger, and frustration are normal, but are not helpful when coaching. No matter what happened in the past, this is where you are now. Worrying about the future only causes additional stress. Try your best to remain in the present moment. Consider writing in a journal to sort through your feelings.

Accept the Present: Try to remain in the present moment. It becomes easy for both teachers and students to think of the myriad of tasks to accomplish in a day, but advisory time provides a break for students from past mistakes and future worries. Journal writing also helps students sort through their feelings.

Accept the Present: We are where we are. Whatever each individual circumstance may be, accept what is beyond control and what can be controlled. Focus on things that can be controlled, such as mindset and perspective.

Encourage: During the healing journey, patients need cheerleaders. You are a source of hope and light during this process and a little support can make a large difference.

Encourage: During the high school journey, students need support. As an advisor, you provide a source of hope, which makes a difference.

Encourage: Reach out to people and connect with them. It is possible for people to become lonely and isolated during the pandemic, and a phone call to check that someone is okay makes a difference.

Gather Information: Ask open ended questions, and listen to student answers. As an advisor, use reflective statements to acknowledge student feelings . If students need additional assistance, refer them to the appropriate resource such as college counseling or the school psychologist.

Gather Information: Numerous news resources exist for information. Find a reputable source and learn from it. Take periodic breaks from the news to avoid information overload, or search for stories of people helping others.

Gather information: The medical professionals such as doctors, physical therapists, occupational therapists, nurses, and speech therapists are here to help you. Ask questions, and listen to their instructions. Consider bringing a notebook with you to write down information so you don't have to remember it.

Practice Patience: As high school students continue their journeys through life, they need supportive adults as role models. Often, the most significant goals cannot happen overnight. Empower students by celebrating progress, no matter how small. Students have numerous people giving them advice, so active listening proves valuable in a role as advisor.

Practice Patience: Even during feelings of pandemic fatigue, know that this era in time won't last forever. It will take time for places to open, people to receive vaccines, and for the virus to be controlled.

Practice Patience: Healing is a journey. No one can wave a magic wand and provide an immediate cure. Celebrate progress, no matter how small.

Self-Care: In order to take care of your loved one, take care of yourself too. You can better help someone else when your own needs, such as hunger and sleep, are met too.

Self-Care: In order to take care of your students, take care of yourself too. You can better help someone else when your own needs, such as hunger and sleep, are met.

Self-Care: Make sure to find moments for self-care. Dealing with the constant reminders of wearing masks, social distancing, washing hands, and cleaning can be exhausting, so find time for healthy moments of comfort.

Chapter 8
Reflections of Anxiety Narratives

ABSTRACT

This narrative discusses a research study using both qualitative and quantitative methods to illustrate the connections between writing and healing. College students who answered survey questions about their health reported anxiety as a concern. Writing in journals became a method of coping with anxiety, which led the research to evolve into a social action project of managing stress and eliminating the stigma surrounding anxiety. Resources to help anxiety include exercise, nutrition, and belonging to a supportive community.

PANDEMIC ANXIETY

We conducted the research for this chapter several years before the pandemic began, but the strategies we implemented for helping people cope with anxiety continue to make a lasting impact. According to the Centers for Disease Control and Prevention (CDC):

The COVID-19 pandemic has had a major effect on our lives. Many of us are facing challenges that can be stressful, overwhelming, and cause strong emotions in adults and children. Public health actions, such as social distancing, are necessary to reduce the spread of COVID-19, but they can make us feel isolated and lonely and can increase stress and anxiety. Learning to cope with stress in a healthy way will make you, the people you care about, and those around you become more resilient. (https://www.cdc.gov/coronavirus/2019-ncov/daily-life-coping/managing-stress-anxiety.html)

We continue to share this research to help anyone experiencing pandemic anxiety, which includes surviving the pandemic and coping as life after the pandemic slowly returns to resembling life before the pandemic. Although life may look similar, people transform as a result of their experiences.

DOI: 10.4018/978-1-7998-9051-5.ch008

CURRICULUM INQUIRY USING RESEARCH NARRATIVES

Curricular change begins when researchers develop ideas with the purpose of implementing enduring effective change. It is one thing to notice a problem, another to solve it. Researchers can benefit from envisioning ideas from different perspectives and borrowing ideas from other fields. The field of city planning follows a research process that leads to implementation of detailed plans; city planning shares similarities with the qualitative interpretive research fields of narrative inquiry and curriculum inquiry, since both rely on narratives to illuminate issues. Illuminating issues can lead to bringing purpose to life, whether a city planner looks at a piece of land and uses plans to create a new housing development or an educational researcher looks at data indicating college students experience stress and anxiety and uses plans to create a curriculum of healing.

Education endures multiple curricular incarnations throughout the decades, since the only constant in the curriculum of schools remains change. Marshall, Sears, and Schubert (2000) discuss the evolution of curriculum and provide the history that "more than any other philosopher, John Dewey influenced the thought of curriculum scholars throughout the twentieth century, and at the century's end curriculum questions remain easily related to his definition of education. The enduring curriculum question thus becomes, "What adds meaning and direction or purpose to experience?" (p. 2). The question still remains today. What experiences bring purpose to life?

While researchers often study texts or programs from an existing curriculum, the stories of the people participating in a curriculum add another dimension to the inquiry process because looking at policies and procedures cannot take the place of witnessing the implementation of such policies and procedures when adding people to the process. Marshall, Sears, and Schubert (2000) believe, "through biography as curricular text we can see how individuals reconstructed themselves and their work, including the need to reread past decisions and changes" (p. 199). An idea may appear one way in theory on paper, but watching the idea unfold in practice may tell a different story. Educators want their stories to possess purpose; students may repeat the words of an excellent teacher years after that teacher's lifetime.

This curriculum inquiry research story alternates from the perspectives of the researchers being both participants and observers. Narrative inquiry is the qualitative interpretive discipline which encourages researchers to use first person when describing events and intertwine their own narratives with the narratives of the research participants. Clandinin and Connelly (2000) define narrative inquiry and explain, "it is a collaboration between researcher and participants, over time, in a place or series of places, and in social interaction with milieus. An inquirer enters this matrix in the midst and progresses in this same spirit, concluding the inquiry still in the midst of living and telling, reliving and retelling, the stories of the experiences that make up people's lives, both individual and social" (p. 20). Therefore, in narrative inquiries, researchers learn about a story, report on the story, and subsequently seek to offer their own contribution to the story already in progress. The sharing of stories serves as the methodology as Clandinin and Connelly elaborate, "in our work, we keep in the foreground of our writing a narrative view of experience, with the participants' and researchers' narratives of experience situated and lived out on storied landscapes as our theoretical methodological frame" (p. 128). Think of it as the researchers reading a poem and then adding their own verse at the end. The researchers are changed by the research setting and also change the setting by being part of it.

Curriculum inquiry uses narratives to study an existing curriculum and determine how the stories of the participants can lead to curricular change. Connelly and Clandinin (1988) discuss, "curriculum inquiry is a process in which teachers read and study curriculum materials in the same way that they would read and study potentially interesting texts" (p. 151). Simply studying curriculum materials, however, does not lead to change. According to city planner and former Florida Atlantic University president Catanese (1996), "for too many years we have not dealt with the most important lesson from the real world, which is that implementation is the most important part of planning" (p. 295). In order to implement lasting change as a result of research, researchers can learn from the process implemented by city planners. Harper (1996) explains, "when I was in graduate school I remember being surprised to learn that the planning process is almost identical to the scientific method of research I had already studied" (p. 194). Like narrative inquiry, city planning uses stories to frame problems and discover solutions. Learning stories and receiving feedback from the constituents impacted by the solutions becomes an essential part of the process because neither cities nor schools are empty places. Both contain people whose lives become transformed either positively or negatively by the implementation of change. Hoch (1995) elaborates, "we use elements of narrative and rhetoric to compose our stories. In planning tales, we usually combine logic and rhetoric, argument and poetics" (p. 295). The same description applies to any story told, whether a citizen writes a letter to a city planner or a student writes a journal entry in a classroom. Both writing processes involve the venting of feelings.

Change occurs not just with a process, but also with people. Change takes courage and requires a transformative leader to step up and lead the way. In order to use research to create curricular change, it helps the transformative leaders to participate in the change process instead of directing others to implement the change. Heifetz (1994) believes, "leadership is both active and reflective. One has to alternate between participating and observing" (p. 252). The extended metaphor of a dance is used to illustrate the concept. To put it in other words, if you are chaperoning a school dance and are on the dance floor dancing the line dance The Electric Slide with the students, you know what it feels like to participate in the dance but can't see the entire picture. If the dance floor has a balcony where you can climb up to the top and look down, you see the entire picture of the dance but are detached from participating. Heifetz uses a ballroom dance example instead of The Electric Slide, but the philosophy remains the same since "to discern the larger patterns on the dance floor – to see who is dancing with whom, in what groups, in what location, and who is sitting out which kind of dance – we have to stop moving and get to the balcony" (p. 253). One of the researchers conducting the study discussed in this chapter needed to learn this lesson because the research took place in her classroom. She needed to alternate between living the subjective experience with her students and maintaining an objective distance. She also relied on the insights of her co-researcher, a medical consultant and physical therapist, because he could see the study from a different perspective and help her switch between the roles of researcher and professor.

HEALING VALUE OF WRITING

This research project began as a study to find connections between writing and healing. The authors of this research study previously conducted another research study and discovered that patients at a physical therapy clinic who used a strong positive writing voice on short answer survey questions demonstrated greater healing gains on existing objective physical therapy measures. The results illustrated writing can influence physical healing.

Other previous studies illustrated the link between writing and health. In a 1983 study, psychologist Pennebaker (1997) assigned college students at Southern Methodist University to one of four writing groups where they would vent about their emotions related to a trauma, write the facts of the trauma, write the facts of the trauma while venting about emotions, or write about superficial topics; he discovered that students in the writing group who both wrote the facts of the trauma while venting about emotions visited the student health center fewer times than students in the other three writing groups and concluded, "writing about their deepest thoughts and feelings about traumas resulted in improved moods, more positive outlook, and greater physical health" (p. 34). A follow up study where Pennebaker collaborated with doctors from the Ohio State University College of Medicine to draw blood samples from college students before and after they wrote revealed that "people who wrote about their deepest thoughts and feelings surrounding traumatic experiences evidenced heightened immune function compared with those who wrote about superficial topics" (p. 37).

Writing professor DeSalvo (1999) concurs with Pennebaker's research and elaborates, "the more people described positive emotions in their writing, the more likely they were to be healthier afterward. But describing negative emotions either excessively or very little or not at all correlated with poorer health. Describing negative emotions in moderation correlated with improved health" (p. 60). Social work researcher and professor Brown (2012) also corroborates Pennebaker's research and explains, "when people shared their stories and experiences, their physical health improved, their doctor's visits decreased, and they showed significant decreases in their stress hormones" (p. 82). Conner (2008) uses her experiences as viewing writing as a spiritual practice to discuss Pennebaker's research through the lens of improved academic performance for college students and reports, "successive research projects demonstrated that students who wrote in an open, meaningful way developed a more positive outlook on life, experienced reduced anxiety and depression, had an improved ability to fight infection with more active T-lymphocytes (the agents in the body that fight cancer), and had lower heart rates. They also - this is my favorite - received better grades" (p. 59). All of the analyses lead to the conclusion that writing leads to healing.

Writing also helps improve depression and anxiety. Helgoe, Wilhelm, and Kommor, (2005) discuss the implications of writing from the perspective of the medical community and elaborate, "'therapeutic journaling,' or writing down your feelings and concerns, has been associated with reductions in symptoms of depression and anxiety. In fact research by James Pennebaker found that immune function was enhanced for study subjects who wrote about their deepest feelings as compared to subjects instructed to write about trivial matters" (p. 260). Pennebaker's research illustrating writing leads to healing even resonates beyond the academic community. In the popular magazine *Oprah,* Kamenetz (2013) discusses Pennebaker "who had found that students who wrote about the worst thing that had ever happened to them felt sadder initially, but six months down the road were visiting doctors less frequently" (p. 140). She used the study as inspiration to discuss how writing helped her and stated that as a result of writing, "I felt no fear or hesitation, just deep gratitude – and an eagerness to write the next chapter" (p. 141). But can writing benefit writers who write about topics other than traumas?

Writing helps people process emotions so they can heal both physically and emotionally from difficult experiences. As DeSalvo (1999) explains, "the act of linking feelings with troubling events, then, makes our bodies display responses associated with yoga and meditation. This explains why writers who stop work soon feel out of sorts – why they become edgy, irritable, anxious, even depressed. This explains, too, why people who begin writing report feeling a greater sense of well-being – why they become calmer, more capable of coping with stress, more serene, even when facing life's challenges, than they'd been before" (p. 23). However, the writing questions on the survey the researchers used at the physical therapy clinic did not ask patients to write about traumatic experiences; instead, patients wrote about their perspectives and goals for healing. Furthermore, through personal experiences with their own writing as well as through informal observations and conversations with high school and college students in English classes, the researchers observed that students benefit from writing about topics other than traumatic ones. In fact, while the occasional student wants to explore a deep emotional issue in writing, most students write on less emotional topics and still report feeling more peaceful after writing. Gruwell (2007) writes of her students, the students known as *The Freedom Writers*, "writing became liberating, as each student discovered they had a story and found comfort in the computer. Although they couldn't change the cast of characters, the computer became their confidant, their therapist, and their outlet, and many of them hoped that they could rewrite their endings" (pp. 151-152). Could the act of completing the writing process have healing benefits for patients regardless of the topic discussed?

RESEARCH METHODS

For this research study, Florida Atlantic University students in the College of Education who chose to volunteer completed two surveys. One survey was a writing survey designed by the researchers, and the other survey was a health survey called the HRQOL (Health Related Quality of Life) survey, a general health survey in the public domain and able to be used by researchers without securing permission or paying copyright fees. The two surveys were stapled together to eliminate the need to match up surveys. Students completed the surveys anonymously, meaning specific responses could not be traced back to individual students. Students received a consent form explaining that completing and returning the survey indicated consent to participate in the research study. The consent form also contained phone numbers for the student health center and student counseling center in case students wanted to discuss a physical or emotional health issue with a professional after writing.

Survey administration took place on February 4, 2014 and February 5, 2014. The researcher informed her two classes that met on February 4 and her one class that met on February 5 that they would have the opportunity to volunteer to participate in a research study, with participation not being connected in any way to the class grade. The class then proceeded as normal with a writing workshop that takes place every semester as part of normal classroom practices. As part of the writing workshop, students were asked to write on post it notes how they felt both physically and emotionally before writing, with a score of 1 being excellent and a score of 5 being poor. At the conclusion of the writing workshop, students were asked to write on post it notes how they felt both physically and emotionally after writing. For example, when the professor completed this activity, her scores were as follows:

Before writing: Emotional = 1, Physical = 3
After writing: Emotional = 1, Physical = 2

Emotionally, she loves teaching and writing, so she felt great before writing, she enjoyed writing in her journal, and continued to feel great after writing. Physically, she had a headache at the beginning of writing, during writing didn't notice it as much, and felt better after writing. She shares her own examples to illustrate the process students experienced, even though students reported only the numbers ranking how they felt, not the reason why they assigned a specific number to their physical and emotional feelings.

Students chose a topic to write about for the first writing session and wrote for ten minutes about the topic. Students were then given the opportunity to read aloud all or part of their writing and share it with their classmates if they chose, but sharing was optional and students were not required to share if they didn't want to read their writing aloud. Several students in each class used the opportunity to share their writing. The process was repeated three more times. For each of the three following writing sessions, students could either continue to write about their first topic or choose a different topic. Each writing session lasted ten minutes, and at the end of each session students had the opportunity to share their writing. The professor participated in the writing workshop and read aloud her writing at the end of each session. Between the second and third writing sessions, the class took a dance break to stand up and stretch. Some students chose to complete dance moves from the popular dances YMCA and The Electric Slide even though there was no music, while others used the two minute break to simply stretch their arms over their heads. Writing then resumed.

At the conclusion of the writing workshop, the professor distributed the surveys while reminding the students that participation was optional and responses would remain anonymous. The professor then left the room so she would not see who completed surveys and who didn't. A manila envelope was left on a desk in the classroom and students placed surveys in the envelope when finished. A volunteer student from each class retrieved the professor from the hallway after all students who chose to participate placed the surveys in the envelope and class proceeded with a discussion of additional writing strategies and stress management techniques.

SURVEY RESULTS AND ANALYSIS

On the writing survey, for each of the four writing sessions, each student who completed the survey was asked to list the writing topic chosen, describe in one word how he or she felt about the topic, and describe the topic as emotional or neutral. Each student was then asked to answer two yes/no questions, with one question asking if he or she chose to share his or her writing by reading it aloud and the other question asking if he or she completed journal writing outside of the writing time in class. The professor wrote about twelve topics instead of four because she completed the writing in all three of her classes. Her topics and how she described them were: love of photography (emotional), first year of teaching (emotional), describing chair arrangements in the classroom (neutral), love of teaching (emotional), required exams (emotional), graduation (emotional), her aunt and role model (emotional), finding her way as a teacher (emotional), required exams (emotional), deeper themes of Disney movies (neutral), required exams (emotional), her writing process (neutral).

On the health survey, students were asked to answer general questions about their health by circling numbers. An example of a question on the Health Related Quality of Life Survey (2011) was:

Would you say that in general your health is:

1. Excellent 1
2. Very good 2
3. Good 3
4. Fair 4
5. Poor 5
   (https://www.cdc.gov/hrqol/hrqol14_measure.htm)

Other questions asked students about specific health issues, such as:

During the past 30 days, for about how many days have you felt worried, tense, or anxious?

Number of days (space for number)
None
Don't know/Not sure
Refused

(https://www.cdc.gov/hrqol/hrqol14_measure.htm)

While the HRQOL contained numerous other questions, the one about feeling worried, tense, or anxious is included here because that question provided the most significant information for the research study.

When scoring the surveys, each survey received a number from 1-64, because 64 subjects chose to participate in the research study. Results were then entered in a table under each survey number to easily keep track of the data. Results are listed in the following summary, and a detailed analysis follows the numbered list to illustrate how a study intended to illuminate connections between writing and healing led to the discovery of anxiety reported by college students and the design of a social action project to help students manage stress.

1. Correlations in SPSS showed no significant relationship between:
    a. Writing about emotional topics and overall health (HRQOL)
    b. Writing about neutral topics and overall health (HRQOL)
    c. Emotional topics and emotional change (pre/post writing)
    d. Emotional topics and physical change (pre/post writing)
    e. Neutral topics and emotional change (pre/post writing)
    f. Neutral topics and physical change (pre/post writing)
    g. Emotional change (pre/post writing) and physical change (pre/post writing)
2. One sample chi square showed equal probabilities of sharing vs. not sharing when compared to general health, as well as equal probabilities of writing at home vs. in class when compared to general health.

Observations: The act of writing is not influenced by topic, whether or not students share, or whether or not they write outside class. This could be a good thing because students receive equal benefits from writing regardless of other factors. The only thing all subjects have in common is they wrote in journals.

3. Physical change during writing:

43 subjects reported no change in the way they felt physically pre/post writing, 15 felt better and 6 felt worse.

Observations: Most students reported excellent or good health to begin with, meaning there was nothing to improve or change. The few who reported severe physical pain would not see it cured by writing; they need to see a doctor. Writing may have caused an increase or decrease in physical health if students relaxed during writing, causing their muscles to be less tense, but there may be other factors such as uncomfortable desks in the classroom. Interestingly, numbers of how students felt pre/post writing did not always correspond to the overall health score on HRQOL, meaning students could have good health overall but had a bad health day or vice versa.

4. Emotional change during writing:

28 subjects reported no change in the way they felt emotionally pre/post writing, 26 felt better and 10 felt worse.

Observations: Some students reported excellent or good health to begin with, meaning there was nothing to improve or change. The increase or decrease in emotional health can be explained by choice in topic; overall, the students who used optimistic words to describe their writing felt better and the students who used pessimistic words felt worse. Also, sometimes when writing about a difficult topic, the writer feels worse initially but better over time.

5. On the HRQOL question that asked during the last 30 days, how many days have you been worried, anxious, or tense, only 5 students responded 0 days, or none of the time. Some used words like all days, parts of every day, and 11 students responded 30 days, or all of the time. The next most common number was 10 days (9 students) followed by 20 days (4 students) and the rest of the students gave varying responses.
6. Most common other health complaints were lack of sleep, low energy, and sadness/depression. Most students who reported a large number of days with lack of sleep also reported a large number of days with low energy. Exactly half, 32 students, reported no physical symptoms but the most common physical symptom reported by 13 students was back and neck pain, which can be a physical manifestation of emotional stress.

Observations: Students are experiencing anxiety and stress, and better methods of managing stress are needed.

7. A significant correlation in SPSS was found between the first word students used to describe their emotions about writing and the number of anxiety days reported on the HRQOL. The correlation was found using the following steps:

    a. Converted the number of anxiety days each student experienced each month into a scale with 20-30 days = high anxiety, 10-19 days = mid anxiety, and 0-9 days = low anxiety.
    b. Scored anxiety using a scale where 1=high anxiety, 3=mid anxiety, 5=low anxiety. The few students who left the question blank received the neutral response of 3.
    c. Looked at the first word students used to describe their feelings about their first writing topic.
    d. Scored the word using the same artistic writing scale rubric used for other writing surveys such as the survey used at the physical therapy clinic, with 1=negative, 3= neutral, 5=positive. The few students who left the question blank received the neutral response of 3.
        - The correlation between the numerical anxiety scale and the positive artistic writing is significant, meaning a trend exists where students who use more positive language have less anxiety.
        - The table below (Table 1) illustrates the significant correlation discussed above.

Table 1. Correlation between more positive language and less anxiety

		Positive Artistic First Word	Anxiety Numeric
Positive artistic first word	Pearson Correlation	1	.265*
	Sig. (2-tailed)		.035
	N	64	64
Anxiety numeric	Pearson Correlation	.265*	1
	Sig. (2-tailed)	.035	
	N	64	64
*. Correlation is significant at the 0.05 level (2-tailed).			

Observations: These results dovetail with the results of the previous study at the physical therapy clinic because students who used a positive writing voice demonstrated lower anxiety.

8. Students with high anxiety typically chose to write about school issues before other topics.

Observations: Listing the topics each student chose to write about is a qualitative notation without quantitative statistical analysis in SPSS, but it was interesting to notice a trend that the first topic students who reported higher anxiety wished to explore in writing focused on school issues such as upcoming exams, current field experience internships, and plans after graduation, while students who reported lower anxiety chose a broader range of topics such as family, favorite books, current events, and other issues unrelated to school experiences.

THE SIGNIFICANCE OF FIRST IMPRESSIONS

Initial analysis of the data from the 64 subjects who completed the survey echoed the findings of previous studies: Writing is healing. Writing also seems to have benefits for people who take the time to put pen to paper regardless of the topic chosen. However, the more important observation existed in the fact on one of the health questions asked on the Health Related Quality of Life Survey (HRQOL), all but five subjects reported experiencing anxiety or stress. This research study did not begin with the intent of studying anxiety in college students, but consequently, the results caused the research to evolve into a social action project to help college students cope with stress and anxiety. Diagnosing a problem raises questions and the need for answers in the form of providing solutions.

As previously mentioned, the results of this research study dovetail with the previous research study the researchers conducted at the physical therapy clinic. College students who used a positive writing voice demonstrated lower anxiety and stronger emotional health, just like physical therapy patients who used a positive writing voice throughout their treatment interventions demonstrated higher recovery gains for objective measures on pre-existing physical therapy surveys. The results illustrate that a strong positive writing voice can help people heal both physically and emotionally.

Voice in writing was assessed using a writing rubric that incorporates both the technical and artistic dimensions of writing. The technical dimension of writing reflects specificity, while the artistic dimension reflects voice. Romano (2013) believes a successful rubric reflects both artistic (holistic) and technical (required) elements of writing and explains when examining writing, "the rubric helps me pay attention to its totality. The holistic portion allows me to open myself to what the paper is doing, to feel it, just as I want to feel other crafted writing I read. The required elements remind me to examine how well students executed specific skills, strategies, and genres I've taught" (p. 167). The artistic dimension of the writing rubric highlighting voice correlated with the amount of anxiety, as students who demonstrated a more positive writing voice showed lower anxiety.

Writing teachers and theorists believe that the first thoughts are the truest thoughts, because the more people write, the more they self-censor. As Goldberg (1986) argues, "first thoughts have tremendous energy. It is the way the mind first flashes on something" (p. 9). That is why the focus of the student writing on the survey became the first topic they chose to write about and the word they used to describe that topic. Most students wrote about multiple topics, but the first topic represents what is really on their minds and how they feel about it. Goldberg (1990) believes, "we need to learn to accept our minds. Believe me, for writing, it is all we have" (p. 53). First thought writing can illuminate a writer's true feelings. When beginning to write about a topic, frequently writers will have a flash of insight that causes them to be honest with themselves when writing. Some writers will continue to reflect on their honest feelings as they continue to write, but other writers will start to question their ideas, worry about what others may think even if no one else is reading the writing, or feel vulnerable and not remain as open to their thoughts when continuing writing. Goldberg (2013) explains, "these moments are a flash, an insight when we see through the confusion of our constant thinking to something clear" (p. 30). Writing captures the insightful moments that illuminate honest first impressions before the writer revises due to second thoughts.

As students participated in the writing workshop, they had time to think about their writing, listen to their classmates' read writing, and add to their original writing. Any of these factors could cause students to censor their own unique writing voices, even though the student writing was not collected for the survey and if students did not choose to share no one else saw or heard the writing. Sometimes writers reread their own words and want the story to be different from what actually happened, not to lie but to make the truth sound better, make more sense, or hurt less. DeSalvo (1999) believes, "we resist chaos narratives. We resist reading them. Sometimes we resist writing them, penning a neater, more hopeful though fraudulent version of events we've survived. We want narratives that demonstrate the resilience of the human spirit. We don't want to admit defeat" (p. 197). Mistakes happen in life, but since we are the authors of our own individual stories, we often chose to cast ourselves as the hero rather than admit sometimes our best thinking got us to a place we don't want to be. But before the doubt that leads a writer to second guess those first thoughts creeps in and tells a new story, the writer's true voice reveals itself. And as Graves (1994) writes, "it is a writer's voice that gives me the best sense of his or her potential" (p. 82). Just like with the physical therapy patients, the college students were using their writing voices to tell stories. We had to figure out what stories.

THE AGE OF ANXIETY

Because the majority of college students surveyed reported experiencing stress and anxiety, we as the researchers decided to help university administrators brainstorm potential strategies to help the students. In order to implement effective solutions to this situation that will improve health for college students, it helps to first understand the problem. Nurse practitioner Clark (2006) explains that, "Anxiety conditions appear as a result of cumulative stress over time" (p. 2). The terms anxiety and stress may be used interchangeably, but they are different. Helgoe, Wilhelm, and Kommor (2005) elaborate, "stress implies external pressure, whereas anxiety describes an internal experience" (p. 26). A different medical practitioner named Clark (2018), a psychologist, believes, "I think of anxiety as the experience that arises from conflict about future unavoidable pain as well as the perceived threat to something we care about. It is also that sense that something isn't quite right, that we've neglected something important, and even sometimes a sense of dread" (p. 35). Therapist Bidwell Smith (2018) provides the definition that, "anxiety comes from the Latin word anxius, which means a state of agitation and distress. This distress is often felt on a deep level, in both the mind and the body. It is the sense of danger but not always a specific one that you can identify" (p. 19). People who experience anxiety feel it mentally, emotionally, and physically.

Agreement exists among practitioners in the medical field that some anxiety can actually be helpful. Clark (2006) argues, "mild anxiety can be a good thing. Without it, you'd be constantly drifting off to sleep, probably couldn't hold a coherent discussion or achieve any of your goals. Mild anxiety is necessary for learning to take place" (p. 15). Helgoe, Wilhelm, and Kommor (2005) concur and add, "anxiety is considered healthy when it motivates us to take action in the name of accomplishment" (p. 22). Finally, psychologist Carmichael (2021) adds, "anxiety's healthy function is to stimulate preparatory behaviors, or to signal that there are emotions or situations that need our attention. By giving this extra energy the right format before it becomes frantic, frenetic, or stagnant, it can become a gift rather than an obstacle" (p. 11). However, anxiety frequently crosses the line and becomes unhealthy. Perry and Winfrey (2021) explain, "it is the controllability, pattern, and intensity of stress that can cause problems" (p. 83). Stress/anxiety over a long time is not healthy. This is called chronic stress. Chronic stress can cause physical symptoms such as headaches, potential weight gain, inability to concentrate, inability to sleep, increased risk for a stroke and/or heart attack, and depression (https://www.helpguide.org/mental/stress_signs.htm). There are different types of stressors which cause stress. External Stressors can be pain, weather, working conditions, abusive relationships. Internal Stressors can be physical or psychological such as infections, inflammation, worrying. (https://umm.edu/health/medical/reports/articles/stress)

In the field of education, the most common reference to anxiety is test anxiety. As English teacher Johnson (1998) advises teachers, "you don't have to make your exams easier in order to improve grades and student motivation in your classroom; you do need to reduce the stress and anxiety your students feel about taking exams" (p. 26). Unfortunately, numerous teachers get pulled into the vortex known as standardized testing and professional obligations eclipse personal wellness. Clark (2006) cautions, "as anxiety increases, your perception of what is going on around you decreases" (p. 16). Many people find themselves trapped in this cycle. Increased anxiety leads to decreased perception, which in turn leads to increased anxiety. When experiencing anxiety, it becomes important to remember what remains within control. Clark (2018) explains, "being so afraid of the experience of anxiety can fool us into believing we can't handle it – a fear that is always based on an illusion. We may not want to handle it, but that's not the same thing. We can" (p. 97). College students can become especially vulnerable to anxiety as they struggle to make decisions about their future.

Another author named Johnson (2009) writes about anxiety from the perspective of a minister and observes, "contrasting the past to the present, the not knowing to the knowing, it creates a totally different point of focus. Before I was anxious; now I am free. Why? Because now I know the outcome. When we know the outcome, we're not nearly as constrained by the process of getting there. To be sure, we are free to rise above the moment and savor the intricacies of the journey" (p. 15). The fact that the next chapter in life remains unwritten can make the journey simultaneously exciting and anxiety provoking.

People may say they have fear of the future, but fear and anxiety are different. Clark (2006) elaborates, "although you may not know the difference between anxiety and fear, the two terms refer to entirely different feelings. Fear is usually directed at an external danger" (p. 11). Conversely, "anxiety has no such easily recognizable source and is often called an unexplained discomfort" (p. 11). However, Helgoe, Wilhelm, and Kommor (2005) highlight the similarities instead of the differences between anxiety and fear by stating, "anxiety is fear without a clear threat. Whereas fear is a natural reaction to an obvious, literal threat to your physical well-being, anxiety often feels abnormal and without use or function" (p. 4). It is also easy to discuss anxiety from the outside looking in at the issue instead of experiencing it. What may seem abnormal to people who haven't experienced anxiety is a normal part of the day for people who live with anxiety. Journalist Smith (2012) describes his personal experiences with anxiety and believes, "and yet to talk about anxiety as directionless and formless and fear as focused and specific only says how the two experiences are different, not how they're related. It also suggests in a backhanded way, that fear is normal, a hardwired Darwinian response, and that anxiety is abnormal, a sort of postindustrial, urban affliction. No experts say this outright, or even at all" (p. 124). Stossel (2013) also shares his personal experiences with anxiety as well as advice from his therapist and elaborates, "yet enough of us do suffer from anxiety that perhaps writing about my own ought not to be an occasion for shame but an opportunity to provide solace to some of the millions of others who share this affliction. And maybe, as Dr. W. often reminds me, the exercise will be therapeutic. 'You can write yourself to health,' he says." (pp. 28-29). Anxiety also appears as a stage in the grieving process for people experiencing loss. Therapist Bidwell Smith (2018) explains, "grief-related anxiety is most often a result of trying to suppress or avoid the strong emotions that come with loss" (p. 49). Unlike other countries which have long mourning periods, the United States has a culture which seems to imply that people need to hurry up and grieve to get on with life. It takes more than a few bereavement days from work to truly honor and grieve a loss.

FBI profiler and security expert DeBecker (1997) describes a nonmedical perspective on fear and explains, "worry, wariness, anxiety, and concern all have a purpose, but they are not fear. So anytime your dreaded outcome cannot reasonably be linked to pain or death and it is isn't a signal in the presence of danger, than it really shouldn't be confused with fear" (p. 286). Echoing the sentiment that anxiety decreases when the outcome of a situation becomes more certain, DeBecker continues, "predictions in which you have high confidence free you to respond, adjust, feel sadness, accept, prepare, or to do whatever is needed. Accordingly, anxiety is reduced by improving your predictions, thus increasing your certainty. It's worth doing, because the word anxiety, like worry, stems from a root that means "to choke," and that is just what it does to us" (p. 292). To feel more certain about predictions encompassing the way people could potentially behave and the resulting outcomes, DeBecker reminds people to use intuition. Intuition represents the first flash of insight that DeBecker believes is often correct. The first mental insight, just like the first thought in writing, is more accurate because second thoughts do not have time to occur.

FOR THE GIRLS

Because more female students than male students completed this survey, it became enlightening to examine factors that may cause college women to experience stress and anxiety. Self-defense expert Baty (2003) references DeBecker's research and advises, "whatever your fears are, the goal is to become proactive" (p. 201). The context of that quote encourages women to take ownership of their own safety, but it nevertheless highlights another interesting observation about the college students who reported anxiety. Because the survey responses remained anonymous, there is no way of knowing if students who indicated high anxiety were male or female. However, the majority of students from the potential pool of respondents were female. This is due to the population composition of the College of Education. With a few exceptions, in most education classes women outnumber the men. Therefore, while the anonymity of the responses prevents this next observation from being stated as a clear fact, it is a safe bet to assume that more women than men completed surveys.

Twenty years ago, educators sounded the alarm that girls endured more stress and anxiety than boys did because antiquated notions of stereotypical gender roles from past generations refused to dissipate. Sadker and Sadker (1994) conducted extensive research in classrooms and made the disturbing observation, "as the snapshots continue, the underlying gender messages become clear. The classroom consists of two worlds: one of boys in action, the other of girls' inaction" (p. 42). The Sadkers painted a troubling portrait of girls sitting back in the classroom while boys volunteered to share their ideas. Sadly, twenty years later Sandberg paints the same troubling portrait of women sitting back in conference rooms while men volunteer to share their ideas. Sandberg (2013) urges women to lean in and make their voices heard without being afraid to speak up because "fear is at the root of so many of the barriers that women face. Fear of not being liked. Fear of making the wrong choice. Fear of drawing negative attention. Fear of overreaching. Fear of being judged. Fear of failure" (p. 24). Twenty years later, the same conversation still takes place.

Even though society should have evolved to the point where a woman can live any life she wants to live, women still experience the pressure of mixed messages. Popular magazines with a target audience of women reveal the messages portrayed on one page emphasize accomplishments while the messages portrayed on the next emphasize appearance. Cohen-Sandler (2005) discusses the effects stress can have on girls and reports that parents and teachers often do not recognize signs of distress because "many signs of stress are so common that they are accepted as the normal, even expected, cost of leading busy, productive lives" (p. 13). But consequences occur when being busy and productive transforms into being overscheduled and overwhelmed. Cohen-Sandler continues, "with a distinct lack of downtime, girls are less able to relax, sleep, read for pleasure, and exercise. This undermines their ability to combat both anxiety and depression. Similarly, without the benefit of solitary activities such as writing in journals, reading, and creating music or art, girls can't soothe themselves as well" (p. 17). Moreover, while Cohen-Sandler concluded through her research that all teens need strategies for coping with stress, girls need more help than boys since "what I discovered is that all girls, even highly functioning ones, can be toppled into crises by a constellation of circumstances: temperament, personality style, past history, school dynamics, and community cultures" (p. 23). Boys are not immune to sociocultural pressures, but Pipher (1994) states that with girls, "calmness is replaced by anxiety" (p. 23). She argues that girls become vulnerable to silencing their own voices because as they try to answer life's questions of their place in the world, "American culture has always smacked girls on the head in early adolescence" (p, 23). And the mixed messages linger for college women. If they have a career, will time run out to have children? And why when they win awards does someone always compliment their cute shoes before their intelligence?

Writing proved healing for girls to process conflicting feelings and mixed messages. The blank page of a journal also gives them space to find their voices. As Barbieri (1995) asks, "for isn't every girl's voice worth saving?" (p. 28). English teacher Barbieri devoted class time for writing so her students, all girls, could share their stories. Shandler (1999) read Pipher's research and developed her own project encouraging girls to share their stories, in the process discovering that "invited to speak honestly, girls told treasured and hidden stories. They wrote to communicate, to heal themselves, and to help other girls. With intelligence, they reflected on the most important experiences in their lives. Sometimes, their stories made me laugh. More often, they made me cry" (p. xv). Writing led to healing because it enabled the authors to identify their feelings, name their fears, and have an audience for their stories. It provided another method of becoming proactive by naming fears and processing them.

As a therapist, Pipher (1994) encouraged patients to express their pain through writing and other creative outlets as she describes, "I teach girls to sit with their pain, to listen to it for messages about their lives, to acknowledge and describe it rather than to run from it. They learn to write about pain, to talk about it, to express it through exercise, art, dance or music" (p. 257). Writing highlights the source of the stress and while writing about a problem may not solve it, it may prevent the author from living in denial of the pain. And denial can lead to anxiety. As DeBecker (1997) explains, "denial is a save-now-pay later scheme, a contract written entirely in small print, for in the long run, the denying person knows the truth on some level, and it causes a constant low-grade anxiety" (p. 10). Through writing about issues and discussing them, perhaps both men and women can alleviate anxiety caused by outdated social pressures and crazy busy lives full of stress so that twenty years from now but preferably much sooner, a different conversation takes place.

ANXIETY AND HEALTH

Regardless of the factors which cause an individual to have anxiety, anxiety influences that person's health. It can help people to comprehend the impact anxiety and stress have on their bodies; it can also help people to know methods for managing anxiety and stress. Clark (2006) states, "anxiety has physical, emotional, mental, even spiritual effects" (p. 12). Emotional distress often leads to physical symptoms. Tindle (2013) discusses her medical research and concludes, "depression, anxiety, and chronic pain are classic examples of chronic "whole body" stressors. Based on the research and my clinical experience, I believe that certain attitudes can be chronic whole body stressors, too. Over time, learning to blunt our own tendencies toward negative automatic responses may reduce overall wear and tear on our bodily organs" (pp. 103-104). She provides the example that a thought about something that causes stress can lead to anxious feelings followed by physical queasiness. Rankin (2013) also discusses her medical research and shares the belief that stress can create illness, elaborating that, "intuitively, we know this, and when we're stressed out, we crave relaxation. But too often, we go about it the wrong way, seeking out unhealthy forms of stress relief like alcohol, tobacco, and illegal drugs, which only exacerbate the problem. There are, however, healthy ways to elicit the relaxation response – such as meditation – that are the best medicine we can take for the treatment of life's stresses" (p. 147). Exercise is also a great way to decrease stress levels. According to the Mayo Clinic (2011) it can decrease depression, increase dopamine, improve self-esteem, improve confidence, decrease risk of stroke, decrease risk of type 2 DM, help you fall asleep quicker, decreases risks of certain types of cancer, helps with arthritis (http://www.mayoclinic.com/health/exercise/HQ01676).

Sometimes when people crave relief from the stressors in life, they don't always make the best decisions. Despite the fact that an apple is a healthier nutritional choice than a cookie, in a moment of pain people may not see the value of making short term sacrifices for long term gains. It may seem fulfilling at the moment eating an unhealthy food item when stressed, yet there are many more long-term health factors you should consider first before making this a routine for coping. Unhealthy eating and physical inactivity can lead to four of the six leading causes of death along with other diseases including: heart disease, diabetes, obesity, hypertension, stroke, osteoporosis, and many cancers. The cancers include colon cancer, prostate cancer, mouth cancer, throat cancer, esophagus cancer, lung cancer, and stomach cancer (http://www.cspinet.org/nutritionpolicy/nutrition_policy.html#eat).

Other times, making life changes that may lead to less anxiety may seem like an insurmountable obstacle. Rankin (2013) continues, "can't quit your stressful job? Not ready to leave your unhappy marriage? Haven't found the love of your life yet? Not interested in going to church? That's okay. I'm not suggesting you have to do everything I've covered in this book in order to be optimally healthy. But I am suggesting that if you're exposed to stressors you either can't change or aren't ready to change, you must prioritize activities that include the relaxation response as a way to counterbalance the stresses in your life" (p. 153). In theory, it may be easy to think of following a stressful activity such as a long commute to work with a relaxing one such as reading a novel, but some people find it difficult to relax. Life coach Beck (2008) conducted her own experiment to see how her thoughts influenced her physical health and describes, "hooked up to that brain-mapping computer, I learned that just remembering times of great fear and then repeating my 'surrender mantras' brought my anxiety-related beta waves down, down, down. Gradually, this taught me how to calm myself. After all those hours of brain-training, hooked up to the mapmakers' computer, I'm less anxious overall" (p. 96). By being able to see how her calm thoughts she called surrender mantras influenced her neurological patterns, Beck learned the value of living in the moment, facing her fears, and letting go of things beyond her control.

Nevertheless, when parts of life feel beyond control, it can be difficult to let go. Numbing the pain through anything that provides a temporary high or just staying too crazy busy to reflect about life becomes easier than facing fears. Brown (2012) discusses the need for people to numb their pain and explains, "the most powerful need for numbing seems to come from combinations of all three – shame, anxiety, and disconnection" (p. 138). Often people feel embarrassed by their stories, especially when the story presents the storyteller in a less than perfect light. No one is alone in this world, but when you make a mistake, fail to reach a goal, or live with pain, it is easy to think no one else has ever felt what you feel. Brown adds, "shame enters for those of us who experience anxiety because not only are we feeling fearful, out of control, and incapable of managing our increasingly demanding lives, but eventually our anxiety is compounded and made unbearable by our belief that if we were just smarter, stronger, or better, we'd be able to handle everything" (p. 139). A lack of connection also contributes to feelings of isolation and loneliness.

With social media and modern technology, it should be easier for people to stay in touch with each other than ever before. Yet how many times do we send a text or an email instead of picking up the phone and calling someone? Social media sites often encourage an individual to share only events worth bragging about without showing the real person behind the screen. College students have more ways of connecting to others than ever, but sometimes feel more alone than their parents and grandparents who remember what it was like not to constantly have a phone in front of them. As Brown (2012) explains, "with disconnection it's a similar story. We may have a couple hundred friends on Facebook, plus a slew of colleagues, real-life friends, and neighbors, but we feel alone and unseen. Because we are hardwired for connection, disconnection always creates pain" (p. 139). Does this disconnection contribute to the anxiety the college students reported? Only future research will tell. But for now, we can use the information we have to implement practices that will lead to increased connection and decreased stress.

THE PROBLEM: IMPLEMENTING STRATEGIES FOR COLLEGE STUDENT SUCCESS

Highlighting an issue such as stress and anxiety raises awareness of it, but brainstorming potential success strategies will not lead to change unless people implement the strategies. While the following strategies focus on helping college students, like the students who were the subjects of this research study, anyone can use these strategies to create a curriculum of community. In discussing community, once again the city planning process mentioned previously can provide a template for implementing change.

As city planner Johnson (1997) believes, "planning for cities begins when we look around us and say, 'this could be different!'" (p. 1). The same applies to planning curriculum change for college students. We as transformative leaders need to believe that the way things are can be different. Johnson explains the planning process, the same process used to design the curriculum change solutions. He continues, "we could think of planning for a given geographic area as a cycle with three major stages. In the first stage, governmental and private planners set goals and criteria to guide the succeeding steps" (p. 10). Later, "in the second stage in the cycle, planners select actions that give the goals tangible form" (p. 10). And finally, "third, planning leads to implementation of the choices" (p. 10). And just as in planning a city, planning to help college students requires a community vision to implement a detailed plan. As Harper (1996) states, "the visioning process may also result in guidance for the comprehensive plan goals and objectives. If there is a community vision, the plan can become an implementation tool" (p. 196). The university community needs to build a vision and work together to meet the needs of its students. Faculty members and university leaders have struggled with the same problems as our students; perhaps we still struggle with the same problems our students do. Regardless of our own experiences, we need to take action.

Kinematics professor Kepler (1973) discusses a physics principle of motion and explains, "kinetics is the study of forces acting on rigid bodies in motion and the effect of such forces in changing the motion" (p. 1). The same physics principle applies to curriculum change: We need to be the force that changes the motion of people. We can use our expertise to share our knowledge and lead the way to create change. We can become the understanding role models students, especially students confronting anxiety, need. College students experiencing anxiety need resources to make healthy choices, a safe supportive community, and a space to share their stories.

THE SOLUTIONS: MAKING HEALTHY CHOICES

Each person's life represents a series of decisions. Behaviors, whether they include the amount of exercise, food choices, or writing about feelings, all influence health. If the choices do not lead to health and happiness, it's never too late to make new choices. On the topic of stress, Juhan (1998) states, "it is clear then that neither the extreme of altogether avoiding stress nor the extreme of altogether ignoring it are really very helpful to the individual who wants to live a long and productive life. The real point is to learn how to handle stress, how to sustain our efforts without burning out, how to keep the nose to the grindstone without grinding it off" (p. 302). However, in order to incorporate the consistently changing medical field while simultaneously dovetailing academic theory with practical advice for the readers of this chapter, websites respected by numerous medical professionals that reflect current practices intertwine with texts from the fields of writing and medicine to present an eclectic approach of using methods that promote healthy behaviors. Juhan (1998) elaborates on this theme of behavior choices enhancing health by sharing the example of a ballet dancer preparing for a recital because "the dancer, if she is to be a successful professional, has no choice but to confront each symptom and discover the way to work through it, not by ignoring nor avoiding its causes, but rather by learning to form a working relationship with the stresses of her activity. She trains herself to produce strength at every point where a weakness develops" (p. 302). Too often, people think of having anxiety as a weakness, but methods exist for coping with it and living a healthy life.

Solutions to the problems discussed in this research utilize a myriad of resources from the fields of writing and medicine to illustrate the benefits of choosing health and limiting stress. Consider identifying sources of stress and implementing the strategies discussed. After all, theories about healthy living must become a lifestyle in order to achieve elite and effective results. It is possible to take initiative and manage stress. Don't lose hope.

Solution #1: Finding A Healthy Lifestyle

One solution to help with stress and anxiety is to live a healthy lifestyle. Medical doctor Winner (2008) provides the reminder, "anxiety disorders and depression are medical conditions. It should not be viewed as weakness to take medication for these problems, any more than it is weakness to take medication for diabetes" (p. 214). The solutions discussed can provide relief from stress and feelings of anxiety. Nevertheless, they cannot take the place of advice from a supportive medical professional such as a physician, physical therapist, psychiatrist, or counselor. There is no shame in seeking medical help, talking to a medical professional, or taking medication to help with anxiety.

It remains essential to acknowledge the connection between stress and health. As Handler (2013) states, "stress can make you sick" (p. 175). Through her research of interviewing doctors, Handler learned, "looking back at a stressful situation tends to create stress in the present moment" (p. 175). It therefore becomes important to remember that recovery takes time, and people suffering from anxiety may notice slow progress and may not feel better immediately. Pennebaker (1997) learned from his writing study, "as it turned out, writing about horrible things made people feel horrible immediately after writing" (p. 34). Over time, however, feelings improved. College students often struggle to find themselves and may change their belief systems. This can lead to anxiety and depression because as Pennebaker discusses, "when beliefs about the world are threatened, traumatized individuals experience intense anxiety, depression, or denial because their worlds don't make sense. With time, individuals may reorient their lives in order to force new experiences into their existing belief systems. Alternatively, peoples' original belief systems may gradually return by their having positive experiences" (p. 76). For college students, they may define a trauma as being homesick, preparing for a test, or feeling uncertain about a career choice. That doesn't mean their problems are more trivial than their counterparts experiencing severe illness or a death in the family.

It also helps for people experiencing anxiety to get moving. Clark (2006) explains, "exercise is one of the most effective ways to reduce anxiety, and even panic attacks. Panic is simply the physical and emotional experience of an excessive surge of adrenaline" (p. 102). What's the recommended amount of exercise? The American College of Sports Medicine (2021) recommends the amount of time for each healthy adult to put in for cardiorespiratory exercise is "moderate intensity aerobic physical activity for a minimum of 30 min on five days per week, or vigorous intensity aerobic activity for a minimum of 20 min on three days per week." For resistance exercise it is recommended by the ACSM that "every adult should perform activities that maintain or increase muscular strength and endurance for a minimum of two days per week." How many repetitions for each exercise? The ACSM advises, "8-12 repetitions improve strength and power, 10-15 repetitions improve strength in middle-age and older persons starting exercise, and 15-20 repetitions improve muscular endurance." Including flexibility exercises and balance exercises can also be beneficial (https://www.acsm.org/all-blog-posts/certification-blog/acsm-certified-blog/2020/09/03/acsm-exercise-guidelines-resources). If you are unable to meet all of these minutes it does not mean that you are unhealthy. Gradually work up to it. Over time increase your amount of minutes, followed by increased intensity levels. Even taking a short break to take a walk around campus or play on the swings outside the residence halls enables a person to receive the benefits of exercise. Going to the dining hall for a salad can also have more health benefits than ordering pizza and drinking beer multiple times a week.

Solution #2: Connecting Through Creating Class Community

Another strategy to help with stress and anxiety is to feel part of a supportive community. While students are in the classroom it is important to make the classroom a home away from home. Heard (1995) writes, "we know where we feel most at home" (p. 5). Teachers want to believe that all students leave the classroom and go home to supportive families. Sadly, for some students, the place where they feel most at home is the classroom because once they leave, they confront difficulties at home. For college students, some may be living away from family for the first time in their lives. Nontraditional students frequently juggle families and jobs in addition to classes and the classroom may provide the only respite in a busy day. So teachers and professors need to create classroom communities where students feel safe and supported. Routman (2003) discusses the value of building a strong class community because "no one talks about bonding, and we need to. Curriculum and standards must first connect with the lives and spirits of our children if we're to have any lasting success. Unless we reach into our students' hearts, we have no entry into their minds" (p. 12). Building a community means encouraging students to trust each other and share their voices. The community can then provide a support network for students by providing strength when a community member struggles.

People only have a certain number of hours in a day, so why not make the time spent in the classroom as enjoyable as possible? Most people strive to find balance in their lives, and students in the College of Education who completed surveys for this research study not only have the stress of completing their own assignments for classes, but also the added pressure of designing inspiring lessons for the students who are in their classrooms during required field experiences and later, student teaching. Time management can be difficult for teachers because, even with constant multitasking, there never seem to be enough hours in the day to accomplish all of the learning goals. Routman (2003) encourages teachers to rethink their schedules and states, "the elusive balanced life remains a mirage. Your time is valuable. Spend it in the most meaningful, productive ways possible" (p. 202). She also encourages teachers to get a life outside of school and tells the story of a friend who almost gave up tickets to the ballet to grade papers. Routman told her friend to go to the ballet and be an interesting person because "you can't come to work each day enthusiastic about teaching if all you did the night before was grade papers. You want to be able to have dinner with a friend, go to a movie. Read a book, cook for fun, reflect about what's just happened. We are not only role models for learning but role models for living" (p. 202). Professors of future teachers need to become role models for students to live balanced lives.

This is easier said than done, because most teachers feel like Codell (1999) at the end of the school year who says "of course, I cried. There was so much I wanted to say. But the sands of the hourglass fell, and they left me, single file" (p. 185). There will always be one more lesson that could have been taught, one more comment that should have been said, and one more idea that would have fit fabulously into class if only there was more time. Gruwell (2007) describes this feeling as "I knew going in that my student teaching position was supposed to last only a semester, but as finals approached, I started getting anxious. There were still so many things I wanted to do, so many stories I wanted to read, and so many places I wanted to take them" (p. 35). College of Education students who prepare to student teach may share the sentiment of wanting to prove themselves as excellent student teachers while not having enough time with their students. But regardless of whether they are in kindergarten or college, once students leave the classroom for the last time, they will remember how they felt as part of a strong class community and that strength will sustain them as they begin the next chapter of their careers.

Furthermore, teachers feel responsible for all their students. Gruwell (2009) describes this feeling as, "as my students became more like a family, I was surprised by how difficult a balancing act being a teacher really is. At the end of each day it became more impossible to leave my students' problems in the classroom. Then there was the fact that my social life was beginning to implode, and I was spending way too much of my own money on school supplies" (p. xviii-xix). As teachers, we want to be role models for students to enjoy their time in the classroom without experiencing stress; yet, secretly, we may be about to collapse from the stress in our lives ourselves. English teacher Johnson (2005) advises teachers, "stress is a serious problem all by itself." (p. 132). She encourages teachers to take mental health breaks as needed and shares the reminder, "teaching is difficult work, but if you make up your mind that you truly want to teach, your determination and sincerity will lead you in the right direction" (p. 135).

But why go through experiences alone? Sandberg (2013) discusses her movement to create community support networks and encourage conversation. Her movement, called Lean In because she wants people to face their fears and lean in to life, begins with the idea "you can also create and join Lean In Circles, small peer groups that meet in person for ongoing encouragement and development" (p. 173). Descriptions of successful Lean In Circles appeared in recent issues of *Glamour* and *Cosmopolitan*, two publications more popular with college students than chapters like this one. Creating a Lean In Circle on a college campus can bring its students together.

Sandberg (2014) successfully implemented Lean In Circles on college campuses and encourages college students to start their own Lean In Circles because "when you need help – and we all do – please look for it. No one needs to navigate this world alone" (p. xvii). Whether participating in Lean In Circles or other forums of conversation such as a discussion between classes, college students need to know they are not alone.

Solution #3: Reflecting Through Writing

Another strategy to help with stress and anxiety is to express thoughts and feelings through writing. Psychologist Bidwell Smith (2018) believes, "being able to tell our story has an enormous impact on our healing process and almost always serves to decrease anxiety" (p. 68). To create a strong community, people who belong to the community need to feel they are not alone. Barbieri (1995) discusses her method of using writing to build community at the school where she taught all girls and describes, "I had explained our curriculum for the year. We would write every day on topics of our own choosing, and yes, I would write with them" (p. 18). She discovered that her students used their writing practice time to discuss issues on their minds and asked the question, "should writing be used as therapy for the girls to work out their developmental issues?" (p. 21). After reflection, she concluded that she wanted to provide a safe community for students to write and discuss their writing with each other because, "their writing practice entries brought me back to earth, as I came to know again that the real magic of writing lies in what it can do for the writer. I should have remembered. How many times had I survived stress, crisis and grief by sitting up at night writing furiously? How many times had I written my way out of confusion, anger, or despair? I should have remembered" (p. 27). When there is no one around to listen, or when the author is not ready to share thoughts and feelings with others, writing can help the writer write right through the pain.

Writing cannot solve all the problems that create anxiety, but it can provide an effective coping mechanism. Murray (1985) argues, "writing is therapy. I tried to avoid that issue as a writing teacher, mostly because I had colleagues who accused some of us of using writing as therapy. I can no longer avoid the fact that writing is therapy – for me and for my students. We write because we need to write, and the act of writing rarely solves our problems, but it is a way of dealing with problems and achieving a momentary distance from them. The act of writing about the most painful subjects – in my case the death of a daughter – seems both necessary and therapeutic" (p. 217). Writing does not take the place of a conversation with a supportive emotional therapist, and sometimes talking to a therapist may be the best method to deal with a difficult issue. Fallon (2020) states, "expressive writing, when combined with a therapeutic process, can double or even triple your efforts by helping you multiply the therapeutic process between times you see your therapist" (p. 104). Thus, writing can enhance the experience of therapy. Pipher (2006) who is a therapist, believes in the power of writing and sharing stories, whether in written or conversational form as she states, "stories are the most basic tool for connecting us to one another" (p. 11). Sharing stories serves as another facet of community building and bringing people together to alleviate isolation and loneliness. Pipher (2006) adds, "healing stories give people hope, teach them empathy, and encourage action" (p. 12). In a community of writers, if one person hears another person's story of healing, that person may feel inspired to survive similar circumstances.

Writing can provide an effective method to relieve anxiety. Helgoe, Wilhelm, and Kommor (2005) provide the medical perspective on writing and elaborate, "it may be that, by just putting the feelings on paper, we are able to back away from the intensity of the situation and better evaluate things. Often, we are able to sort out feelings and reach insight and clarity through writing. Also, writing slows us down, which is a real benefit to anxiety sufferers" (p. 260). Nurse practitioner Clark (2006) concurs and adds, "journaling, or journal writing, is a way to establish a permanent record of your thoughts, feelings, and situations that evoke anxiety" (p. 146). By rereading journal entries, it becomes possible for the author to discover the source of the anxiety. Or if the author lacks the distance or expertise to provide a self-diagnosis, a supportive audience such as a counselor can help. This is similar to completing a pain journal of physical pain and sharing it with a physician or physical therapist. Writing helps the writer identify the source of the emotions. Psychologist Clark (2018) believes, "when anxiety is buried in different feelings, it can act as an escalator of those other emotions. I sometimes refer to anxiety as a 'volume control' of other painful emotions; the higher the volume, the higher the anxiety" (p. 180). Writing provides the writer with the opportunity to uncover the stories behind the emotions and begin the process of healing from painful emotions and experiences.

Psychologist Pipher (2006) continues the discussion of the healing benefits of writing by stating, "paradoxically, even though writing is anxiety provoking, it is also therapeutic. Once we are immersed in writing, we forget our anxiety. Focusing on clarity and beauty calms us down" (p. 79). Writing illuminates issues and motivates the author to create change because, as Pipher believes, "stewing in our own stress is not a good way to handle difficulty. Action ameliorates anxiety" (p. 79). If a writer also belongs to a supportive community, the community members will encourage the writer to take steps toward achieving a goal. And any step becomes progress. As Cameron (2002) believes, "most blocked creatives have an active addiction to anxiety. We prefer the low-grade pain and occasional heart stopping panic attack to the drudgery of small and simple daily steps in the right direction" (p. 143). Writing can raise awareness so the writer can determine the real issue and take steps to process any pain instead of turning to unhealthy choices to numb it. Cameron highlights the value of this process and continues, "as we become aware of our blocking devices – food, busyness, alcohol, sex, other drugs – we can feel our U-turns as we make them. The blocks will no longer work effectively. Over time, we will try – perhaps slowly at first and erratically – to ride out the anxiety and see where we emerge. Anxiety is fuel. We can use it to write with, paint with, work with" (pp. 165-166). And when anxiety becomes fuel, it can provide help instead of hurt for the individual experiencing it.

SUSTAINING HEALTHY CHOICES

Each person controls the series of decisions that comprises a life story. The choices made will determine that individual's health story. As Lamott (2005) states, "your problem is how you are going to spend this one odd and precious life you have been issued" (p. 303). Often people feel overwhelmed by life and their choices, which can cause stress. Therefore, the key to healthy choices remains taking initiative by identifying and managing stress. Each individual possesses the power to write the next chapter in his or her story; the commitment to choosing health can lead to more peace and less stress as that unwritten chapter unfolds. As Beck (2008) explains, "in the gym – and in life – the point of endeavor is not sustaining the apex of achievement. The point is falling from that apex and finding our way back, over and over" (p. 217). Engaging in healthy habits represents a journey. Some days will always seem more difficult than others, but the goal becomes to be healthy and learn what triggers unhealthy behavior. Or as Beck (2012) believes, value exists in learning from experiences and making changes because "great artists embrace the full catastrophe of our condition and find beyond it an even deeper truth of peace, healing, and redemption" (p. 243). And know that tomorrow can begin a new chapter.

CONTRIBUTE A VERSE

This research study began with the goal of adding insights to the conversation of writing as healing and led in the unexpected direction of helping college students cope with anxiety and ongoing stresses in life. Psychologist Clark (2018) provides hope for people experiencing anxiety with the explanation, "whether anxiety is experienced loudly as fear, quietly as worry, or physically as stress, it is an undeniable presence and force in all our lives. Getting a handle on what it is, what it feels like for us, and what we call it is fundamental to harnessing it" (p. 38).

Since one of the researchers was also the professor of the students who participated as subjects in the study, even though the student survey responses were anonymous, a strong level of trust existed in the classroom for students to feel comfortable sharing their thoughts in writing on the surveys even though the researchers would never know who wrote what. Perhaps the students can relate to Zimmermann

(2002) who shares, "fear of the future paralyzes us with anxiety" (p. 34). Her advice for coping? She suggests, "take several deep, centering breaths. Now write for at least fifteen minutes" (p. 35). The journal writing continued during class sessions after the conclusion of this research project, which helped students discover the answers they needed. Both researchers provided additional help by sharing stress management strategies.

Every semester, the writing professor/researcher strives to establish a safe community in her classroom. As DeSalvo (1999) writes, "by sharing our stories under the safest conditions, we learn from one another that we need not engage in shame and self-hatred. They are the result of what happened to us, of what we survived. In time, we can learn to transform those feelings; we can learn to value ourselves and love ourselves" (p. 169). Because students found the courage to share, the responsibility now becomes that of the university community to use the information to increase student retention and decrease student stress. Heifetz (1994) writes of transformative leaders, "their lives would be less stressful if they did not care" (p. 252). But we have to care and make a difference. We as leaders also need to manage our own stress so we can help students manage theirs. Heifetz cautions, "to lead and yet sustain the personal stresses that come with leading requires inner discipline" (p. 252). University leaders can also benefit from the stress management techniques discussed in this chapter and can simultaneously take care of themselves while taking care of students. Anyone experiencing anxiety can find hope remembering the words from Clark (2018), that, "anxiety is not in control – we are – and this is the hope. You are in control" (p. 350). Let's build a community vision for change, where everyone works together with the purpose of helping college students succeed. Through this method, research can become the catalyst for additional conversations.

That's the long term goal. The short term goal echoes the sentiment of Gruwell (1999), who writes, "I encouraged the Freedom Writers to use a pen as a means of revolution. Through their writing, they discovered they shared a common identity, which united them into a community that connected them, not separated them from the world" (p. 276). The goal is for every student to write in a journal and belong to a class community. Doing so will help them find their purpose in life. This chapter ends with the same question in which it began. The question still remains today. What experiences bring purpose to life? Walt Whitman (1855) gives us the answer in his poem *O Me! O Life!* "That you are here – that life exists and identity, that the powerful play goes on and you may contribute a verse" (p. 341).

Make your verse a good one.

ACKNOWLEDGMENT

This chapter was co-authored by Dr. Eric Wanner, Director of the Physical Therapy Department at Palm Beach Sports Medicine and Orthopaedic Center. Eric loves research, and I enjoyed collaborating to designing a unique survey featuring both numerical subjective and written subjective questions to assess goal setting for physical therapy patients. Eric and I also conducted research to assess anxiety in college students and recommended effective methods for coping with anxiety, such as exercising, nutrition, writing, and belonging to a supportive community. We continued our collaboration by using health coaching to supplement physical therapy treatment plans for both staff members and patients at a hospital. I feel proud of our lasting contributions to interdisciplinary research that helped numerous people and remain grateful for Eric's talent of condensing my overly wordy first drafts into the most essential ideas.

The preceding chapter contains excerpts from the following previous IGI publications:

Bird, J.L., & Wanner, E.T. (2020). Narratives of anxiety. In *Using narrative writing to enhance healing* (pp. 185-237). Hershey, PA: Information Science Reference.

Bird, J.L., & Wanner, E.T. (2015). Research as curriculum inquiry: helping college students with anxiety. In V.C.X. Wang (Ed.), *Handbook of research on scholarly publishing and research methods* (pp. 273-295). Hershey, PA: Information Science Reference.

REFERENCES

ACSM Staff. (2021). *ACSM exercise guidelines.* American College of Sports Medicine. Retrieved from https://www.acsm.org/all-blog-posts/certification-blog/acsm-certified-blog/2020/09/03/acsm-exercise-guidelines-resources

Barbieri, M. (1995). *Sounds from the heart.* Heinemann.

Baty, K. (2003). *A girl's gotta do what a girl's gotta do.* Rodale.

Beck, M. (2008). *Steering by starlight.* Rodale.

Beck, M. (2012). *Finding your way in a wild new world.* Free Press.

Bidwell Smith, C. (2018). *Anxiety: the missing stage of grief.* Hachette Books.

Brown, B. (2012). *Daring greatly.* Gotham Books.

Cameron, J. (2002). *The artist's way* (2nd ed.). Tarcher/Putnam.

Carmichael, C. (2021). *Nervous energy.* St. Martin's Essentials.

Catanese, A. J. (1996). Lessons learned. In B. W. McClendon & A. J. Catanese (Eds.), *Planners on planning* (pp. 287–295). Jossey-Bass.

Centers for Disease Control and Prevention. (2011). *Health Related Quality of Life.* Health Related Quality of Life Surveillance Program. Retrieved from https://www.cdc.gov/hrqol/hrqol14_measure.htm

Centers for Disease Control and Prevention. (2021). *Coping with Stress.* U.S. Department of Health & Human Services. Retrieved from https://www.cdc.gov/coronavirus/2019-ncov/daily-life-coping/managing-stress-anxiety.html

Clandinin, D. J., & Connelly, F. M. (2000). *Narrative inquiry.* Jossey-Bass.

Clark, A. H. (2018). *Hack your anxiety.* Sourcebooks, Inc.

Clark, C. C. (2006). *Living well with anxiety.* HarperCollins.

Codell, E. R. (1999). *Educating Esme.* Algonquin Books.

Cohen-Sandler, R. (2005). *Stressed-out girls.* Viking.

Connelly, F. M., & Clandinin, D. J. (1988). *Teachers as curriculum planners.* Teachers College Press.

Conner, J. (2008). *Writing down your soul.* Conari.

DeBecker, G. (1997). *The gift of fear*. Little, Brown and Company.

DeSalvo, L. (1999). *Writing as a way of healing*. Beacon Press.

Fallon, A. (2020). *The power of writing it down*. Zondervan.

Goldberg, N. (1986). *Writing down the bones*. Shambhala.

Goldberg, N. (1990). *Wild mind*. Bantam.

Goldberg, N. (2013). *The true secret of writing*. Atria.

Graves, D. (1994). *A fresh look at writing*. Heinemann.

Gruwell, E. (2007). *Teach with your heart.*

Gruwell, E. (2009). *Teaching hope.*

Gruwell, E.Freedom Writers. (1999). *The Freedom Writers diary.*

Handler, J. (2013). *Braving the fire*. St. Martin's Griffin.

Harper, A. N. (1996). Tooling up for effective planning. In B. W. McClendon & A. J. Catanese (Eds.), *Planners on planning* (pp. 190–198). Jossey-Bass.

Heard, G. (1995). *Writing toward home*. Heinemann.

Heifetz, R. A. (1994). *Leadership without easy answers*. The Belnap Press of Harvard University Press.

Helgoe, L. A., Wilhelm, L. R., & Kommor, M. J. (2005). *The anxiety answer book*. Sourcebooks, Inc.

Helpguide. (2013). *Stress symptoms, signs, causes*. Retrieved from https://www.helpguide.org/mental/stress_signs.htm

Hoch, C. (1995). Teaching ethics and planning theory. In S. Hendler (Ed.), Planning ethics (pp. 281-300). New Brunswick, NJ: Rutgers.

Johnson, B. (2009). *But now! Awakening faith in an age of anxiety*. Essence Publishing.

Johnson, L. (1998). *Two parts textbook, one part love*. Hyperion.

Johnson, L. (2005). *Teaching outside the box*. Jossey-Bass.

Johnson, W. C. (1997). *Urban planning and politics*. American Planning Association.

Juhan, D. (1998). *Job's body*. Station Hill.

Kamenetz, A. (2013). Power of the pen. *Oprah, 14*(12), 140–141.

Kepler, H. B. (1973). *Basic graphical kinematics* (2nd ed.). McGraw Hill.

Lamott, A. (2005). *Plan B: further thoughts on faith*. Riverhead.

Marshall, J. D., Sears, J. T., & Schubert, W. H. (2000). *Turning points in curriculum*. Merrill/Prentice Hall.

Mayo Clinic Staff. (2011). *7 benefits of regular physical activity.* Mayo Clinic. Retrieved from http://www.mayoclinic.com/health/exercise/HQ01676

Murray, D. M. (1985). *A writer teaches writing* (2nd ed.). Houghton Mifflin.

Nutrition Policy Staff. (2013). *Why good nutrition is important.* Center for Science in the Public Interest. Retrieved from https://www.cspinet.org/nutritionpolicy/nutrition_policy.html

Pennebaker, J. W. (1997). *Opening up: the healing power of expressing emotions.* The Guilford Press.

Perry, B. D., & Winfrey, O. (2021). *What happened to you?* Flatiron Books.

Pipher, M. (1994). *Reviving Ophelia.* Grosset/Putnam.

Pipher, M. (2006). *Writing to change the world.* Riverhead.

Rankin, L. (2013). *Mind over medicine.* Hay House.

Romano, T. (2013). *Fearless writing.* Heinemann.

Routman, R. (2003). *Reading essentials.* Heinemann.

Sadker, M., & Sadker, D. (1994). *Failing at fairness.* Charles Scribner's Sons.

Sandberg, S. (2013). *Lean in.* Alfred A. Knopf.

Sandberg, S. (2014). *Lean in for graduates.* Alfred A. Knopf.

Shandler, S. (1999). *Ophelia speaks.* HarperCollins.

Smith, D. (2012). *Monkey mind: a memoir of anxiety.* Simon & Schuster.

Stossel, S. (2013). *My age of anxiety.* Alfred A. Knopf.

Tindle, H. (2013). *Up: how positive outlook can transform our health and aging.* Hudson Street Press.

University of Maryland Medical Center. (2014). *Stress.* Retrieved from https://umm.edu/health/medical/reports/articles/stress

Whitman, W. (1993). O Me! O Life! In *Leaves of grass* (p. 341). Random House. (Original work published 1855)

Winner, J. (2008). *Take the stress out of your life.* Da Capo.

Zimmermann, S. (2002). *Writing to heal the soul.* Three Rivers Press.

KEY TERMS AND DEFINITIONS

Anxiety: Different clinicians have different definitions of anxiety, and someone who lives with anxiety will describe it from a different point of view than a clinical definition in a textbook, but the general consensus is that anxiety is chronic fear or stress that can result in panic attacks and a person feeling an inability to cope with life's stressors.

Artistic and Technical Writing: English teachers design rubrics which incorporate both artistic and technical writing when evaluating student essays. Artistic writing is the writer's tone of word choice, also known as voice, while technical writing is the writer's specificity of word choice.

Community Development: Designing a place where people feel welcomed and supported, whether it is a neighborhood, a classroom, or a network of colleagues who provide support for an individual.

Curriculum Inquiry: A form of narrative inquiry made popular in the field of research by F. Michael Connelly and D. Jean Clandinin, curriculum inquiry is a qualitative interpretative form of research that focuses on the telling, retelling, and sharing of stories through the lens of curriculum to implement program changes.

HRQOL (Health Related Quality of Life) Survey: A general health survey in the public domain and able to be used by researchers without securing permission or paying copyright fees.

Lean in Circles: Sheryl Sandberg's movement to encourage community support and discussion groups that motivate participants to face their fears and lean in to life.

Planning Process: Used in the fields of city planning as well as curricular change, this process encompasses the following steps: survey, analysis, plan, implementation, and feedback.

Writing as Healing: Numerous studies have been conducted investigating the influence of writing on physical and emotional health. James Pennebaker is a leader in the field which explores the health benefits of writing.

Writing Voice: Voice in writing highlights a writer's word choice and tone to compose a journal entry or other written composition that reflects the writer's personality. Every writer has a unique writing voice, just like each person has a unique speaking voice.

Chapter 9
Reflections of Spiritual Narratives

ABSTRACT

This narrative illustrates the connections between spirituality, writing, and health. It does not promote a specific religion but demonstrates strength people gain from believing in a higher power. Prayers with hospital patients and the search for connections more than coincidences illustrate how people find and maintain hope and faith when presented with tragic events such as the recent pandemic. Each reader may find encouragement while reflecting on and following an individual spiritual path.

FAITH NARRATIVES

Spirituality enhances health. To preface this narrative, the stories shared do not advocate the following of specific religious beliefs. Some people find comfort in a religious community of worship. Other people find spirituality by taking walks in nature. I share my experiences through the lens of my spirituality, but encourage you to follow your own religious or spiritual beliefs to find strength during difficult times. Regardless of what you believe, may you find encouragement in the following examples.

In the coronavirus era, I want to keep my faith, both my spiritual faith and my faith in modern medicine. Medicine and spirituality converged for me when I spent time volunteering for the pastoral care team at my local hospital. In my roles as health coach and Stephen Minister, I observed the connections between spirituality, health, and healing. My past experiences give me faith in the present moment as medical teams race to control the coronavirus, and a future filled with hope.

I wrote the following narrative a couple years before the pandemic, when I could still walk the hospital hallways freely. The pandemic closed the hospital to all except the most essential workers, and I pray for the safety and health of all who cross the entryway to save lives. I planned to use my pastoral care narratives in a collection that the hospital, understandingly, never published due to the severity of the coronavirus. I hope the narratives illustrate the role prayer plays in healing, as people with loved ones still in hospitals use prayer to sustain them.

DOI: 10.4018/978-1-7998-9051-5.ch009

I sling my lanyard with my badge around my neck and walk into the hospital. My first stop is the chapel, where I say a prayer for all the patients I will see today. I hope I can provide some comfort to them. During my rounds, I always thank the nurses, physical therapists, and occupational therapists for the work they do to help patients. I have no idea how to teach a patient exercises or give them medicine, and I appreciate the members of the hospital family who know how to save a life. The team members also thank me for my prayers. Prayers give patients hope, and a positive attitude can help patients heal.

I completed my health coach internship at the hospital and serve as a Stephen Minister for my church. With my full time job as a high school English teacher, I don't have as many hours to spend volunteering at the hospital as I would like. However, I have the goal of making a difference in the time I have with patients.

My training as both a Stephen Minister and a health coach reinforces the power of listening and learning patient's stories. In addition to my roles as high school English teacher and health coach, I serve as a Stephen Minister at my church. Haugk (2000) defines, "Stephen Ministers are lay Christians carefully recruited, selected, trained, commissioned, and supervised for lay caring ministry" (p. 17). With my role as a Stephen Minister, I use the same skills of reflective listening and partnering with people on their healing journeys as I do as a health coach. The difference with Stephen Ministry is that people may be experiencing a spiritual crisis instead of a health crisis, and I also have prayer as a resource. While I write about Stephen Ministry from the perspective of my experiences, the writing practices I describe are not meant to be seen only from the perspective of Christian faith.

Sometimes I only have five minutes with a patient, but I believe my path was meant to cross with the lives of the patients I meet. For most patients, I will not know the sequels to their stories or what happens to them after they leave the hospital hallways. I pick up my list of patients who will soon transform from names on a page to a mosaic of stories I feel blessed to be part of, even if only for a moment.

One of my favorite stories is when I prayed with two members of the same family who were at the hospital for two different reasons. The mother was recovering from a medical procedure on one floor of the hospital and felt concerned about her daughter, who was recovering from a different procedure on the floor above her. As soon as I left the mother's room, I went upstairs to pray with the daughter and relay a message from her mother. The daughter was comforted, and then I returned downstairs to tell the mother her daughter was okay. The mother felt comforted and finally slept.

Not every story is as heartwarming. One day I was called to the emergency room to comfort a family whose loved one collapsed suddenly from a heart condition and was rushed to the hospital. The patient was a wife, mother, and daughter, and I met her devastated family in the waiting room. I juggled cups of water for them and offered prayers. Every person in the family had a different coping strategy from screaming to crying to attempting to be stoic for the others and not show emotion. The doctors did the best they could, but I never found out if the patient, who was in critical condition when I left for the day, lived or died.

Another day a nurse asked me to stay with a patient who just learned her cancer was untreatable. The patient was remarkably optimistic although her family had to leave her room so they could cry. Her wish was to die quickly so she and her family wouldn't suffer, but I reminded her she still had time for more conversations with her loved ones.

One patient admitted she was bored and loved that I arrived when I did so she could tell me all about her children and her volunteer work. Another patient supervised a youth group at her church and we had a long conversation about God's plan for us. Yet another patient wanted to know what happens when we die, and we discussed books written by people who had near death experiences.

I enjoy being part of a team where everyone is focused on working together to help their patients. I once prayed for a patient and the nurse in the room asked to stay and listen to the prayer. One day I paused in the doorway of a room, not wanting to interrupt the doctor who was talking to the patient. The doctor motioned for me to join her. She looked at the patient and said of me, "she can help you." The patient was dealing with a variety of addictions and didn't know what to do next.

There is an outstanding group physical therapy class held in the mornings for patients to do their exercises together and share their stories. Inspirational quotes play on the television screen while patients receive education and encouragement about their exercises. I was invited to share some motivational words with the patients, and I try to remind them that healing is a journey. Patients often want to feel better overnight, but if each day they feel better than the day before, that is progress.

Sometimes family members need as much help as the patients. A team of excellent medical professionals consistently monitor the patients, but visiting family members often welcome prayer and words of encouragement. Being a caregiver for a loved one is not an easy responsibility, and often family members ask me to pray with them while the patient takes a much needed nap.

Even if it is only for a short amount of time, I enjoy playing a small role in the stories of patients' lives. One patient studied music during his hospital stay because he became determined to perform in a music concert a few weeks later with a famous Broadway performer. Another patient wanted to share how she couldn't wait to return to teaching. She wanted to be a role model for her students and show them if she could overcome adversity, they could too. If a patient is reluctant to talk, a book on a bedside table often becomes a way for me to connect with them. When patients find out I teach literature and writing, they enjoy discussing contemporary novels or the latest celebrity gossip magazine. Discussing a fictional character's struggles can often help patients discuss their own emotions.

I can't help but wonder how the stories of the patients continue once they leave the hospital. I watched in awe as a physical therapist and occupational therapist helped a patient take her first steps after she thought she wouldn't be able to walk again. And then I never saw the family again. "You came into my life just when I needed you," one patient told me, and that is what I believe whenever my path crosses a patient's path. I won't know the rest of the story. All I can do is hope that my time with each patient made a difference in some way.

So I feel gratitude for the patient entertaining a large group of visitors who had to be reminded to rest, the patient who told me to return after she watched her favorite singer on television, the patient who was excited to write in her journal, the patient and his wife who wanted to discuss religion, the patient who was in pain but was more concerned about his wife's health, the patient who wanted to discuss literature, the patient who wondered if writing could lead to healing, the patient who was optimistic even after experiencing complications in surgery, the patient who wrote notes to remember what to tell her medical team, the patient who still needed to talk even when confused by pain medication, the patient who wanted to have a long conversation about life after death, the patient whose daughter refused to leave her while she was in pain, the patient who constantly told jokes to the medical team, the patient who quoted Shakespeare, and the patient who couldn't find her glasses. All of them, along with all the other patients whose stories touched my life, helped me as much as I helped them. I am reminded that life is short and people don't always get the time they think they will have, but life is also long and thanks to impressive medical care, there will be another day to write a new story. Some patients cope with their diagnosis with grace and dignity while others whine and complain, but they all need compassion.

Thus, I continue to sling my lanyard around my neck to meet the next group of patients who wish to share their stories with me.

HEALTH COACHING INTERNSHIP (2014)

I begin my hospital internship to earn certification as a health coach specializing in using writing as healing. To think the English teacher who still takes an alternate route through the high school hallways whenever the biology class dissects something earned a place in a hospital orthopedic unit amazes me. I smooth the skirt of my coral dress, feel thankful I wore ivory ballet flats because I will walk a significant amount, and try not to get stuck in the broken elevator.

I meet my first patient while Eric, a physical therapist, takes notes. He will complete the patent's physical evaluation while I will ask her open ended questions which focus on her emotional state of mind. Eric completes his evaluation first while I watch and take notes. When my turn arrives, I sit in a chair next to the patient and focus my attention on her.

REFLECTION (2021)

I recently threw away the ivory ballet flats because the soles finally fell off the shoes. As an English teacher, I love metaphors, and compare the broken soles of the shoes to the broken souls during the pandemic. Adjusting to this pandemic world required resilience and sacrifice. Families cannot see their loved ones in the hospital. Patients struggle with the coronavirus in the hospital and later at home, if they survive the illness. I receive thanks from my students' parents for being a teacher during this pandemic era, and try to make my classroom a safe space while worrying I am not making as much of a difference as the medical professionals saving lives. So the only thing I can do is use my spiritual gifts to share hope and help others. I provide writing strategies to my students and also share wellness strategies I learned during my health coaching training. I also share the wellness strategies, importance of patient narratives, and the value of spirituality with you, the reader, with the hopes such knowledge helps you or someone you love.

HEALING THROUGH SPIRITUALITY

By serving as a Stephen Minister at both the hospital and my church, I know that prayer does not replace traditional medical care. Occasionally someone describes a healing miracle, but such stories make news because they don't happen every day. Bessey (2019) encourages, "I pray that you would remain open to participating in your own healing, even if it comes to you in ways that you resent and fear at first. Just because it's new to you doesn't mean God isn't already waiting there for you in the doctor's office, in the therapist's room, on the page, in the conversation, in the solitude" (p. 210). I like the image of God waiting for us when we need to be in the waiting room of a medical facility, but we need to show up and participate by following medical advice.

During the pandemic, I started the ritual of walking around my neighborhood in the mornings before school as the sun rises. On Saturdays, I still walk at the same time, but because I don't have to hurry home to get ready for school, my ritual includes stopping at a fountain next to a local assisted living facility to pray. I wonder how the residents inside deal with isolation; had my grandparents been alive during the pandemic they probably would have drawn strength from all they previously survived in their lives. Prayer gives me the same strength. I feel blessed to know I can call family and friends, but sometimes I share the sentiment of Doyle (2016) who shares, "but most often, the listener makes the pain harder for me by trying to make it easier for her" (p. 146). Sometimes I don't want to burden people I love with my pain. Sometimes I don't want to be cheered up or given advice. Sometimes I just want to vent to God. And then I stand up, not minding if I got wet from sitting at the base of the fountain because I appreciate the cleansing symbolism of the water, and walk away with hope for the day.

SPIRITUAL NARRATIVES

Two years ago, while waiting at an airport, I wrote a prayer book (Bird, 2019). I wrote the prayers as inspiration for my life, and feel happy they helped other people too. Readers thanked me for giving them peace. I wrote a prayer for each week of the year and with each prayer included a Bible passage, a short vignette from my life, and prompts for journal writing. Spiritual writing provides healing as well as the opportunity for prayer and reflection.

When I write prayers in my journal, I let the words flow. Bernstein (2018) describes the experience of spiritual writing as, "I find it very powerful to put pen to paper and write my prayers in my journal. When I write them down, I feel like I'm releasing my internal suffering and inviting an invisible force to heal me" (pp. 105-106). When I wrote my prayer book, I didn't intend for anyone else to read it. When praying with the church choir one Sunday morning (before the pandemic prevented us from performing), several people asked me if I could write down my words so they could read the prayers anytime. I interpreted the moment as a nudge from God to share my gifts of prayer and writing. I find purpose in free flowing prayers, and I find value in clearly stating my intentions. Bernstein (2016) suggests, "write your faith statement, and don't edit a word. Write down whatever comes out. Don't judge what you write, and don't try to make it perfect. Just let it flow" (pp. 121-122). My faith statement: I find purpose and meaning in sharing my prayers and writing to help others heal by finding coaching and teaching moments.

Several writers compare writing to the chemical process of alchemy. But if alchemy symbolizes transformation, it becomes spiritual. Doyle (2020) believes, "life is alchemy, and emotions are the fire that turns me to gold" (p. 51). Hatmaker (2020) uses a similar metaphor and shares, "for me, the practice of putting pen to paper creates an alchemy hard to duplicate any other way" (p. 213). Synthesizing ideas and emotions leads to transformative alchemy in life.

During this pandemic era, life seems senseless. Writing prayers can bring both comfort and order to the chaos. Lyons (2019) recounts, "I snuck downstairs in the middle of the night to unload the burdens of my heart on my laptop. Writing was the only way I knew to process what God might be doing in my life" (p. 27). The pandemic taught me even when a significant amount of life lurks out of my control, I discover what I can control, such as my attitude or the lessons I teach in my classroom, and do something about it. Whether writing prayers or free writing about life, writing brings comfort. Ashcroft and Olsen (2012) recommend, "don't try to be profound on the pages of your journal; just be yourself. This is about you, your heart, your guts, your relationship with God. All you have to do is start writing" (p. 141). Journal writing, just like life, doesn't fit a pattern. My current journal contains artwork, quotes written on post-it notes, and writing in five different colors of ink. Most likely no one else could decipher it, but it makes perfect sense to me. TerKeurst (2020) writes, "my journals weren't linear like spreadsheets or crystal clear like photographs. They were more like abstract art made up of words that probably wouldn't make sense to others" (p. 98-99). Indeed, journals become works of art which tell the stories of our lives.

My life story:
As a daughter of a city planner, I saw the importance of communities to help people.
As a teacher, I saw the impacts of stress on students.
As a patient with an autoimmune disease, I saw the results of reworking my lifestyle.
As a health coach, I saw the benefits of a positive attitude for patients.
As a Stephen Minister, I saw the value of faith in the unseen.
As a writer, I saw the evidence of capturing narratives on paper.
And I realized the value of narratives because stories provide a snapshot of life.

Perhaps the most challenging part of pandemic times became granting myself permission to enjoy moments of fun. How can I laugh while removing Lucy the cat from a puzzle I attempt to complete when people suffer in the hospital? How dare I take a class of students outside to read a book in the sunshine when healthcare workers struggle to save lives? Most adults don't find time in their lives to laugh. As Beck (2003) writes, "consider that a typical small child laughs over four hundred times a day. For the average adult, the number is a paltry fifteen" (p. 152). During the pandemic, it becomes important to find moments of joy amidst the chaos. From my role as pastoral care volunteer, I witnessed heartbreak and suffering. I improved by no longer feeling sick when looking at blood, but no one (most of all myself) wants me holding a scalpel to save a life. So I save the emotional lives of the teenagers I teach by giving them a moment outside with a great work of literature. We still wear our face masks, but our souls can breathe for a moment. Arioto (2019) shares, "so instead of overthinking them, overplanning them, or pretending I can control them, I am focused on having more fun with the days I am given" (p. 18). I agree with the great advice to not take life so seriously, even in the middle of a pandemic. But while I enjoy moments of fun, I honor the hospital patients and the medical professionals who care for them. I learned the following lessons from being a health coach in the inpatient orthopedic wing of the hospital and working with physical therapy patients, as well as from being a Stephen Minister and praying with other patients experiencing a variety of illnesses. My hope is that the patients who recover from the coronavirus will find this information helpful as part of the recovery process, while anyone looking for hope during a difficult time can find a passage or phrase which provides comfort.

When stories are shared, sometimes they become open to interpretation. Gilbert (2015) recalls a time when a reader misinterpreted the words she wrote and elaborates, "whatever her emotional motive, though, she had embroidered herself into my story and erased my actual narrative in the process. Strange as it seems, I submit that it was her absolute right to do this. I submit that this woman has the God-given right to misread my book however she wants to misread it. Once my book entered her hands, after all, everything about it belonged to her, and never again to me" (p. 125). Works of literature will always have a variety of perspectives and opinions. The same applies to people's personal narratives. Personal narratives become open to interpretation when reviewing a life story. Looking back, I see how moments in my life led me to my current path.

My dad is a city planner who is one of only several hundred people in the country to have the highest credential in the field. As a kid, I didn't care about my dad's credentials; I loved the field trips. Dad and I would get into the car and drive to study various pieces of land. What did the land look like? What potential did it have? Harper (1996) writes of the city planning process, "as a plan is adopted, the implementation tools must be made available, and their use must be encouraged at the right times and places" (p. 196). The same exact statements apply to health coaching. As clients adopt a plan, the tools to implement that plan must be made available in order for that plan to be successful. The city planning process of survey, analysis, plan, implement, feedback also perfectly describes the health coaching process. When planning a city or planning a person's life, trust the process.

My mom was a teacher, hospital volunteer, and probably would have been a health coach had the training existed when she was helping patients at an Ohio hospital. After her death, I had to write a new story for my life. I chose to find the positive in a devastating experience by helping people as a teacher and health coach. Every time I found myself getting stuck along the road of life, I reminded myself that I was doing exactly what my mom would want me to do by surpassing all of my goals and living my life as a positive person. One of my family members refers to me as a Health Sherpa; Sherpa mountain guides help climbers find their way, but the climbers still have to strap on their backpacks and do the work. It gives me pride to serve as a health coach and help other people surpass their goals. Oprah Winfrey (2014) reminds us, "the hardest experiences are often the ones that teach us the most" (p. 141). I feel I can better walk with others on their journeys because of the journey I lived.

SPIRITUALITY AND HEALTH COACHING

Just like health coaches are not psychologists, they are also not ministers either and cannot take the place of a confidential spiritual counselor if a patient requests a session with hospital clergy. I will always let the patient conversations lead the way. If a patient is receptive to writing or asks to pray, I have the expertise to provide additional resources to the patient. As a health coach, I make referrals to colleagues with other areas of expertise, such as consulting with physical therapists or other medical professionals.

While some patients may prefer to write their thoughts, other patients may prefer to speak their thoughts in prayer. Writing teacher Georgia Heard (1995) states, "all writing is in a sense prayer – a sending out of hope, a thanksgiving, a celebration, a song sent into the wind that we hope someone will hear" (p. 113). Regardless of a patient's religious beliefs, a sense of purpose is something health coaching has in common with spirituality. Spiritual beliefs and health coaching can help people connect the seemingly disconnected threads of their lives and find meaning in them. Haugk (2012) states, "victories are results of many actions well executed; or in other words, victories come as a result of process" (p. 141). If patients have a sense of purpose and can mentally time travel into the future to imagine achieving their health goals, the goals they set become part of their larger life's purpose as they make the choice to heal. Arterburn (2011) explains, "though we acknowledge that there are many ways to be healed, the choice to heal, whether it is physical, spiritual, or psychological, is a personal choice each person must make" (p. 54). Healing becomes a journey.

For patients, the journey to healing involves being vulnerable and finding the courage to share stories with people who can help. Brown (2012) explains, "from the field of health psychology, studies show that perceived vulnerability, meaning the ability to acknowledge our risks and exposure, greatly increases our chances of adhering to some kind of positive health regimen" (pp. 39-40). It becomes easier to share when a patient has a health coach and other compassionate clinicians who listen to a patient's hopes, dreams, and fears without judgment. Hale (2021) describes therapists when observing, "we all need someone to talk to, and we all have things we could use an unbiased person to help us work on" (p. 207). Health coaches are not therapists but do practice the same skills of active listening and not judging. Helldorfer and Moss (2007) remind practitioners, "an integral part of healing is the quality of human contact a patient experiences during the time they are with us" (p. 193). When a patient knows someone accepts his or her story, the next chapter of the story can begin to be written. To some people, this symbolizes a spiritual connection; to others, it means a stronger sense of awareness. Helldorfer and Moss continue, "the spiritual side of life is always present. The spiritual side of life is embedded within, and not separate from, the ordinariness of everyday life" (p. 295). A health coach provides a supportive presence while the client walks through such experiences.

WRITING HEALING NARRATIVES

Research by Pennebaker (1997) revealed, "not only are there benefits to health, but writing about emotional topics has been found to reduce anxiety and depression, improve grades in college, and, as we have seen, aid people in securing new jobs" (p. 40). Pennebaker discusses the health benefits of writing and concludes, "as we have found in many of our studies, you may feel sad or depressed immediately after writing. These negative feelings usually dissipate within an hour or so. In rare cases, they may last a day or two. The overwhelming majority of our volunteers, however, report feelings of relief, happiness, and contentment soon after the writing studies are concluded" (p. 42). Pennebaker and Chung (2010) highlight concrete physical health benefits of Pennebaker's research and elaborate, "writing or talking about emotional experiences relative to writing about superficial control topics has been found to be associated with significant drops in physician visits from before to after writing among relatively healthy samples" (p. 16). Therefore, research demonstrates that writing can heal people not only emotionally but also physically. Evans (2010) reports, "wellness and writing are connected in ways yet to be fully researched and exploited, but the literature of several disciplines declares that for many people wellness and writing are connected in ways useful for emotional, physical, and spiritual health" (p. 3). New discoveries continue to emerge illustrating additional influences of writing on emotional, physical, and spiritual healing. Fallon (2020) elaborates, "writing comes from that place – from the thoughts and feelings you didn't even know you had. The ones buried beneath your consciousness. The ones with the greatest leverage to improve your physical health, to change your habits and patterns, to break old ties, to build new neural connections and forge a new path forward" (pp. 52-53). Writing illuminates a narrative so the writer can process and comprehend it. Once we have a draft of a story, we can decide what needs to be revised.

When illness or injury cause life to feel out of control for patients, writing provides a centering experience and reminds the patient what remains within control, even if the only thing a patient can control becomes perspective. Trusting the first impression in writing feels like praying if the writer chooses a spiritual narrative, or writing may become a practice of processing information and feelings. Goldberg (1986) discusses that when writing, writers need to trust their first impressions and not censor their thoughts because "to do writing practice means to deal ultimately with your whole life" (p. 3). To deal with life means being honest with oneself. As Heard (1995) explains, "in writing, I try to tell the truth" (p. 119). Writers write about an event, but then choose how to interpret their narrative when rereading their stories. An interpretation ranges from positive feelings of acknowledging the story happened and moving forward, to negative feelings of remaining stuck in the story.

Regardless of the writer's attitude, he or she must own the story and write honestly, even if no one sees the story but the writer. Lamott (1994) elaborates, "you set out to tell a story of some sort, to tell the truth as you feel it, because something is calling you to do so" (p. 31). When writers write the truth, it leads to awareness of the stories they tell themselves. Experiencing illness or injury for a patient may last temporarily, or may affect a patient permanently. A year after the pandemic began, medical teams learn about the long term effects of the coronavirus. Whether a patient experiences the coronavirus or another illness or injury, accepting reality becomes important for recovery. Files (2016) explains, "the details that show up when you write may not match those of any of the other players in the drama, but they are your truth" (p. 79). Because each person views a story through the lens of experience, while a story may seem true to the author, a person's subjective interpretation may differ from objective facts. DeSalvo (1999) believes, "for our writing to be healing, we must encounter something that puzzles, confuses, troubles, or pains us" (p. 93). Regardless of whether someone became a patient during the pandemic, the pandemic offers numerous opportunities for writers to wrestle with news stories which puzzle, confuse, trouble, or cause pain. Writing provides a reason to turn off the news for awhile, because it helps to take a break from distressing narratives and feeling empathy overload. Heard (1995) believes, "I do all I can to clear out my life, but in the end there are obligations, distractions, and messes, and I write anyway" (p. 19). Sometimes I don't feel like writing, but it helps to write anyway.

When I don't feel like writing, it helps to not overthink. Goldberg (2000) describes this process as "first thoughts have their own structure, move in their own rhythm, rise full-muscled from the bottom of the mind. They appear and disappear, present themselves and fade away unless we try to smother them, frightened by their power and truth, or smash them into polite second or third thoughts" (pp. 30-31). The first response to a prompt such as "How are you feeling?" is often the truest and most honest response before a person's self-censor can reevaluate and change the perspective. Honesty about true feelings can seem difficult, but becomes necessary for receiving physical, emotional, and spiritual help. Sharp (2000) suggests, "whatever it takes, don't think, don't second-guess, don't edit. This exercise must come as directly as possible from your head to the page, traveling without censorship" (p. 18). I recently reread an old journal entry from the middle of the pandemic. It expressed frustration, anger, hope, and also the desire to let go and turn the things I couldn't control (like the pandemic) over to God. Rereading the intensity of the raw emotion surprised me, but I said what I needed to say at the time I wrote those words so I could continue to cope with pandemic life. Lamott (1994) advises writers, "you need to start somewhere. Start by getting something – anything – down on paper" (p. 25). Brown (2015) agrees, "what you write doesn't have to be a sweeping narrative. It can be a bulleted list on a Post-it note or a simple paragraph in a journal. Just get it down" (p. 86). Writing with strong honesty and pure emotion will continue to help as the world emerges from the pandemic. People will need to continue reflecting on their experiences as the virus subsides, because hope mixes with uncertainty as everyone wonders what life after the pandemic will look like. Faith in a higher power helps during uncertain times.

HEALTH AND SPIRITUALITY

In her medical practice, Rankin (2013) tells her patients that in addition to receiving care from medical providers, they need to do their part in their own healing because "you need radical self-care, not just in your health habits, but in the rest of your life" (p. 163). Writing can encourage patients to process their emotions, help patients set goals for their healing, record symptoms and identify activities that cause pain that can help physical therapists, physicians, or other medical practitioners implement the most effective treatment plan.

When a person writes about how he or she feels both physically and emotionally, the writing illustrates patterns in life and in health. As Sharp (2000) says of writing thoughts and feelings, "this writing does not need to be interesting, or funny, for anybody. Think of it as a record book of your life, day by day.

Assume that no one will ever see them. This will open you up and help the truth to appear on the page" (p. 18). While it is true that writing for an audience of only oneself provides the writer with the chance to vent about feelings, if that writer keeps a pain journal but lacks the medical knowledge to know what the symptoms mean, it becomes time to trust medical professionals and share. Pipher (2006) discusses the value of connection and explains, "writing to connect is 'change writing,' which, like good therapy, creates the conditions that allow people to be transformed" (p. 8). If an individual completes a pain journal of the intensity of pain felt, when it is felt, and what actions were taken when the pain was felt, it keeps that individual from forgetting what to tell a doctor, physical therapist, emotional therapist, or other medical specialist. Stephen Ministers, pastoral care volunteers, and members of the patient's own faith community can discuss feelings of pain with the patient to provide support and spiritual healing.

This type of connection between patient who writes and medical professional who reads and diagnoses can lead to health transformations. DeSalvo (1999) states, "for when we deal with unassimilated events, when we tell our stories and describe our feelings and integrate them into our sense of self, we no longer must actively work at inhibition. This alleviates the stress of holding back our stories and repressing or hiding our emotions, and so our health improves" (pp. 24-25). She discusses the value of sharing writing and elaborates, "when we share our writing, someone else knows what we've been through. Someone else cares. Someone else has heard our voice. Someone else understands. We learn that we are no longer alone and that we no longer need be alone" (p. 213). When faced with pain or illness, an individual may feel scared and alone. A caring person who knows the story and also has the medical expertise to provide help and healing provides a reminder that no one is alone and everyone has someone on his or her team to provide support during the healing journey. A caring person who knows the story and also has the spiritual expertise to provide prayer and comfort provides a similar reminder that no one walks this life's journey alone.

NARRATIVES OF HOPE AND HEALING

Gaining clarity about an experience that occurred, whether a physical pain narrative from a patient or an emotional pain narrative from a person experiencing challenges in life, becomes a step on the path to healing. Seeing thoughts and feelings on paper serves the dual purpose of gaining clarity and releasing feelings. Brown (2015) believes, "writing can be an extremely powerful tool for uncovering the story we're making up" (p. 218). Sometimes people believe a story to be true because they are emotionally connected to it, but writing can help uncover the facts and strip a story down to its basic essence so a person can see if the story is really factually true or emotionally what is perceived to be true. Cameron (1998) states, "I write to tell myself the truth, the whole truth, and nothing but the truth. I write, not to make art, but to make sense" (p. 109). By trusting first impressions when writing, writers learn the truth of what is in their hearts and minds and what they may need to address before moving forward. When people own their stories, they feel more in control of their lives. Brown (2010) believes, "the willingness to tell our stories, feel the pain of others, and stay genuinely connected in this disconnected world is not something we can do halfheartedly" (p. 21). No matter what has happened to in the past, each day brings a new opportunity to write a new chapter in a life story.

Writing does not have to be about a trauma, but for some patients the circumstances that led them to seek medical treatment can feel like a trauma, so it helps to express such thoughts and feelings in writing. Dalebout (2016) explains the most important thing in journal writing is honesty, "but sometimes letting it out is messy. And messy writing is often the most healing writing" (p. 39). My messiest writing often feels like a direct conversation with God. Files (2016) encourages, "let the writing serve its true purpose: to lead you to your truths" (p. 83). Admitting the truth about the stories we tell ourselves leads to accepting the narratives and reframing them if necessary. In her medical practice, Tindle (2013) conducted research about outlook and searched for a way to capture the script her patients told themselves because "if we can briefly slow down our internal dialogue long enough to take a look at it, we gain yet another window into our current outlook in action and catch glimpses of a new outlook" (p. 111). Journal writing helps English teachers determine the stories students tell themselves; consequently, writing provides the same benefit for professionals in the medical field. Writing teacher Cameron (1998) believes, "when there is something we are not telling ourselves, our writing points that out" (p. 140). Therefore, writing helps medical practitioners learn their patients' stories.

Learning the stories patients tell themselves leads to behavior change and empowerment. Bernstein (2016) explains, "our own interpretation determines our perception of the reality we experience" (p. 24). For example, if a patient's writing reflects a negative attitude, a physical therapist, health coach, physician, or other medical professional helps the patient set new goals and rewrite the narrative. Similarly, a Stephen Minister or other spiritual leader walks with a person on the journey of rewriting the narrative.

Writing helps people rewrite their stories and create a next new chapter of health and hope. Tindle (2013) reports, "even the brightest bulbs sometimes flicker. Being an optimist doesn't necessarily mean you're the brightest bulb on the Christmas tree. It means you keep your bulb burning brightly and steadily enough to light up your own path – and maybe the path of others – to better physical, mental, and spiritual health" (p. 72). Rankin (2013) adds, "if you're a pessimist prone to unhappiness, don't despair. According to happiness researchers, things like optimism and happiness can be learned, and you can enjoy the physical and mental health benefits as a result" (p. 138). A positive attitude brings healing benefits and helps people feel hopeful about their healing journeys.

If the stories people tell themselves create stress, writing helps the author craft a new narrative. Enayati (2015) feels perspective can alleviate the stress people experience since "we may have a story of stress that does not serve us, but we have the power to choose our perceptions, to choose different stories, more aligned with reality, that do serve us better. We can choose a narrative that helps reframe the stressors that besiege and overwhelm us as catalysts that become our strengths and guides" (p. 32). People may find themselves stuck in their stories, blaming themselves for what caused their current condition, and making themselves feel worse. Brown (2015) explains, "there's growing empirical evidence that not owning and integrating our stories affects not just our emotional health but also our physical well-being" (p. 67). It therefore becomes important to not only own the story, but demonstrate self-compassion. Brown (2012) explains, "we must also remember that our worthiness, that core belief that we are enough, comes only when we live inside our story" (p. 132). Writing allows for a story to be relived and reinterpreted in order to change the narrative's perspective.

FINDING STRENGTH THROUGH SHARING STORIES

Whatever an individual's story may be, it influences health. Rankin (2013) discusses this issue from a doctor's perspective and elaborates, "when you work in a hospital, you often hear inspiring stories of optimism linked to disease remission and pessimism associated with disease progression" (p. 127). She also observes, "the body is the physical manifestation of the sum of your life experiences" (p. 173). Tindle

(2013) shares this belief that outlook influences health and explains, "we – meaning people in general, but also the larger medical and scientific community – may understand that there is some relationship between outlook and physical health" (p. 14). Rewriting a life story and starting on the path to a healthier lifestyle means people must meet themselves where they are. Individuals must forgive themselves if they aren't happy with their life choices and know the ending of that life story remains unwritten. Brown (2012) discusses her research on shame and vulnerability by explaining, "when we bury the story we forever stay the subject of the story. If we own the story we get to narrate the ending" (p. 80). This means celebrating past accomplishments and taking steps in the present to achieve future goals.

Thinking about a goal already achieved can provide motivation when tackling a new goal. Brown (2010) provides the reminder, "owning our story can be hard but not nearly as difficult as spending our lives running from it" (p. 6). Many people do choose to run from their stories and numb physical and emotional pain with unhealthy results. This behavior causes Brown (2012) to observe, "Americans today are more debt-ridden, obese, medicated, and addicted than we ever have been" (p. 138). Individuals often worry about what other people think. Those individuals may feel the need to be perfect, when just being themselves is more than enough for the people who truly care about them. Each individual should know that the people who deserve to be in his or her life are the ones who will listen to a story while providing acceptance and support, no matter what the story may be. Often people who are perfectionists are harder on themselves than anyone else could ever be. Furthermore, Brown (2010) shares, "the stories of our struggles are difficult for everyone to own, and if we've worked hard to make sure everything looks 'just right' on the outside, the stakes are high when it comes to truth-telling. This is why shame loves perfectionists – it's so easy to keep us quiet" (p. 39). Articulating goals provides strength to achieve them and transform negative thoughts to positive affirmations.

FINDING STRENGTH THROUGH WRITING

People all have moments in life where they feel lost, alone, and uncertain. Whether these feelings exist because of an emotional trauma, ongoing stress, or simply the feeling of having too many things to do and not enough hours to do them, life can feel overwhelming sometimes. Too often, people don't cope with such feelings in a healthy manner. They head to the local bar or the mall and add a hangover or credit card debt to their list of problems. Everyone has a favorite coping mechanism, so why not use writing as a method for processing thoughts and feelings?

Goldberg (2007) discusses the value of writing and says, "you have to speak. That's why you put the pen in your hand to begin with: in order to not blank out or turn your back" (p. 33). Writing provides a method of saying what needs to be said to a blank piece of paper. A notebook won't judge or talk back, thus giving the author the freedom to write anything and everything that may cause stress. Journal writing becomes whatever the author wants and needs it to be. Journal writing might be a schedule of a day to see if the majority of time is spent on activities that do not provide happiness. Journal writing might be a letter to someone who has died or a letter to someone who is alive that will never be sent. Journal writing might be a list of gratitude declaring everything appreciated in life. Journal writing might be a prayer for what is needed. Journal writing might be a list of past accomplishments or future goals. It then becomes the decision of the author whether or not to share the writing with an audience.

People all have things that scare them and things they are afraid to feel. An individual may be afraid to admit he or she doesn't like something about life because then change is required, and this takes courage. Writing, however, brings a sense of control to life. Goldberg (2000) advises writers to put pen to paper and see where the writing leads since, "you keep your hand moving, you stay in there, you move closer and closer to the edge of what scares you" (p. 86). A writer can always write, "I don't know what to write about" until inspiration occurs. Romano (2004) believes, "there is so much in our lives we cannot control. We can, however, control our writing" (p. 218). Admitting feelings is better than locking emotions inside. That creates stress, which leads to health problems.

Writing experts have differing opinions about whether or not writing is a form of therapy. Goldberg (1990) believes, "it's not therapy: it's the root of literature, direct connection with your mind" (p. 69). Conversely, Cameron (1998) counters, "without my writing, I would not have seen this dynamic. If this sounds as if I am saying writing is therapy, let me be clear that I feel writing is something therapy often is not; writing is therapeutic" (p. 94). Regardless, when writing about a difficult issue, it may help to share that writing with someone. Medical professionals will interpret physical symptoms or emotional issues and provide advice for how to help heal. Spiritual guides will provide prayer and hope.

When sharing writing, it helps to find a trusting audience. Sometimes, I finish writing and speak my words aloud for only myself and God to hear. It helps. Lamott (1994) believes the right audience is essential for writers to feel comfortable sharing their writing and suggests, "if you look around, I think you will find the person you need" (p. 171). Finding a person to trust with thoughts and feelings makes sharing easier and helps the confidant provide help after learning the story. In my role as a Stephen Minister, I listen to a person's story without trying to fix anything. A supportive audience helps see patterns in one's life that the author cannot because either the author lacks information or feels too close to the situation to see clearly and achieve clarity. Heard (1995) believes larger patterns emerge when studying seemingly small events because, "by looking at the small, everyday circumstances and happenings, we find ideas to fill volumes" (p. 12). Sometimes small circumstances, whether they result in notes in a journal discussing pain symptoms or observations about behavior patterns, can fit into a larger picture that symbolizes a life story. Cameron (1998) shares, "what writing brings to a life is clarity and tenderness" (p. 83). Writing illuminates events and make sense of them. However, when trying to make sense of a life story, people need to forgive themselves for their mistakes. Everyone makes them, and writing illuminates behavior patterns. Goldberg (1986) shares the reminder, "we have trouble connecting with our own confident writing voice that is inside all of us, and even when we do connect and write well, we don't claim it" (p. 154). It is never too late to make different decisions if existing behavior patterns don't help.

FINDING STRENGTH IN SPIRITUALITY

Believing in something provides hope for endeavors endured in life. As Cameron (2002) explains, "life is what we make of it. Whether we conceive of an inner god force or an other, outer God, doesn't matter. Relying on that force does" (p. 64). When people go through a difficult time, it helps them to know they are not alone in the world. Rankin (2013) discusses the health benefits of spirituality and describes, "in addition to the relaxation responses induced by supportive community, faith in a higher power may also induce positive emotions, which counteract stress and contribute to the state of physiological rest necessary for the body to repair itself" (p. 89). Of course, people don't have to go to church in order to stop and reflect on life experiences. Tindle (2013) calls this practice contemplation and elaborates, "note that contemplative practice, just like the other techniques we're discussing, does not necessarily mean that you instantly feel better. Rather it means that you remain 'sober' enough to see your way to the next step, which may be to exercise or to ask for spiritual help, or identify another way to safely metabolize your tension" (p. 110). Becoming emotionally sober means being aware of thoughts and feelings and most importantly, asking for help when needed. That help may be prayer or a hug from a friend, or the knowledge that life's path does not need to be a solitary journey.

Regardless of an individual's beliefs, the science of healthy living and spirituality can coexist. Alexander (2012) discusses how he reconciled the science of his medical training with his spirituality after he spent time in a coma and believes, "certain members of the scientific community, who are pledged to the materialist worldview, have insisted again and again that science and spirituality cannot coexist. They are mistaken" (p. 73). Similarly, Neal (2012) discusses the connection between spirituality and healing after she reconciled her spiritual experiences with her scientific orthopedic surgery training and elaborates, "although the medical profession has recently, and somewhat tentatively, recognized the spiritual component of healing and of dying, patients have experienced this connection throughout the ages" (p. 25). She continues, "I encountered many patients during my training who wanted to tell me about their spiritual experiences. It was usually done apologetically and with a tone of embarrassment, as they did not want to offend me and did not think 'medical people' would listen or believe. Science and spirituality were presumed to be incompatible" (p. 25). Spirituality leads to individuals feeling more confident, which can lead to increased health.

Often people feel stress when searching for the answers to life's questions. Cameron (2002) feels, "there is a path for each of us. When we are on our right path, we have a surefootedness. We know the next right action – although not necessarily what is just around the bend" (p. 194). Uncertainty about life leads people to look for signs along the way in the form of coincidences as the puzzle pieces of life fall into place. Rushnell (2012) believes that coincidences aren't really coincidences and states, "additional signposts for you, providing you allow yourself to see them, will be godwinks, the messages from above that pop up like little coincidences all along your way" (pp. 149-150). Regardless of personal beliefs, the most important thing is to have faith in something.

FINDING GRATITUDE IN GODWINKS

During the pandemic, I asked questions of God. How did this happen? Why did this happen? The questions seem similar to questions I asked God during other losses in my life. Arterburn (2011) believes, "You lack a unifying understanding of why all these unrelated pieces are hanging together in your life. If so, the choice to serve may be the choice that puts it all together for you" (p. 370). People in various health professions often end up where they are because of their own personal experiences. Often people who have experienced physical or emotional pain in their own lives find careers in healing professions because they want to help others through similar experiences. Once we write new chapters in our own stories, we can turn around and help others on their healing journeys.

Helping others feels counterintuitive; during difficult times I just want to retreat and not leave my house. Demonstrating hermitlike behavior, however, becomes the fastest route to a dark spiral of emotions. Graves (2001) believes, "I've found there is energy in preparing to help others" (p. 39). So I remove my cat from my lap and myself from the couch and try to make a difference. I may not know the answers to all my questions, but I demonstrate the same faith as Hale (2018) who writes, "It was time to accept, once and for all, that God was enough. That my life was enough. That I was enough" (p. 129). Who I am in this moment is enough.

Whenever I attempt to make sense of life, I wonder if I will see a Godwink. Beck (2001) writes that the word synchronicity "is sometimes used to mean a coincidence so remarkable it seems beyond chance" (p. 234). Godwinks are moments beyond coincidences that symbolize signposts from God showing people the right path. Rushnell (2012) defines a Godwink as, "your destiny will not arrive in a limo to pick you up. Determining where you want to go in life is your job. And once you do – once you pull yourself from the curb and head in whatever direction your inner compass is telling you to head – the signposts will unfold…godwinks, all along the way. That's a promise" (p. 73). Godwinks enable people to see patterns in their lives. Godwinks provide hope for people unsure where the path of life may lead next or why certain things happen. Hale (2014) believes, "call it synchronicity or fate or, as I call it, divine order; every moment of your life pushes you toward your greater calling" (p. 12). In a moment we may not know why something happens, but the reason why it happened becomes clear later. During the pandemic, however, I needed to admit some things may not become clear, or maybe I won't know the answers to my questions about why such things happen for a long time.

Writing helps illuminate my purpose in life. Rushnell (2012) writes, "I have a thesis that Divine Alignment, as well as godwinks, occur with greater frequency when you are actively involved in tasks that you believe God wants you to be doing: when you are stepping out in faith heading for what you believe to be your destiny" (p. 129). Faith helped me through the difficult times in my life, but I also possessed the fearlessness to use the pain I felt to inspire others when giving up would have seemed easier. Beck (2012) writes, "count on it: whatever you're suffering is leading you toward your life's purpose." (p. 243). I want to use my experiences to help other people with their journeys. I want to make the lives of other people better because their paths crossed mine. Hale (2015) offers the advice, "I urge you to save some room for the unexpected. Stay open to plot twists, to edits, to rewrites, to uncertainty" (p. 194). Uncertainty feels unsettling, but in literature, moments of uncertainty occur just before the best plot twists.

Despite uncertainty, it becomes important to show love and kindness for other people. Almost everyone has witnessed life change in some way by the pandemic. Goff (2012) shares, "living a life fully engaged and full of whimsy and the kind of things that love does is something most people plan to do, but along the way they just kind of forget" (p. xiii). When the pandemic forced life to change, love mattered. Showing up for my family, even on a video chat, made a difference. I remembered fun and whimsy. I put the holiday decorations back up for my birthday in May, because why not? Why not try to find fun and whimsy and joy and laughter in the midst of sadness? Some days such little moments of joy kept me sane. Goff (2020) reminds, "I want you to become fully awake to your biggest and most worthwhile ambitions by becoming fully awake to yourself and your God-given purposes" (p. xiii). I became even more aware of my purpose as a teacher, because my role in the pandemic could provide students with hope. Helping them find hope helped me find it too. Bob Goff recently gave a video message to my church and asked the question of what you would do with twenty seconds of insane courage. To paraphrase the titles of his books, I would remind myself that love does dream big and I should keep following my life's purpose.

Life feels stressful and chaotic at times, and Godwinks bring order to the chaos, especially during a pandemic. As Heard (1995) writes, "synchronicity draws recognizable patterns on a sometimes chaotic universe. Writers need to pay attention to these synchronistic moments and events" (p. 104). These Godwink moments provide faith that the puzzle pieces of life will eventually fit together, maybe not in the current moment, but someday soon. Zimmermann (2002) reminds us to trust the journey because "the stars have lined up, and we had nothing to do with it. Some call it grace; some call it synchronicity; some call it serendipity; some call it a connection with the divine; some call it coincidence; some call it luck. If we stay open to life, unexpected gifts begin to appear" (p. 160). Sometimes we don't know why things happen. We don't get something we want, or a prayer goes unanswered. But looking back and mapping the Godwinks of an experience can show that perhaps not getting the thing we originally wanted led to something better down the road. Or as Hale (2013) powerfully states, "on the journey of life, sometimes it takes losing our way to find ourselves" (p. 177).

And sometimes losing our way can help us find our greater purpose in life.

ACKNOWLEDGMENT

The preceding chapter contains excerpts from the following previous IGI publications:

Bird, J.L. (2020). Narratives of patient care. In *Using narrative writing to enhance healing* (pp. 157-184). Hershey, PA: Information Science Reference.

Bird, J.L., & Wanner, E.T. (2020). Narratives of spirituality. In *Using narrative writing to enhance healing* (pp. 1-39). Hershey, PA: Information Science Reference.

Bird, J.L., & Wanner, E.T. (2020). Narratives of anxiety. In *Using narrative writing to enhance healing* (pp. 185-237). Hershey, PA: Information Science Reference.

Bird, J.L. (2017). Writing healing narratives. In *Healthcare community synergism between patients, practitioners, and researchers*. Hershey, PA: Information Science Reference.

REFERENCES

Alexander, E. (2012). *Proof of Heaven*. Simon and Schuster.

Arioto, M. (2019). *Have more fun*. Zondervan.

Arterburn, S. (2011). *Healing is a choice*. Thomas Nelson.

Ashcroft, M., & Olsen, R. (2012). *My one word*. Zondervan.

Beck, M. (2001). *Finding your own North Star*. Three Rivers Press.

Beck, M. (2003). *The joy diet*. Crown.

Beck, M. (2012). *Finding your way in a wild new world*. Free Press.

Bernstein, G. (2016). *The universe has your back*. Hay House.

Bernstein, G. (2018). *Judgment detox*. North Star Way.

Bessey, S. (2019). *Miracles and other reasonable things*. Howard Books.

Bird, J. L. (2019). *Prayers in the key of narrative*. Kindle Direct.

Brown, B. (2010). *The gifts of imperfection*. Hazelden.

Brown, B. (2012). *Daring greatly*. Gotham Books.

Brown, B. (2015). *Rising strong*. Spiegel & Grau.

Cameron, J. (1998). *The right to write*. Tarcher/Putnam.

Cameron, J. (2002). *The artist's way* (2nd ed.). Tarcher/Putnam.

Dalebout, K. (2016). *Let it out*. Hay House.

DeSalvo, L. (1999). *Writing as a way of healing*. Beacon Press.

Doyle, G. (2016). *Love Warrior*. Flatiron Books.

Doyle, G. (2020). *Untamed*. The Dial Press.

Enayati, A. (2015). *Seeking serenity*. New American Library.

Evans, J. F. (2010). Introducing wellness & writing connections conference papers. In J. F. Evans (Ed.), *Wellness & Writing Connections* (pp. 3–10). Idyll Arbor, Inc.

Fallon, A. (2020). *The power of writing it down*. Zondervan.

Files, M. (2016). *Writing what you know*. Allworth.

Gilbert, E. (2015). *Big magic: creative living beyond fear*. Riverhead Books.

Goff, B. (2012). *Love does*. Nelson.

Goff, B. (2020). *Dream big*. Nelson.

Goldberg, N. (1986). *Writing down the bones*. Shambhala.

Goldberg, N. (1990). *Wild mind*. Bantam.

Goldberg, N. (2000). *Thunder and lightning*. Bantam.

Goldberg, N. (2007). *Old friend from far away*. Free Press.

Graves, D. (2001). *The energy to teach*. Heinemann.

Hale, M. (2013). *The single woman*. Thomas Nelson.

Hale, M. (2014). *I've never been to Vegas but my luggage has*. Thomas Nelson.

Hale, M. (2015). *Beautiful uncertainty*. Thomas Nelson.

Hale, M. (2018). *You are enough*. FaithWords.

Hale, M. (2021). *Don't believe the swipe*. Revell.

Harper, A. N. (1996). Tooling up for effective planning. In B. W. McClendon & A. J. Catanese (Eds.), *Planners on planning* (pp. 190–198). Jossey-Bass.

Hatmaker, J. (2020). *Fierce, free, and full of fire*. Nelson Books.

Haugk, K. C. (2000). *When and how to use mental health resources*. Stephen Ministries.

Haugk, K. C. (2012). *Christian caregiving*. Stephen Ministries.

Heard, G. (1995). *Writing toward home*. Heinemann.

Helldorfer, M., & Moss, T. (2007). *Healing with heart*. Moss Communications.

Lamott, A. (1994). *Bird by bird*. Anchor Books.

Lyons, R. (2019). *Rhythms of renewal*. Zondervan.

Neal, M. C. (2012). *To Heaven and back*. WaterBrook Press.

Pennebaker, J., & Chung, C. K. (2010). Expressive writing, emotional upheavals, and health. In J. Evans (Ed.), *Wellness and writing connections* (pp. 11–52). Idyll Arbor.

Pennebaker, J. W. (1997). *Opening up: the healing power of expressing emotions*. The Guilford Press.

Pipher, M. (2006). *Writing to change the world*. Riverhead.

Rankin, L. (2013). *Mind over medicine*. Hay House.

Romano, T. (2004). *Crafting authentic voice*. Heinemann.

Rushnell, S. (2012). *Divine alignment*. Howard Books.

Sharp, C. (2000). *A writer's workbook*. St. Martin's Press.

TerKeurst, L. (2020). *Forgiving what you can't forget*. Nelson Books.

Tindle, H. (2013). *Up: how positive outlook can transform our health and aging*. Hudson Street Press.

Winfrey, O. (2014). *What I know for sure*. Hearst Communications.

Zimmermann, S. (2002). *Writing to heal the soul*. Three Rivers Press.

KEY TERMS AND DEFINITIONS

Expressive Writing: Writing that is exploratory and focuses on meaning and first impressions.

Godwink: A moment where synchronicity occurs in the form of a coincidence; instead of being interpreted as a coincidence the event is perceived as a message from God.

Narrative Writing: Writing that shares a story. Narrative writing is frequently told from a first-person perspective.

Spirituality: Regardless of religion, spirituality and a belief in a higher power can lead to increased health and provide both hope and strength for patients.

Writing as Healing: Numerous studies have been conducted investigating the influence of writing on physical and emotional health. James Pennebaker is a leader in the field which explores the health benefits of writing.

Writing Voice: Voice in writing describes how a writer uses word choice and tone when writing a journal entry or other composition that reflects the personality of the writer. Just like each person has a unique speaking voice, each writer has a unique writing voice.

Chapter 10
Reflections of Healing Narratives

ABSTRACT

This narrative discusses research illustrating how writing assists patients in healing from both emotional and physical pain. An English professor and physical therapist collaborated to design a survey that uses writing prompts to assess goal setting for physical therapy patients. Advice for patients, such as keeping a pain journal of symptoms to share with a medical professional, demonstrates how writing helps the healing process while leading to collaboration between a patient and the medical team.

PAIN NARRATIVES

Being a patient feels exhausting. Patients not only experience pain or illness, but also the stress of advocating for effective care while navigating a medical system. While I have not experienced being a patient with the coronavirus, I have witnessed numerous people I know fight the virus. I also saw numerous specialists several years before the pandemic as a patient who eventually experienced remission from the autoimmune disease Sjogren's syndrome. Periodically my neck pain sends me back to physical therapy. Transforming a pain narrative or illness narrative into a narrative of health and healing requires overcoming obstacles. I share the story of my feelings as a patient and the lessons I learned from my experiences to provide inspiration and hope.

PART I: INTRODUCTION TO WRITING AS HEALING (2012)

During the past few years, my life settled into a predictable and comfortable pattern. Each semester my students read wonderful works of literature and created poems, scenes from characters' perspectives, mix CDs, artwork and various other innovative projects based on those wonderful works of literature. They wrote detailed rationales explaining their project choices and shared their masterpieces with classmates on presentation day. This was a day where I always skipped meals because several people in the class

DOI: 10.4018/978-1-7998-9051-5.ch010

usually brought food for a genre connected to the text. My life and teaching progressed in a splendid manner until another twist of fate in my life led me to see multigenre writing as more than an academic research project. Multigenre writing became a way for me to help heal my physical pain. This is a story of using writing as healing told from the perspectives of both the patient and the physical therapist; the lessons learned from this experience led to additional research and advice to help others.

I used the theory of narrative inquiry and the practice of multigenre writing to analyze my story of life as a patient. Romano (2000) argues, "theory about narrative thinking provides scholarly underpinning for multigenre writing" (p, 18). Both multigenre writing and narrative inquiry support the telling of stories as research. They encourage researchers to look not only outward at others but also inward at themselves and hold a mirror to their own lives.

In the qualitative interpretive research field of narrative inquiry, when we tell our life stories to other people, we choose how we frame and share information. We don't just share our stories with other people; for better or worse, the stories we retell ourselves can influence our perception of life. Clandinin and Connelly (2000) explain, "therefore, difficult as it may be to tell a story, the more difficult but important task is the retelling of stories that allow for growth and change" (p. 71). If I keep telling myself the same story, I am never going to change.

During my physical therapy for neck pain, if I told myself the story, "I am in a lot of pain right now," it would force me to dwell on how much I hurt. I needed to rewrite that story as, "I am in a lot of pain right now, but I am getting better." Even though I felt intense physical pain, my goal became to approach each therapy session with a positive attitude and a willingness to complete the lesson plan of exercises designed for me to help me feel better. Connelly and Clandinin (1988) suggest writing down stories and to "keep an open mind and try to see what patterns emerge" (p. 37). When I wrote down the stories of how I felt, it led to the creation of a neck pain journal and a new perspective on healing. For this reason, Clandinin and Connelly (2000) believe that "autobiography and memoir are recognized forms of research texts" (p. 101).

Sometimes, however, we can't see the patterns of our own stories and need others to help us view the story from a new perspective.

THE IMPORTANCE OF WRITING WHILE IN PAIN

My physical therapist, Dr. Eric Wanner, always took the time to answer my endless questions about why my neck felt a certain way and what exercises I could do to make it feel better. He also would not let me get away with telling him I felt fine when I didn't. It helped him plan my exercises and treatment if I assigned my pain level a number at the beginning of each session and gave some examples of what I did between sessions to make the pain feel better or worse.

One particular week I looked at the yellow flurry of post-it notes on which I wrote all my observations about my pain I wanted to tell Eric so I didn't forget anything. When presented with chaos my reaction becomes to organize everything. Because of the pain, just teaching my classes became a large effort leaving me with no energy to write any interesting articles. I missed writing. Cameron (1998) believes, "there is something very right about simply letting yourself write. And the way to do that is to begin, to begin where you are" (p. 5). So I grabbed a sheet of paper and assigned a high and low numeric value to my pain level for each day. I also wrote down what I was doing to cause the pain. Of course, my writing voice needed to shine through on paper. Instead of being content to write, "I did my exercises today,"

I wrote, "9:30pm + home from work late + still need to do second set of exercises = Neck Exercise Disco Dance Party!! Turn on Kylie Minogue CD for motivation and actually have to remind myself to slow down the exercises."

My neck pain journal entertained me, but I couldn't make any sense of why my neck hurt at certain times and not others. I didn't know how Eric was going to react to my writing, but Goldberg (2007) states, "trust what you put down, even if the editor or critic inside you says it's wrong or you made a mistake" (p. 2). In the past I placed drafts of my writing in progress on display for an entire class of students without even thinking about it, so an audience of one physical therapist shouldn't have worried me. This writing, however, seemed more personal. Goldberg (2000) argues, "someone who edits your work – at any level – is giving you their mind, just as in your writing you have given them yours" (p. 189). Sharing my writing required a combination of vulnerability and trust. I couldn't eliminate things, because each piece of the neck pain puzzle might make more sense when all the pieces were examined as a whole.

I gave Eric a copy of my neck pain journal at my next physical therapy session. I don't remember the exact conversation, but it went something like this:

"This is your copy. I decided to write everything down in a neck pain journal."
"I like it."
"Really?"
"Looks like your neck hurts whenever you look down for a long period of time, and when you are under a lot of stress."

It impressed me that within minutes Eric looked over my writing and found a pattern to my neck pain. He adjusted the treatment plan that session and my neck felt better.

FUTURE TRENDS AND FUTURE RESEARCH: ERIC'S PERSPECTIVE

While Jen was a patient of mine, she always expressed her interest in research and how she wanted to do something related to her multigenre writing in a medical type of setting. I myself, have a great interest in research, and thought that this idea could really lead to something positive with my patients. We decided to make this happen and designed a survey together to try to see how patients view different aspects of physical therapy during their treatments. This research is currently being done, but would not be possible if it was not for the writing that Jen did herself.

We both hope to do more research in the future to try to enable people to be able to freely express their feelings during a healing process, and see if it affects their recovery in a more positive way. When patients have a positive view during their recovery the thought is that they will be more willing to do their home exercises, try harder while in physical therapy, and thus accelerate their healing process. Hopefully this will open up the minds of clinicians on how to give each patient the best chance toward a full recovery.

FUTURE TRENDS AND FUTURE RESEARCH: JEN'S PERSPECTIVE

While Eric was my physical therapist we always discussed research and writing. At the end of my treatment, I knew I would not miss the neck pain, but I realized how much I was going to miss those conversations. I enjoy research and my students and I discuss how writing helps people heal emotionally. Until I lived the experience, I didn't realize that expressing my feelings could also lead to physical healing. I also thought this idea could lead to something positive for other patients and like Eric said, we decided to make this happen.

We used Eric's expert knowledge in medicine and mine in writing to design a survey that provides a unique perspective of how patients view their physical therapy treatments. We both hope our current research project leads to more research and more writing that enables patients to share their feelings and enhance the recovery process for each patient.

RESEARCH REFLECTIONS

Eric used Jen's writing to help her heal, and they decided to continue to learn from each other through writing, research, and creating a survey that uses writing to assist the healing process. The survey features both numerical subjective questions, where patients are asked to rate how they feel by circling a number, and written subjective questions, where patients are asked to respond to a prompt by providing a short written answer. The writing prompts are scored using a rubric similar to the rubrics used by writing teachers when evaluating students' papers. The rubric designed to assess patient writing in the survey splits the writing into the technical (specificity of word choice) and artistic (tone of word choice) dimensions of writing. As discussed by Romano (2013), "I divided the rubric in half: a holistic part that was my gut reaction to the paper as a reader who longed to be informed, moved, and carried away by the power of written words" (p. 160). That describes the artistic part of writing. Romano continues, "In the second half of the rubric, I turned my attention to specific parts of the paper I wanted students to write" (p. 162). That describes the technical part of writing.

In designing our research and implementing our survey, we wanted to answer the question if there was a relationship between a patient's positive outlook when writing down his or her feelings and the patient's recovery process. As of this writing our research remains ongoing and we plan to study this topic further, but our initial study revealed that patients who used more positive language when responding to short answer writing prompts on the survey we designed showed higher objective improvements on existing physical therapy measurements such as the DASH (Disabilities of the Arm Shoulder Hand), LEFS (Lower Extremity Functional Scale), NDI (Neck Disability Index), and Modified Oswestry (for back pain). We wanted our research and writing to continue to help the patients at Eric's clinic and the students in Jen's classroom.

Jen

As Eric once said, I help patients learn to conquer fragile moments in life with writing. He helps patients regain the ability to do what they want to be able to do again, and this holistic approach of emotional and physical health intertwines for our unique approach to health education.

I almost didn't write the neck pain journal that started this research story. Patients are supposed to go to medical facilities and follow established protocols, not ask their clinicians to spend extra time reading writing. During each of my physical therapy sessions for neck pain, Eric, my physical therapist, asked me to assign a number to the pain I felt in my neck. I would tell him the number of how I felt that particular moment, but maybe an hour or two earlier I would have said a different number. How was I supposed to remember all those numbers? When faced with a dilemma, I turn to writing. So on a sheet of paper, I wrote not only the number of how I felt at any given time, but also the activity I did to cause me to feel that number. I didn't know Eric well, so I had no idea how he would react if I showed him my journal. I took a leap of faith and shared my writing, because maybe there was something in those notes that could help him solve the mystery of my neck pain. Not only did Eric read every word, he encouraged me to write more and used my writing to adjust my treatment. I never would have healed from physical pain if I hadn't told the story of what was causing my symptoms, and I appreciated that the person who could help me heal wanted to hear my story.

Eric and I discussed academic articles we read during my treatment sessions, and I enjoyed those conversations that made physical therapy actually fun. On my last day of physical therapy, Eric asked me if I wanted to write something about my experiences. Why hadn't I thought of that idea? I'm happy he did. We wrote about my neck pain journal and wondered if my experiences with writing as healing could help other patients.

My mom died young of a carotid artery aneurism. After her death my dad found a journal of possible symptoms she kept and never shared with anyone. I will never know if her story would have ended differently if she shared her writing with someone in the medical field, but maybe I could help other patients rewrite their stories.

My neck pain journal also brought me back to a topic I loved. During my first couple years teaching at Florida Atlantic University, I focused on entertaining my students with various ideas; discussing the connections between Katy Perry's songs and literary inferences became a smash sensation with college undergraduates. I missed research, however, so when I returned to researching writing I rediscovered my purpose in life.

During this process I enjoyed working with Eric, who shared my passion for the topic. Sometimes collaborating with others can be frustrating when people won't complete their share of the work, but working with Eric has been easy and fun because we have the same strong work ethic and dedication to the research. Eric and I brainstormed ideas for the survey we designed and sent emails back and forth. He always responded to my ideas with a combination of positive comments and questions that made me think about more ideas. He even read my long emails that had Roman Numeral subheadings for each topic! We designed a survey we named after ourselves, *The Wanner-Bird Healing Survey for Pain Recovery*. I looked forward to seeing how patients would respond to our combination of numeric and written subjective questions.

Eric

As Jen discussed earlier we had an idea to do research together to collaborate ideas from two different fields. Physical therapists usually look more toward what recent research shows with objective tests and measures, and are just now starting to look at patients' expectations in physical therapy with measures such as the SETS survey (Stanford Expectations of Treatment Scale). Research was performed by Younger, Gandhi, Hubbard, and Mackey (2012) that looked at the expectation patients had in physical therapy (whether positive and negative) called the SETS (Stanford Expectations of Treatment Scale). It showed that patients that had a more positive expectancy did better than patients with negative expectancy (p. 767). With this mentality, patients will be willing to do all of their exercises in physical therapy and have a better chance for a full recovery. Even if one falls just short of the goal, that patient may get to a place he or she never dreamed.

After performing our research, I realized that physical therapists do not use the writing concept as much as they should. With our research, it showed that patients who used more artistic writing scored higher objectively on pre-existing physical therapy measures depending on their body part that was injured. We used the DASH (Disabilities of the Arm, Shoulder and Hand), NDI (Neck Disability Index), Modified Oswestry (for back pain), and LEFS (Lower Extremity Functional Scale) as our objective measures to compare with our survey.

It seemed to be clear that as patients had higher artistic writing scores, they also seemed to be objectively improving at the same rate. Also, patients who set clearer goals for themselves improved the most objectively as well. People seem to perform better when striving to reach a goal. Schunk (1990) discusses research performed where subjects that set higher goals tended to have higher self-efficacy. According to the findings, "when students perceive satisfactory goal progress, they feel capable of improving their skills; goal attainment, coupled with high self-efficacy, leads students to set new challenging goals" (p. 71). Patients also seem to do better with writing by allowing them to truly express how they feel. Becoming more aware of what is helping or hurting their recovery process makes them more accountable to do their recommended home exercises and makes them work harder while in physical therapy.

When we came to this realization, we wrote about our findings and ideas to help others get better with a few publications and presentations along the way. Our goal is to share with as many people as possible our groundbreaking research findings to help them either recover from an injury using our tactics in addition to what the physician recommends, or even in life in general.

When talking about sharing your life with a medical professional it may seem like a crazy idea. Most people believe they don't have enough time to ask their physician or physical therapist questions about their life. Most people allow stress to eat away at them until nothing is left. But what if you actually decided to take the risk like Jen did and discuss pertinent information about your life? When does your pain feel the best? When does your pain feel the worst? These questions are actually key elements for people in the medical field to be aware of in order to find contributing factors to the patient's symptoms. Writing will help bring awareness to your situation prior to your medical visit and is actually very beneficial. It might even remind you to ask certain questions since writing down ideas helps you remember.

As my past patient, Jen actually wrote about her symptoms in a table format when she was feeling at her best and worst each day along with what she was doing at those times. She did not know if it related or not but wrote about it anyway. If she would have only written about some of the times she was feeling bad or good along with what she was doing at those times it would have made it harder for me to see trends in her symptoms. She wrote freely and I was able to modify my treatment program along with making recommendations for her ergonomic factors such as propping papers on a stack of books while grading them to allow her to become pain-free. Writing can lead to healing!

WRITING AS HEALING

Research studies demonstrating that expressing emotional writing can lead to physical healing began with Pennebaker (1997), who conducted a research study that showed "people who wrote about their deepest thoughts and feelings surrounding a trauma evidenced an impressive drop in illness visits after the study compared with the other groups" (p. 34). Fallon (2020) elaborates about Pennebaker's research, "researchers found that even months after the experiment was over, the participants' immune systems were still stronger than their control group" (p. 19). More studies confirmed the results of the original, as Enayati (2015) reports, "study after study bore out Pennebaker's thesis that putting negative experiences into words has positive physical and psychological effects" (p. 73). Brown (2015) adds, "what's important to note about Pennebaker's research is the fact that he advocates limited writing, or short spurts" (p. 87). Short answer responses effectively lead the writer to process emotions and eliminate both physical and emotional stress.

Writing also does not have to be about a trauma to be beneficial to the writer. Pennebaker and Smyth (2016) conclude, "writing can be an inexpensive, simple, albeit sometimes painful way to help maintain our health" (p. 80). The pain they refer to is that sometimes people may feel worse short term after writing if they explore an emotional topic, but long term they feel better by releasing their emotions because "writing moves us to a resolution. Even if there is no meaning to an event, it becomes psychologically complete" (p. 152). Writing can also release physical tension in the body when emotional tension is released onto the page. Files (2016) advises, "so, patients, get out thy notebooks and heal thyselves" (p. 102). Writing provides an outlet to help patients discuss their narratives and help them eliminate emotional barriers that may impede physical healing.

DIALOGUE JOURNALS

One method patients and their medical practitioners can use for writing as healing is through dialogue journals. Unlike a private journal intended to be seen by only the individual writing in it, a dialogue journal is meant to be a written conversation between two or more people. It looks like an email conversation, only on notebook paper. The value of writing conversations is that it gives both authors time to reflect on ideas. Patients and family members can write their questions in a notebook so they do not forget them. The physical therapist or other medical practitioner uses the questions and any other observations to modify the treatment plan if necessary. The patient benefits from writing down their questions between treatment sessions so they don't forget what they what to ask once the therapist arrives. Vacca, Vacca, and Mraz (2014) provide the definition, "as is the case with response and double-entry journals, students keep an ongoing record of learning as it happens in a notebook" (p. 299). Patients are therefore able to track their learning as it takes place so the medical practitioner has a record of progress and family members have a record of insights to help them care for their loved one. As Romano (1987) writes, "readers peer into the writer's very soul" (p. 41). Some people express themselves better in writing instead of speaking. Dialogue journals open the door for such conversations. But during the healing process, the patient needs to trust that a medical practitioner is used to discussing sensitive medical information.

Such support can lead patients and their medial practitioners to exchange ideas in writing. Audience becomes essential for a writer. Negative comments cause writers to put their pages away and never share their words with anyone except themselves; conversely, positive comments can provide a source of encouragement for the writer. Sharp (2000) explains, "you hand your work over to Person X and then wait, hating the waiting, praying for a good review, hoping that Person X will be honest and kind" (p. 136). For Jen, she wanted Eric to be an audience for her writing but also needed to be her own audience and reflect on what she was feeling. In this way, writing is a mirror that reflects a writer's true feelings. Goldberg (2000) argues, "writing is an immediate mirror: it reports back to you. You can't fool anyone, especially yourself" (p. 218). Sharing writing takes risk. A writer never truly knows how an audience will react until the words are shared. Jen found the courage to share her neck pain journal with Eric. He not only read it but liked it and found a pattern to her neck pain. She felt better, and he encouraged her to write more while modifying his treatment plan to best help her. Jen and Eric enjoyed their collaboration, and it became the first chapter in a longer narrative.

ERIC'S REFLECTIONS

One idea seemed to branch off to another until something beneficial to all patients was made for the medical setting. We truly reached a milestone in the medical field with this survey and I strongly believe that it will lead to much more research in the future. This survey has true potential to help others during their recovery process by getting the results that they are striving for. This survey allows others to freely write throughout their physical therapy sessions and be more self-aware of why they are feeling the way they are. It implements accountability that the patient must assume to get optimal results. It allows the patients to set goals knowing that if one strives for a very strong goal, coming just short of it could lead to miraculous results. It allows the physical therapist to look over the patient's thoughts on paper that they may not divulge to the therapist in regards to: how they are currently feeling, how close they feel they are to reaching their goals, and any barriers they may perceive which could prevent them from achieving their goals at a set time.

This survey is unique since it is the first time a physical therapist and an English professor came together and designed a survey for a physical therapy clinic in hopes that it could facilitate patients' full recovery in addition to normal physical therapy sessions. This entire process that Jen and I had to go through was time consuming, yet easily manageable with us both sharing a strong work ethic in this project and having the passion to make sure it would be a success. We both want to help as many people as possible in life. With physical therapy I help the patients regain the ability to do what they want to be able to do again, and Jen helps patients learn to conquer fragile moments in life with writing. Combining our thoughts into a survey I believe, is a very holistic approach for all patients in the physical therapy world.

I truly believe there is more to a patient than just pain and what they can do; the patient's personality and what they are going through in life must be accounted for, and I think our survey does a good job with this. We are both aware that we cannot discuss our thoughts with everyone individually in the physical therapy clinics, but knowing that the survey has the potential to help is fulfilling.

After rereading what Jen and I wrote, I always think of how I can best transfer this style into my practice. I became a better clinician doing this, realizing that if I allow a patient to truly express themselves to me, they will be more willing to listen to my advice and be more compliant with their physical therapy exercises. If patients are more compliant with their exercises for physical therapy it allows them to have a quicker recovery time and leads to elite results. Our survey allows for this to happen even when the clinic is very busy. It allows patients to be more at ease, while simultaneously assessing where they currently are and what goals they want to achieve. I believe that writing helps people express how they truly feel with less pressure put on them. Writing helps people set goals that they can strive for and achieve. Writing helps people come to realizations of certain things that could be affecting their health and their recovery process. Writing helps show one's true personality and how an individual is able to cope with different elements in life. Hopefully our survey will transfer over into all clinics for physical therapy and allow everyone to have the chance to really strive for their goals! Hopefully it will lead to several more research studies as well as showing the importance of patient goal setting in the medical field!

JEN'S REFLECTIONS

I'm proud of us and this research! We designed a survey about goal setting for patients. We also set our own goals for our research, achieved them, and worked very well together. It was fun for me to see how we challenged each other in positive ways to do our best work. I knew Eric shared my dedication to the project, so whenever he thought of a wonderful idea it motivated me to develop my own wonderful ideas too.

I also appreciated how we listened to each other's ideas. We learned from each other. I found myself caring more about medicine because Eric felt passionate about it, and I hope my passion for writing inspired him too. I felt free to create because I always knew Eric would do his part of the work. Because I knew someone else depended on my contribution to the project, I was never going to give up on this research. We spent a lot of time working on this, but when something is fun it doesn't feel like work at all and that's the best part.

I loved it when Eric wrote that I help patients conquer fragile moments in life through writing. During the difficult times in my life, I viewed writing as a type of therapy. Writing about my experiences helped me process my thoughts and feelings. I also had the opportunity to witness my students experience the same writing process. In class, I give students writing prompts on various topics and time to write. Students enjoy the writing time, but more important to them is the sharing time, when they can choose to share what they wrote with their classmates. The sharing times built class community and provided a comfortable environment for discussion.

If I asked my students to share, I needed to share too. Sharing takes courage, but I discovered my writing meant more to me when I shared it than when I just left it in my notebook with myself as the only audience.

Eric helps his physical therapy patients return to what they want to do again not just by providing them with appropriate exercises that are well researched, high level manual skills as needed, and a treatment plan, but also by taking the time to learn their life stories. Writing is a way for people, whether they are students in my classroom or patients at Eric's clinic, to share their life stories. By writing, the authors of the stories often see events from a different perspective, just like Eric and I have a different perspective on our writing after rereading our original conversation with each other.

PART II: CONNECTING MULTIGENRE WRITING TO MEDICINE (2014)

I experienced both physical and emotional tension when I began experiencing migraine headaches two years after writing the original chapter about my neck pain journal. I had just started my health coach certification program at Duke Integrative Medicine. The irony was that I was training to counsel patients on dealing with their own health issues while experiencing one of my own. I was supposed to be listening to the stories of other people, not adding another one of my stories to the collection. How I viewed my story would influence my healing.

JEN'S JOURNAL

I cannot believe I am going to be a physical therapy patient again. The irony is that I have no neck pain, but I can't live with these migraines. My cousin Robin asked if stress was causing them, but I'm relaxed and content with my life. Seriously, in the past few days I've made egg salad, a pizza, a vegetable dish, and an apple crisp. When I create edible meals it means I am not stressed. Since Eric is now working at the hospital he can't be my physical therapist, so he is recommending that I see his colleague Ryan. I'm really hoping this pain doesn't get so bad that I end up in the hospital, although there were a couple nights when my head hurt bad enough to consider it. Ryan was Eric's student awhile ago and Eric has complete confidence in Ryan's ability to relieve my symptoms. Robin's going to physical therapy with Ryan too so we will have fun (and provide Ryan with hours of entertainment) scheduling our physical therapy sessions together and cheering each other on when doing exercises. It's exciting knowing that I will be going to a very good physical therapist in a clinic right across the street from where I live. There are too many other patients Eric and I need to save with our research and writing for me to be in the hospital! Although Eric and Ryan are constantly reminding me I need to take care of myself before I take care of other people. The weird thing is that my original neck pain journal led to this research and writing journey, but now I can't even keep a pain journal. The pain is ALL THE TIME! AHHHHHH!!!!

Now if only I could sleep……

BACK TO SLEEP

Lucy the cat knows
Whenever Jen can't sleep, Lucy is there
She curls up next to her person and starts purring
Lucy's brother Andy runs around in a circle chasing his tail
He stops his game and joins Lucy to start a chorus of purrs
Jen's breathing slows and for a moment forgets her pain
Thanks to pet therapy

ANIMALS PROVIDE COMFORT

Dr. David Dosa, a geriatrician, witnessed the story of Oscar the cat when checking on patients at a nursing home. Oscar, a cat who lived in the nursing home, sensed which elderly patients were the sickest and about to die, so he would visit their rooms, curl up next to them on their beds, and provide comfort. Dosa (2010) reports that "I'd like to think Oscar embodies empathy and companionship. He is a critical cog in a well-oiled and dedicated health care team" (p. 218). Animals may not have medical training, but they know when they are needed.

ERIC'S PERSPECTIVE

The beauty of this situation by having Jen go through these symptoms, she will have more of an understanding what my patients may be going through when coaching them. Having an understanding of what patients feel versus memorizing from a textbook what they should be feeling makes a significant difference. If patients understand that you went through a similar situation that they are going through, they will be much more willing to listen what you have to say and actually be compliant for what you recommend. Jen will also be able to explain things more accurately from a firsthand perspective. Will writing about headaches always cure it? No. It depends on the situation for what's causing it, but it could lead to physicians and physical therapists making more accurate diagnoses for the patient. On top of that, when patients write about their symptoms including their outlook it has been shown to decrease their stress levels, increase self-awareness, and increase goal setting which in turn can speed up their recovery process. This eclectic approach is where healthcare should be going.

JEN'S PERSPECTIVE

Healthcare does need an eclectic approach. The Wheel of Health from Duke Integrative Medicine (2010) encourages patients to reflect on multiple dimensions of health including movement, exercise and rest; nutrition; personal and professional development, physical environment; relationships and communication; spirituality; mind-body connection; and mindful awareness (p. 5). This makes health become a comprehensive plan that focuses on the person, not just the disease. I didn't want to be a patient and experience pain again, but it is amazing seeing both sides of the story from perspective of patient and health coach. It is going to make me a better clinician. Eric and I have learned about the power of writing to influence healing from our research. I love that I am going to be able to use my writing training to help patients in a clinic as well as students in a classroom. However, I've learned that writing is not the only answer. My cousin Robin loves writing, but music motivates her more. So a "PT CD mix" of music to motivate her to do her at home exercises inspired her more than a journal. Other patients may want to use painting, watching sitcoms, or reading an inspirational book as resources to help them heal. I also had to adjust my own expectations. With my original neck pain journal, I wrote information that helped Eric find patterns to my pain. With my migraines, creating that style of journal didn't work because the headaches were constant, so my notes to Ryan about how I felt after each physical therapy session helped him the most. Clinicians achieve success with treatment plans by individualizing them for each patient.

ACROSTIC POEM ABOUT MIGRAINES

Maddening
Intolerable
Gigantic
Relentless
Agitating
Inflexible
Nonstop

Endless

CONVERSATIONS IN PHYSICAL THERAPY CLINICS

In order for physical therapists to effectively treat patients, it helps them to know their patients' stories. This helps the physical therapist properly diagnose patients, determine their prognosis, and development an appropriate intervention. By learning patients' stories, physical therapists can also help patients set goals. Randall and McEwen (2000) discuss the value of physical therapists collaborating with patients to write patient-centered functional goals and elaborate, "physical therapists who incorporate a patient-centered approach to writing functional goals may see a change in how they interact with their patients and the decisions they make regarding patient care. Therapists may spend more time getting to know their patients and the self-care, work, or leisure activities that are important to them" (p. 1202). Clinicians need to believe in the value of goal setting and take time to discover a patient's story. When the patient sets out goals it brings them more onboard to achieving them and increases accountability for the patient.

Most patients want to know that their clinician understands them and cares about them as individuals, not just names on charts. As Croft (1980) explains, "the therapist does not need to accept each patient's beliefs and values as his own in order to be empathetic toward that patient. What is important is that the patient has something to say that is important to him at that time. The therapist, then, needs to convey to the patient that nothing at the moment is more important to him than listening to and helping the patient as much as possible" (p. 1034). Because when a patient is in pain, having an empathetic clinician who listens becomes essential. This can also increase the patient's outlook for their recovery process, allow the patient to become more optimistic, work harder at reaching their goals, and increase their compliance. All of those combined leads to a quicker recovery!

HEADACHE JOURNAL

For any patient in pain, it can help clinicians make a diagnosis if the patient keeps a journal of symptoms. Dr. Hagen and the Mayo Clinic Staff (2001) recommend that for recurrent headaches, keep a headache diary and include the following factors: severity, frequency and duration, related symptoms, location, family history, and triggers (p. 83). But don't feel you need to follow a specific format if a different writing style works for you.

JEN'S JOURNAL

Pain free for four days after Wednesday's PT session!!! Yay!!! Dull headache started Sunday after church when I looked down while praying (oh, the irony…..) I know the fast neck movement triggered it, but it is still only a dull ache instead of a sharp pain. Have not needed pain medicine indomethacin in a week and this morning neurologist said that if the cortisone shot and PT is working I can stop taking pain medicine unless needed. I forgot what it is like to be pain free!!!

AND IN THE END

Jen and Robin both healed from their pain with Ryan's help. Jen and Eric worked at the same hospital and researched the benefits of health coaching for physical therapy patients. Concluding a narrative inquiry feels similar to leaving the theater before the end of a play, but then the researcher must have faith there will be other stories to tell and other chapters to write.

PART III: JEN'S REPRISE OF PAIN IN A HAIKU (2019)

Wake up with headache
Occipital neuralgia
Pain journal again
And in the Beginning

Occipital Neuralgia. Inflamed nerves which cause headaches. Once again, my headaches and neck pain required medical attention. This time, however, an MRI scan revealed a herniated disc in my neck which also pressed on a nerve. Hence, the headaches and neck pain. Usually I feel positive, but this seemed overwhelming. I followed the advice of Arioto (2019), who believes, "life is short, too short to spend our time dwelling on mistakes or what we don't have. Too short to feel like a shell of a human being, going through the motions but never really living" (p. 175). I needed to stop dwelling on the pain and start focusing on my treatment plan to fix it. But first, I had to find the energy. Graves (2001) feels, "emotional roller coasters demand energy – high energy – and you need to know how to maximize what gives you energy and minimize what takes it away" (p. 2). Graves discusses teaching in this example, but the same words apply to dealing with a complicated medical situation. I knew I had minimum energy when going to various medical specialists; I knew I had maximum energy when writing. So it made sense to balance something that gave me energy with something that took it away.

Because I had a complex case, I needed to become a prepared patient. In her nursing career working with patients, Goldberg (2019) advises, "a provider's license to practice medicine does not mean that they know you or your body best. They will come to better decisions about how to use their expertise if you meet them in making decisions about your health" (p. 7). So I made the decision: *All right, medical professionals. You will see me. You will know me.*

I chose a new journal, one with black and gold sequins, and started taking notes. When discussing writing as healing, Pennebaker (1997) states, "planning to show your writing to someone can affect your mind-set while writing" (p. 41). Throughout my years of teaching, I watch my students write with more confidence if they practice writing techniques in their journals before showing me the final draft of their essays. Writers write differently when we know we will share our writing. Pennebaker continues, "from a health perspective, you will be better off making yourself the audience. In that way, you don't have to rationalize or justify yourself to suit the perspective of another person" (p. 41). In the case of my pain journal, however, I needed to share it so the medical providers I saw could help me. I wrote my notes in my black and gold sequined journal, typed up the relevant information, and handed it to the receptionist at each medical office. I also kept a copy for myself and I took notes during each appointment. I felt like Niequist (2016), who writes, "brave is articulating my feelings, especially when the feelings are sad or scared or fragile instead of confident or happy or light" (p. 126). Sharing writing made an emotionally and physically painful process easier. I felt scared, but I refused to let my health issues define me.

JEN'S JOURNAL

It's exhausting having a low grade headache all the time, in addition to neck pain. When I finished physical therapy the last time, I thought that would be the end of needing physical therapy. I'm learning that life, like healing, is a journey. I love being a high school writing and reading center director and don't feel stressed, but my neck is telling me a different story. I'm grateful to be at the clinic where Eric is a director working with an outstanding physical therapy team of Dak and David. My new neck pain bullet journals are entertaining Dak, and the entire clinic team creates a fun environment for doing exercises.

HAIKU OF REVELATION

Journal advocate
But when a patient in pain
Writing takes effort

MOMENT OF INSIGHT

For fun, I answered the survey questions Eric and I designed and compared it to my responses when I had headaches five years ago. Interestingly, I wrote similar responses.

August 2014: For the question of being close to achieving my short term goals, I circled a 3 (in the middle) for the numerical subjective question and for the written subjective question wrote: "My goals are still to be healthy and free of migraines! I am optimistic I can follow the treatment plan and get there."

August 2019: For the question of being close to achieving my short term goals, I circled a 3 (in the middle) for the numerical subjective question and for the written subjective question wrote: "I still have the goal of being pain free and realized healing takes time."

Later, when asked to identify obstacles, I admitted (both then and now) I needed to relax. I found it interesting that while my numerical responses stayed the same, my narratives changed slightly. My writing five years ago was more optimistic than my recent writing, but maybe too optimistic? Maybe I'm more realistic now? Since Eric and I designed the survey, more patient education exists about the value of narratives. As a medical practitioner, Goldberg (2019) advises patients, "it's helpful to create a narrative or story around the situation prior to going to the appointment. This will give your symptoms context and provide meaning to the timeline, and you'll naturally equip your provider with key information you may not even realize is relevant" (p. 123). She advises practitioners, "it is vital for medical providers not only to hear but also to help create their patients' narratives" (p. 168). When patients find the courage to share their narratives and when medical practitioners demonstrate the compassion to listen, the collaboration can help the patient's healing process.

Sharing narratives illuminates contributing factors which may interfere with healing. When I reread my journal, I notice I used words like "exhausting" and "stressed" twice as much as words like "grateful." Evidence exists to illustrate the influence of environmental and social factors on stress. As medical doctor Harding (2019) explains, "the essentials of health start with recognizing the role of the hidden factors on stress and their impact on physical and mental health" (p. 143). Looking over my recent pain journal, I finally saw how the puzzle pieces fit together. Fallon (2020) explains, "the reason writing is such a powerful tool for change is because it helps us begin to see things more objectively than we've been able to see them before" (p. 96). My pain journal discussed my symptoms, but what if I looked closer at contributing factors? Harding (2019) elaborates, "here is what I wish I had known when I was starting in medical school and life: our social conditions (hidden factors) profoundly shape our physical and mental health. Kind and loving choices that support emotional well-being and reduce stress may help prevent or delay the onset of many diseases" (p. 193). Paying attention to contributing factors won't replace my physical therapy exercises in helping me feel better, but if I repeat unhelpful stressful life patterns, I won't receive the maximum benefit from the exercises. As Harding (2019) believes, "when new mental or physical symptoms arise, we can check in with ourselves as a first step" (p. 163). And it also helps to share my thoughts with my medical team.

While writing mostly helped me, it also caused me to occasionally overanalyze my symptoms. I needed to remind myself that expressive writing, just like physical therapy, does not involve control but instead trusting the process.

JEN'S JOURNAL

Finally, I can see some hope. Each day, I now have a few headache free hours. I do my exercises at my school's clinic on the days I don't have physical therapy. I'm experimenting with different ways to carry books and papers through the school hallways. My goals are to be pain free and avoid surgery, so I need to commit to lifestyle changes.

JEN'S JOURNAL (A FEW WEEKS LATER)

Tuesday was first headache free day in five months!!!

I'm getting my life back – honestly forgot what it felt like to be pain free!!

JEN'S JOURNAL (A FEW WEEKS LATER)

Overall the best week yet as far as pain levels. No pattern to anything, so I have to stop overanalyzing what might be causing the pain.

Pain level is tolerable if I had to live with it but my goal is still to be pain free!

CONSULTING A MEDICAL PROFESSIONAL

Writing about thoughts and feelings can relieve stress because of the act of putting emotions on paper instead of holding them inside. As Pennebaker (1997) discusses, "although not a panacea, writing can be an inexpensive, simple, and sometimes painful way to help maintain our health" (p. 197). While writing can lead to healing, at times it may feel painful to explore certain topics. People may find themselves writing about an emotional issue that is traumatic, or a physical issue where the symptoms seem confusing. Individuals who have those feelings should share them with someone who can provide help. Nothing a person can read or write will take the place of a conversation with a supportive medical professional.

As the editor-in-chief of *The Merck Manual of Medical Information*, medical doctor Berkow (1997) cautions, "no book can replace the expertise and advice of health care practitioners who have direct contact with a patient" (p. v). Sometimes people may attempt to provide self-diagnosis by reaching for a book or a computer, but that might lead to incorrect information or unnecessarily scary information. The best way to alleviate any concerns is to share them with a doctor, physical therapist, or other medical professional. As medical doctor Rankin (2013) discusses, "patients get well, at least in part, because they believe in the power of modern medicine and expect to feel relief when they see doctors and other health care specialists they trust" (p. 40). It becomes essential for patients to trust their medical professionals. Don't be embarrassed by what a doctor might think. Medical professionals want to help their patients heal, but they can't help if they don't know all the symptoms.

Everyone has a story. Brown (2010) believes, "if we can find someone who has earned the right to hear our story, we need to tell it." (p. 40). Supportive medical professionals earn the right to hear their patients' stories by providing valuable advice; similarly, patients trust their medical professionals to listen to their stories and put the pieces of health puzzles together. Brown (2012) encourages sharing with a supportive audience "because sharing appropriately, with boundaries, means sharing with people with whom we've developed relationships that can bear the weight of our story" (p. 46). If people develop a strong collaborative professional relationship with doctors and other medical specialists in their lives, those medical professionals will take any detail of the stories shared with them to provide support and information for their patients to feel happier and healthier. As Graves (2001) states, "it is in the giving of energy that energy returns to us" (p. 175). Energy given with a record of symptoms for a doctor leads to energy returned in the form of improved health.

PART IV: REFLECTIONS ON RESEARCH (2020)

At the commencement of my writing as healing odyssey, I could not predict the amount I would learn on my journey to become pain free from neck pain I also could not predict the new insights I would have about previous research when becoming a patient again: People feel vulnerable when sharing stories with others, pain changes patient perception, bullet points provide reflection for people who prefer not to write journal entries, it becomes essential to find your motivation, and practicing self-care becomes necessary when feeling pain.

VIBES

I realized I could control the vibe I gave during treatment. In theory, I should act calm whenever I walked into an exam room. In practice, I would sometimes act stressed and anxious. To remember the lessons I learned when confronting chronic pain, I used the acronym VIBES.

Vulnerability helps you.
Identify your emotions.
Bullet journals share information.
Embrace your why.
Self-care matters.

PATIENT LESSON #1: VULNERABILITY HELPS YOU

As a patient, I needed to be my own best advocate. Yes, this specialist is recommending that treatment, but is it the best thing for me? Agreeing to have an occipital nerve block injection in both sides of my neck caused fear with the procedure, and more fear when I still felt pain. Goldberg (2019), a nurse, explains to patients, "vulnerability and distress intensify when we don't know the source of the pain, the symptom, or the side effect" (p. 159). Each time I needed to share my story, I needed to find the courage to share my story. Seeking medical help means being vulnerable. Sitting on an examination table while having my reflexes tested and often having to wear a medical gown does not instill the same confidence I feel when sitting behind my classroom desk, looking professional while wearing my sassy high heels and feeling ready to conquer the world (or at least whatever student dramas unfold that day).

Writing teacher Romano (2015) believes, "in writing we seek to capture some of this experience of living" (p. 4). While those of us who are English teachers see the value of narratives in our lives and our classrooms, most people who seek medical help do not share an English teacher's perspective on writing. It takes vulnerability to share writing with others, whether the person reading the writing is an English teacher looking through a student's journal in a classroom or a physical therapist looking over a patient's insights about pain in a clinic.

Vulnerability often prevents people from speaking, even if they know that sharing information will help them. In her research as a social worker, Brown (2007) describes times when people have told her they share too much with someone and later regret "what I call the vulnerability hangover. The vulnerability hangover directly relates to our fear of vulnerability, and unfortunately, most of us have experienced it" (p. 206). If someone showed vulnerability in the past and experienced rejection, the person will feel even more vulnerable when sharing again. I experienced a moment of vulnerability hangover when I shared my original neck pain journal with Eric, my physical therapist. My thoughts at the time: I have just shared with this physical therapist more about my life than he probably ever wanted to know. Fortunately, Eric responded as a compassionate clinician and actually encouraged me to share more. Anyone on the receiving end of writing needs to demonstrate compassion or the writer will no longer want to share. I feel grateful Eric demonstrated compassion with me as a patient, and I remind myself to demonstrate compassion with my students as a teacher.

PATIENT LESSON #2: IDENTIFY YOUR EMOTIONS

As a patient, I didn't always feel positive. I knew a positive attitude would help me heal, although sometimes pain makes positivity difficult. Physical and emotional pain can eclipse other feelings. Dooley (2019) writes, "I want to live my story, even the hard and long and messy days" (p. 211). I needed to accept the difficult days in addition to the happy ones and give myself permission to feel what I felt.

Making sure to monitor that my mood did not cross into depression, I accepted the occasional sad days and knew some days I would feel happier than others. A medical explanation exists for this as Rankin (2013) explains, "the stress response also reduces serotonin, the most important neurotransmitter responsible for a positive mood" (p. 134). When I feel pain, my internal narrative resembles the following: I'm in pain. Why won't the pain go away? This is so annoying! Therefore, pain clouds my judgement even when I know to maintain a positive attitude, seek medical attention, and write my symptoms so I can help my doctor help me. According to Tindle (2013), one change makes a difference because, "regardless of how dark our own health situation has been and regardless of for how long, even the spark of one idea to do things differently can light our path to better health" (p. 134). So once again, vulnerability becomes necessary because if I can't find the optimism and courage to make that change, I need to ask for help and lean on others to serve as the light in the dark as I progress through my healing journey.

Feeling gratitude keeps me grounded and improves my mood. As Brown (2012) shares from one of her studies, "research participants consistently described both joyfulness and gratitude as spiritual practices that were bound to a belief in human connectedness and a power greater than us" (p. 123). Stopping in the moment of pain to appreciate the red Poinciana flowers on the tree outside my window or the two purring cats, Lucy and Andy, who sit next to me and play with their toy mice as I write these words can be enough to interrupt my negative pain thoughts and redirect them into more positive ones. Anything that provides even a little bit of light or joy, whatever that may be for you, can be enough to get you through the day until you feel better.

PATIENT LESSON #3: BULLET JOURNALS SHARE INFORMATION

As a patient, I learned I did not have much of a doctor's time. Therefore, as much as I liked narratives and sharing my story, I needed to quickly get to the point. My new pain journals contained bold headings and bullet points describing my medical history and symptoms. The specialists I with whom I shared them found the notes helpful because of the details and context.

When rereading the original notes that Eric and I completed, I noticed we used the process of bulleted, organized lists now known as dot journals. According to Wilkerson Miller (2017), "dot journaling helps you record all of the things that are going on in your life, and makes it easy to keep track of everything you want to do in the future" (p. 8). Our note system helped keep track of current patient symptoms and future goals. Since the original research, dot journals, also known as bullet journals, experienced growth in popularity. Carroll (2018) describes a bullet journal as, "it will help you get organized by providing simple tools and techniques that can inject clarity, direction, and focus into your days" (p. 11). Bullet journals provide another resource for patients, since the writer completes a bulleted list instead of a longer narrative in a journal. Patients might find completing a bullet journal easier because it does not take as much time and looks more like a list than a written narrative. Some patients may feel more comfortable sharing observations in a list format.

PATIENT LESSON #4: EMBRACE YOUR WHY

As a patient, I needed to find reasons to stay motivated. Knowing why you want something, not just what you want, leads to achieving a goal. Hollis (2019) explains, "you have to have the leverage – you have to know your why – or you will never make change. You have to know what to focus on, or you will never make progress" (p. 107). I knew my why: I want to kick this pain into oblivion and be healthy so I can do the things I love to do with my family and friends. I needed to keep that goal in front of me on the days when I felt frustrated or the pain felt worse. Soukup (2019) believes, "it's not enough to set big goals; we have to know why they're important to us. Because truthfully? If you don't know your why, your reason may not justify the sacrifices you need to make to get there" (p. 148). The why of this writing and research journey started as a way to help me cope with the emotional pain of losing my mom and later the physical pain in my neck joints. It would have been enough that my writing helped me. But what if my writing could help other people through difficult experiences?

My sense of purpose transformed into using my passion for writing to help others. Leonard (2018) describes her writing experience as, "I picked up my journal to write down thoughts that had come to me while I was walking. My journaling started as random words, disconnected thoughts, and sometimes even sketches. But after a couple days, my thoughts were beginning to take shape" (p. 224). The description of my journal would sound similar, but what if I found the courage to share and find a narrative thread to my random thoughts? I find the courage every day I teach to discuss writing with students; maybe other people would listen too. Hollis (2018) advises people going through pain, "you are a warrior because of the trials you are going through, but don't you dare squander the strength you have earned just because the acquisition of it was painful. Those are the most important stories to share" (pp. 68-69). If my story inspires someone else, the pain I lived through will have purpose and the power to provide comfort for others as they write their narratives.

PATIENT LESSON #5: SELF-CARE MATTERS

As a patient, I needed to let myself feel a range of emotions. I would feel confident when sharing my story in a medical office, but break down and cry when I returned home. I would feel energetic when swimming in the pool to loosen my muscles, but exhausted and needing to rest an hour later because of a headache and neck pain. Soukup (2016) provides the reminder, "we discovered that while we often think balance is something we can do, balance actually happens when we stop doing and just rest" (p. 180-181). I gave myself permission to remove items from my calendar. I became determined to create positive moments during the time I felt well. I invited my dad, stepmom, aunts, uncles, and cousins over for an indoor picnic. I laughed, I cried, and I prayed.

While I respond to others with compassion and appreciate when I receive compassion, I am my own worst critic and don't always show myself compassion. Neff and Germer (2018) elaborate, "although a simple way to think about self-compassion is treating yourself as you would treat a good friend, the more complete definition involves three core elements that we bring to bear when we are in pain: self-kindness, common humanity, and mindfulness" (p. 10). When I am in pain, it feels difficult to remain present, know that other people experience pain too, and show myself kindness. On some days, I feel I still need to learn the value of being kind to myself and practicing self-care. Pink (2018) explains, "imagine what someone who cares about you might say. He would likely be more forgiving than you" (pp. 143-144).

He adds, "but mix understanding with action. Add a few sentences on what changes you can make to your life and how you can improve in the future" (p. 144). Whether setting a goal for a physical therapy treatment plan or another part of life, it becomes important to combine reflection with action.

Eric once told me to "think like a turtle." Similarly, writing often takes time to work. Grant (2016) elaborates, "James Pennebaker has demonstrated that expressing our thoughts and feelings about a stressful or traumatic event is most salutary after we've had some time to process the event, when we're not blinded by anger or consumed by distress" (p. 240). Trying to write in a journal after an injury, life changing event, or other emotional experience may not be effective because processing an event takes time. I couldn't write anything immediately after my mom's death, and I did not arrive with a pain journal during my first physical therapy session with Eric. Writing became part of my emotional and physical healing only after I began to process the original trauma. Sandberg and Grant (2017) explain, "immediately after a tragedy or crisis, journaling can backfire: the event is too raw for some to process" (p. 63). Pain often prevents a person from writing. So if writing doesn't initially work, the pain may be too new; put the notebook down for awhile and pick up a pen again when ready.

PART V: FULL CIRCLE (2021)

Seeing my words in front of me reminded me to stay optimistic about my healing journey and stress less about the process. Dalebout (2016) reports the existing foundation of research as, "though we've witnessed the power of the mind in healing the body again and again in numerous studies on the placebo effect, we still often forget the supremacy of our beliefs" (p. 154). Granted, I couldn't just meditate and write my way to being one hundred percent pain free without the help of my physical therapy team because positive thoughts and a notebook wouldn't change the herniated disc in my neck and my occipital neuralgia. But I will, however, use methods that help me relieve stress in addition to my home exercise plan. Bernstein (2014) believes, "as we release stress in our lives, we help others do the same" (p. 4). When Eric and I gave presentations encouraging the audience to "take initiative and manage stress" (Bird and Wanner, 2013, 2014), I needed to control my stress so I could inspire others to do the same. So I looked back through the notes and reminded myself to take my own advice!

As a researcher, I love the theory of using writing as healing. Life as a patient taught me that while the practice of journal writing is excellent, different styles of journals need to exist. Whether used with patients in a clinic or students in a classroom, writing can illuminate a person's thoughts and coalesce the swirl of ideas in the mind. Medical doctor Tindle (2013) recommends to patients, "we need to come face-to face with our own internal dialogue so that we can learn whether we truly believe the things we are telling ourselves" (p. 95). How to capture a patient's inner dialogue? Write about it. Writing teacher Cameron (1998) shares with writers, "things do come to us through writing, and they are not always so intangible as insights. Moving our hands across the page, we make a handmade life" (p. 28). The survey Eric and I designed built on the existing foundation of research while adding a unique interdisciplinary collaboration and interpretation. We connected our own insights and perspectives with existing research in the field. Medical doctor Harding (2019) describes the lasting impact of Pennebaker's initial research showing the health benefits of writing as, "subsequent follow-up studies show benefits across age, gender, social class, culture, and even personality type in as little as fifteen minutes a day of writing for three days" (p. 137). I discovered the success of the research I did with Eric, Jayne, and others we added to our team exists in the lives of the people who we help by the information we learned and decided to share.

It feels vulnerable to share a story. Even after writing about my experiences in book chapters, I still feel vulnerable sharing my pain narrative, but experts like my physical therapists Eric, Ryan, and Dak always showed willingness to help. I feel vulnerable sharing narratives of my life with you, the reader of this story, but I share my story with the wish it will inspire you to write your own narrative and make it a good one. Lamott (1994) writes, "against all odds, you have put it down on paper, so that it won't be lost. And who knows? Maybe what you've written will help others, will be a small part of the solution" (p. 235). I want my research and writing to continue to help others. I hope to live my life in a way similar to the words of Hale (2018) when she says, "so I urge you to put yourself out there. Be vulnerable. Take a chance. Step outside your comfort zone. Try something new and daring and audacious" (p. 23). I'm grateful that years ago I took a chance and shared my pain narrative with Eric because he helped me and we then used our research and writing to help others.

My purpose in sharing my narrative reflects my life's larger purpose of using my passion for writing, especially narrative writing, to help others. Hollis (2019) explains, "this goal, this mission of yours, this dream, this place that you're headed – this is not a temporary thing" (p. 185). I want to continue to write narratives which educate and inspire because I agree with Hollis (2018) who shares, "writing – for me –is its own kind of worship" (p. 150). As an English teacher, I believe in the value of writing. I agree with Heard (1995) who writes, "writing is an act of faith: faith that what I have to say, how I see the world, are important" (p. 27). I want my students to have faith that writing can lead the way to heal from the past, honor the present, and articulate goals for the future.

It took awhile for me to learn the lesson that healing will always be a journey. Stress from the pandemic triggered a flare of my Sjogren's autoimmune syndrome. I returned to work with my physical therapy team in both 2020 and 2021 when my herniated disc caused more neck pain and nerve pain in my arms. Since I already had a diagnosis, I didn't need to revise my narrative. As a writer, I want to end this writing as healing story with a nice, neat ending. But real life isn't fiction. Life happens. Pain happens. Pandemics happen. People consistently demonstrate resilience as they rewrite their life stories and persevere through pain. I will live more stories as soon as I write this concluding paragraph. Most narratives never have a definitive ending; the end of one narrative leads to the beginning of another.

ACKNOWLEDGMENT

This chapter was co-authored by Dr. Eric Wanner, Director of the Physical Therapy Department at Palm Beach Sports Medicine and Orthopaedic Center. Eric loves research, and I enjoyed collaborating to designing a unique survey featuring both numerical subjective and written subjective questions to assess goal setting for physical therapy patients. Eric and I also conducted research to assess anxiety in college students and recommended effective methods for coping with anxiety, such as exercising, nutrition, writing, and belonging to a supportive community. We continued our collaboration by using health coaching to supplement physical therapy treatment plans for both staff members and patients at a hospital. I feel proud of our lasting contributions to interdisciplinary research that helped numerous people and remain grateful for Eric's talent of condensing my overly wordy first drafts into the most essential ideas.

The preceding chapter contains excerpts from the following previous IGI publications:

Bird, J.L., & Wanner, E.T. (2020). Narratives of spirituality. In *Using narrative writing to enhance healing* (pp. 1-39). Hershey, PA: Information Science Reference.

Table 1. Jen's Neck Pain Journal

Date	Pain Level 1=Low, 10=High	Observations
Summary	Left side pain is gone and I have my range of motion back. The right side pain has been a roller coaster this week. The numbers below are the average for each day; there are moments when it is better or worse but neither lasts very long.	I'm doing my exercises twice a day. I added meditation, more laughter, and a turtle necklace as my personal symbol to slow down. I checked in with a therapist to talk about my mom's death. I love my life and am peaceful with it. Okay, neck, what more do you want from me?!
Mon 4/2	Right Side Pain Level = 3	Better after physical therapy. No rehearsal tonight so time off and rest helped.
Tues 4/3	Right Side Pain Level = 1	High stress day at work with student registration for new semester and lots of stressed out students and colleagues. Doing what feels like 100 things per hour but my neck is better. Scary that neck likes stress!!
Wed 4/4	Right Side Pain Level = 4	Two days of constant stress = neck pain worse. That's kind of a no brainer. Still doing my exercises but feeling frustrated that the pain is worse today. Sleep on my side and know I'm not helping myself but I'm physically and emotionally exhausted.
Thurs 4/5	Right Side Pain Level = 5	Today is the day I wonder if I can live with pain. That lasts for about 10 minutes before I tell myself that I'm not giving up and Eric is not going to let me give up. See news story that meditation helps with pain. Motivate self to keep going.
Fri 4/6	Right Side Pain Level = 2	Feeling better today. Leave work early and hang out at the nursing home with Grandma, who feels that since she is almost 90 she no longer needs to censor anything she says. She always makes me laugh.

Bird, J.L., & Wanner, E.T. (2020). Narratives of research design. In *Using narrative writing to enhance healing* (pp. 40-72). Hershey, PA: Information Science Reference.

Bird, J.L. (2020). Narratives of emotional truth. In *Using narrative writing to enhance healing* (pp. 101-128). Hershey, PA: Information Science Reference.

Bird, J.L. (2020). Narratives of patient care. In *Using narrative writing to enhance healing* (pp. 157-184). Hershey, PA: Information Science Reference.

Bird, J.L., & Wanner, E.T. (2020). Narratives of anxiety. In *Using narrative writing to enhance healing* (pp. 185-237). Hershey, PA: Information Science Reference.

Bird, J.L., & Wanner, E.T. (2020). Narratives of writing as healing. In *Using narrative writing to enhance healing* (pp. 295-338). Hershey, PA: Information Science Reference.

REFERENCES

Arioto, M. (2019). *Have more fun*. Zondervan.

Berkow, R. (Ed.). (1997). *The Merck manual of medical information*. Merck & Co.

Bernstein, G. (2014). *Miracles now*. Hay House.

Bird, J. L., & Wanner, E. T. (2013). Take initiative and manage stress. *Learn Green Conference*.

Bird, J. L., & Wanner, E. T. (2014). Take initiative and manage stress. *Learn Green Conference.*

Brown, B. (2007). *I thought it was just me*. Gotham Books.

Brown, B. (2010). *The gifts of imperfection*. Hazelden.

Brown, B. (2012). *Daring greatly*. Gotham Books.

Brown, B. (2015). *Rising strong*. Spiegel & Grau.

Cameron, J. (1998). *The right to write*. Tarcher/Putnam.

Carroll, R. (2018). *The bullet journal method*. Portfolio/Penguin.

Clandinin, D. J., & Connelly, F. M. (2000). *Narrative inquiry*. Jossey-Bass.

Connelly, F. M., & Clandinin, D. J. (1988). *Teachers as curriculum planners*. Teachers College press.

Croft, J. (1980). Interviewing in physical therapy. *Physical Therapy*, *60*(8), 1033–1036. doi:10.1093/ptj/60.8.1033 PMID:7403279

Dalebout, K. (2016). *Let it out*. Hay House.

Dooley, J. L. (2019). *Own your everyday*. Waterbrook.

Dosa, D. (2010). *Making rounds with Oscar*. Hyperion.

Duke Integrative Medicine Staff. (2010). *Personalized health plan manual*. Duke Integrative Medicine.

Enayati, A. (2015). *Seeking serenity*. New American Library.

Fallon, A. (2020). *The power of writing it down*. Zondervan.

Files, M. (2016). *Writing what you know*. Allworth.

Goldberg, N. (2000). *Thunder and lightning*. Bantam.

Goldberg, N. (2007). *Old friend from far away*. Free Press.

Goldberg, S. (2019). *How to be a patient*. Harper Wave.

Grant, A. (2016). *Originals*. Viking.

Graves, D. (2001). *The energy to teach*. Heinemann.

Hagen, P. T. (Ed.). (2001). *Mayo clinic guide to self-care*. Mayo Clinic.

Hale, M. (2018). *You are enough*. FaithWords.

Harding, K. (2019). *The rabbit effect*. Atria.

Heard, G. (1995). *Writing toward home*. Heinemann.

Hollis, R. (2018). *Girl, wash your face*. Nelson Books.

Hollis, R. (2019). *Girl, stop apologizing*. HarperCollins Leadership.

Lamott, A. (1994). *Bird by bird.* Anchor Books.

Leonard, L. (2018). *Brave love.* Zondervan.

Miller, R. W. (2017). *Dot journaling.* The Experiment.

Neff, K., & Germer, C. (2018). *The mindful self-compassion workbook.* Guilford.

Niequist, S. (2016). *Present over perfect.* Zondervan.

Pennebaker, J. W. (1997). *Opening up: The healing power of expressing emotions.* The Guilford Press.

Pennebaker, J. W., & Smyth, J. M. (2016). *Opening up by writing it down.* The Guilford Press.

Pink, D. (2018). *When.* Riverhead.

Randall, K. E., & McEwen, I. R. (2000). Writing patient-centered functional goals. *Physical Therapy, 80*(12), 1197–1203. doi:10.1093/ptj/80.12.1197 PMID:11087306

Rankin, L. (2013). *Mind over medicine.* Hay House.

Romano, T. (1987). *Clearing the way.* Heinemann.

Romano, T. (2000). *Blending genre, altering style.* Heinemann.

Romano, T. (2013). *Fearless writing.* Heinemann.

Romano, T. (2015). *Write what matters.* Zigzag.

Sandberg, S., & Grant, A. (2017). *Option B.* Knopf.

Schunk, D. H. (1990). Goal setting and self-efficacy during self-regulated learning. *Educational Psychologist, 25*(1), 71–86. doi:10.120715326985ep2501_6

Sharp, C. (2000). *A writer's workbook.* St. Martin's Press.

Soukup, R. (2016). *Unstuffed.* Zondervan.

Soukup, R. (2019). *Do it scared.* Zondervan.

Tindle, H. (2013). *Up: how positive outlook can transform our health and aging.* Hudson Street Press.

Vacca, R. T., Vacca, J. L., & Mraz, M. (2014). *Content area reading* (11th ed.). Pearson.

Wanner, E.T., & Bird, J.L. (2013). *The Wanner Bird healing survey for pain recovery.* Academic Press.

Younger, J., Gandhi, V., Hubbard, E., & Mackey, S. (2012). Development of the Stanford expectations of treatment scale (SETS): A tool for measuring patient outcome expectancy in clinical trials. *Clinical Trials, 9*(6), 767–776. doi:10.1177/1740774512465064 PMID:23169874

KEY TERMS AND DEFINITIONS

Artistic and Technical Writing: Artistic writing focuses on the writer's tone of word choice, also known as voice, while technical writing focuses on the writer's specificity of word choice. English teachers design rubrics that incorporate both artistic and technical writing.

Expressive Writing: Writing that is exploratory and focuses on meaning and first impressions.

Neck Pain Journal: Jen created a journal of what she was doing when her neck felt pain. Eric read the journal and adjusted Jen's treatment plan to make her neck feel better.

Physical Therapy Outcome Measures: Tests used by physical therapists to measure the progress a patient makes, such as such as the DASH (Disabilities of the Arm Shoulder Hand), LEFS (Lower Extremity Functional Scale), NDI (Neck Disability Index), and Modified Oswestry (for back pain). Physical therapists choose which outcome measure to use based on the body part where the patient experiences pain.

Wanner-Bird Healing Survey for Pain Recovery: An original survey designed by Dr. Eric Wanner and Dr. Jennifer Bird. This survey features both numerical subjective questions, where patients are asked to respond to statements by circling a number from 1-5, and written subjective questions that score patients' written responses on a rubric with a score of 1, 3, or 5. The rubric incorporates both the technical and artistic dimensions of writing.

Writing as Healing: Numerous studies have been conducted investigating the influence of writing on physical and emotional health. James Pennebaker is a leader in the field which explores the health benefits of writing.

Related References

To continue our tradition of advancing information science and technology research, we have compiled a list of recommended IGI Global readings. These references will provide additional information and guidance to further enrich your knowledge and assist you with your own research and future publications.

Abu Seman, S. A., & Ramayah, T. (2017). Are We Ready to App?: A Study on mHealth Apps, Its Future, and Trends in Malaysia Context. In J. Pelet (Ed.), *Mobile Platforms, Design, and Apps for Social Commerce* (pp. 69–83). Hershey, PA: IGI Global. doi:10.4018/978-1-5225-2469-4.ch005

Aggarwal, S., & Azad, V. (2017). A Hybrid System Based on FMM and MLP to Diagnose Heart Disease. In S. Bhattacharyya, S. De, I. Pan, & P. Dutta (Eds.), *Intelligent Multidimensional Data Clustering and Analysis* (pp. 293–325). Hershey, PA: IGI Global. doi:10.4018/978-1-5225-1776-4.ch011

Akaichi, J., & Mhadhbi, L. (2016). A Clinical Decision Support System: Ontology-Driven Approach for Effective Emergency Management. In J. Moon & M. Galea (Eds.), *Improving Health Management through Clinical Decision Support Systems* (pp. 270–294). Hershey, PA: IGI Global. doi:10.4018/978-1-4666-9432-3.ch013

Akerkar, R. (2016). Towards an Intelligent Integrated Approach for Clinical Decision Support. In A. Aggarwal (Ed.), *Managing Big Data Integration in the Public Sector* (pp. 187–205). Hershey, PA: IGI Global. doi:10.4018/978-1-4666-9649-5.ch011

Al-Busaidi, S. S. (2018). Interdisciplinary Relationships Between Medicine and Social Sciences. In M. Al-Suqri, A. Al-Kindi, S. AlKindi, & N. Saleem (Eds.), *Promoting Interdisciplinarity in Knowledge Generation and Problem Solving* (pp. 124–137). Hershey, PA: IGI Global. doi:10.4018/978-1-5225-3878-3.ch009

Al Kareh, T., & Thoumy, M. (2018). The Impact of Health Information Digitization on the Physiotherapist-Patient Relationship: A Pilot Study of the Lebanese Community. *International Journal of Healthcare Information Systems and Informatics, 13*(2), 29–53. doi:10.4018/IJHISI.2018040103

Alenzuela, R. (2017). Research, Leadership, and Resource-Sharing Initiatives: The Role of Local Library Consortia in Access to Medical Information. In S. Ram (Ed.), *Library and Information Services for Bioinformatics Education and Research* (pp. 199–211). Hershey, PA: IGI Global. doi:10.4018/978-1-5225-1871-6.ch012

Ameri, H., Alizadeh, S., & Noughabi, E. A. (2017). Application of Data Mining Techniques in Clinical Decision Making: A Literature Review and Classification. In E. Noughabi, B. Raahemi, A. Albadvi, & B. Far (Eds.), *Handbook of Research on Data Science for Effective Healthcare Practice and Administration* (pp. 257–295). Hershey, PA: IGI Global. doi:10.4018/978-1-5225-2515-8.ch012

Anand, S. (2017). Medical Image Enhancement Using Edge Information-Based Methods. In B. Singh (Ed.), *Computational Tools and Techniques for Biomedical Signal Processing* (pp. 123–148). Hershey, PA: IGI Global. doi:10.4018/978-1-5225-0660-7.ch006

Angjellari-Dajci, F., Sapienza, C., Lawless, W. F., & Kavanagh, K. (2016). Human Capital Accumulation in Medical Simulated Learning Environments: A Framework for Economic Evaluation. In M. Russ (Ed.), *Quantitative Multidisciplinary Approaches in Human Capital and Asset Management* (pp. 65–88). Hershey, PA: IGI Global. doi:10.4018/978-1-4666-9652-5.ch004

Anil, M., Ayyildiz-Tamis, D., Tasdemir, S., Sendemir-Urkmez, A., & Gulce-Iz, S. (2016). Bioinspired Materials and Biocompatibility. In M. Bououdina (Ed.), *Emerging Research on Bioinspired Materials Engineering* (pp. 294–322). Hershey, PA: IGI Global. doi:10.4018/978-1-4666-9811-6.ch011

Anton, J. L., Soriano, J. V., Martinez, M. I., & Garcia, F. B. (2018). Comprehensive E-Learning Appraisal System. In M. Khosrow-Pour, D.B.A. (Ed.), Encyclopedia of Information Science and Technology, Fourth Edition (pp. 5787-5799). Hershey, PA: IGI Global. doi:10.4018/978-1-5225-2255-3.ch503

Arabi, M. (2016). Redesigning the Organizational Structure to Reach Efficiency: The Case of Ministry of Health and Medical Education of Iran. In R. Gholipour & K. Rouzbehani (Eds.), *Social, Economic, and Political Perspectives on Public Health Policy-Making* (pp. 257–294). Hershey, PA: IGI Global. doi:10.4018/978-1-4666-9944-1.ch012

Assis-Hassid, S., Heart, T., Reychav, I., & Pliskin, J. S. (2016). Modelling Factors Affecting Patient-Doctor-Computer Communication in Primary Care. *International Journal of Reliable and Quality E-Healthcare*, *5*(1), 1–17. doi:10.4018/IJRQEH.2016010101

Atzori, B., Hoffman, H. G., Vagnoli, L., Messeri, A., & Grotto, R. L. (2018). Virtual Reality as Distraction Technique for Pain Management in Children and Adolescents. In M. Khosrow-Pour, D.B.A. (Ed.), Encyclopedia of Information Science and Technology, Fourth Edition (pp. 5955-5965). Hershey, PA: IGI Global. doi:10.4018/978-1-5225-2255-3.ch518

Audibert, M., Mathonnat, J., Pélissier, A., & Huang, X. X. (2018). The Impact of the New Rural Cooperative Medical Scheme on Township Hospitals' Utilization and Income Structure in Weifang Prefecture, China. In I. Management Association (Ed.), Health Economics and Healthcare Reform: Breakthroughs in Research and Practice (pp. 109-121). Hershey, PA: IGI Global. doi:10.4018/978-1-5225-3168-5.ch007

Ayyachamy, S. (2016). Analysis and Comparison of Developed 2D Medical Image Database Design using Registration Scheme, Retrieval Scheme, and Bag-of-Visual-Words. In N. Dey & A. Ashour (Eds.), *Classification and Clustering in Biomedical Signal Processing* (pp. 149–168). Hershey, PA: IGI Global. doi:10.4018/978-1-5225-0140-4.ch007

Babalola, A. C. (2016). Literacy and Decision Making on Health Issues among Married Women in Southwest Nigeria. In V. Wang (Ed.), *Handbook of Research on Advancing Health Education through Technology* (pp. 191–212). Hershey, PA: IGI Global. doi:10.4018/978-1-4666-9494-1.ch009

Babu, A., & Ayyappan, S. (2017). A Methodological Evaluation of Crypto-Watermarking System for Medical Images. In C. Bhatt & S. Peddoju (Eds.), *Cloud Computing Systems and Applications in Healthcare* (pp. 189–217). Hershey, PA: IGI Global. doi:10.4018/978-1-5225-1002-4.ch010

Bakke, A. (2017). Ethos in E-Health: From Informational to Interactive Websites. In M. Folk & S. Apostel (Eds.), *Establishing and Evaluating Digital Ethos and Online Credibility* (pp. 85–103). Hershey, PA: IGI Global. doi:10.4018/978-1-5225-1072-7.ch005

Bali, S. (2018). Enhancing the Reach of Health Care Through Telemedicine: Status and New Possibilities in Developing Countries. In U. Pandey & V. Indrakanti (Eds.), *Open and Distance Learning Initiatives for Sustainable Development* (pp. 339–354). Hershey, PA: IGI Global. doi:10.4018/978-1-5225-2621-6.ch019

Barrett, T. E. (2018). Essentials for Education and Training for Tomorrow's Physicians. In C. Smith (Ed.), *Exploring the Pressures of Medical Education From a Mental Health and Wellness Perspective* (pp. 230–252). Hershey, PA: IGI Global. doi:10.4018/978-1-5225-2811-1.ch010

Barrett, T. J. (2016). Knowledge in Action: Fostering Health Education through Technology. In V. Wang (Ed.), *Handbook of Research on Advancing Health Education through Technology* (pp. 39–62). Hershey, PA: IGI Global. doi:10.4018/978-1-4666-9494-1.ch003

Berrahal, S., & Boudriga, N. (2017). The Risks of Wearable Technologies to Individuals and Organizations. In A. Marrington, D. Kerr, & J. Gammack (Eds.), *Managing Security Issues and the Hidden Dangers of Wearable Technologies* (pp. 18–46). Hershey, PA: IGI Global. doi:10.4018/978-1-5225-1016-1.ch002

Bhagat, A. P., & Atique, M. (2016). Medical Image Mining Using Fuzzy Connectedness Image Segmentation: Efficient Retrieval of Patients' Stored Images. In W. Karâa & N. Dey (Eds.), *Biomedical Image Analysis and Mining Techniques for Improved Health Outcomes* (pp. 184–209). Hershey, PA: IGI Global. doi:10.4018/978-1-4666-8811-7.ch009

Bhargava, P. (2018). Blended Learning: An Effective Application to Clinical Teaching. In S. Tang & C. Lim (Eds.), *Preparing the Next Generation of Teachers for 21st Century Education* (pp. 302–320). Hershey, PA: IGI Global. doi:10.4018/978-1-5225-4080-9.ch018

Binh, N. T., & Tuyet, V. T. (2016). The Combination of Adaptive Filters to Improve the Quality of Medical Images in New Wavelet Domain. In N. Dey & A. Ashour (Eds.), *Classification and Clustering in Biomedical Signal Processing* (pp. 46–76). Hershey, PA: IGI Global. doi:10.4018/978-1-5225-0140-4.ch003

Bird, J. L. (2017). Writing Healing Narratives. In V. Bryan & J. Bird (Eds.), *Healthcare Community Synergism between Patients, Practitioners, and Researchers* (pp. 1–28). Hershey, PA: IGI Global. doi:10.4018/978-1-5225-0640-9.ch001

Bottrighi, A., Leonardi, G., Piovesan, L., & Terenziani, P. (2016). Knowledge-Based Support to the Treatment of Exceptions in Computer Interpretable Clinical Guidelines. *International Journal of Knowledge-Based Organizations*, *6*(3), 1–27. doi:10.4018/IJKBO.2016070101

Bougoulias, K., Kouris, I., Prasinos, M., Giokas, K., & Koutsouris, D. (2017). Ob/Gyn EMR Software: A Solution for Obstetricians and Gynecologists. In A. Moumtzoglou (Ed.), *Design, Development, and Integration of Reliable Electronic Healthcare Platforms* (pp. 101–111). Hershey, PA: IGI Global. doi:10.4018/978-1-5225-1724-5.ch006

Bouslimi, R., Ayadi, M. G., & Akaichi, J. (2018). Medical Image Retrieval in Healthcare Social Networks. *International Journal of Healthcare Information Systems and Informatics*, *13*(2), 13–28. doi:10.4018/IJHISI.2018040102

Bouzaabia, O., Bouzaabia, R., & Mejri, K. (2017). Role of Internet in the Development of Medical Tourism Service in Tunisia. In A. Capatina & E. Rancati (Eds.), *Key Challenges and Opportunities in Web Entrepreneurship* (pp. 211–241). Hershey, PA: IGI Global. doi:10.4018/978-1-5225-2466-3.ch009

Briz-Ponce, L., Juanes-Méndez, J. A., & García-Peñalvo, F. J. (2016). The Role of Gender in Technology Acceptance for Medical Education. In M. Cruz-Cunha, I. Miranda, R. Martinho, & R. Rijo (Eds.), *Encyclopedia of E-Health and Telemedicine* (pp. 1013–1027). Hershey, PA: IGI Global. doi:10.4018/978-1-4666-9978-6.ch079

Briz-Ponce, L., Juanes-Méndez, J. A., & García-Peñalvo, F. J. (2016). A Research Contribution to the Analysis of Mobile Devices in Higher Education from Medical Students' Point of View. In L. Briz-Ponce, J. Juanes-Méndez, & F. García-Peñalvo (Eds.), *Handbook of Research on Mobile Devices and Applications in Higher Education Settings* (pp. 196–221). Hershey, PA: IGI Global. doi:10.4018/978-1-5225-0256-2.ch009

Brown-Jackson, K. L. (2018). Telemedicine and Telehealth: Academics Engaging the Community in a Call to Action. In S. Burton (Ed.), *Engaged Scholarship and Civic Responsibility in Higher Education* (pp. 166–193). Hershey, PA: IGI Global. doi:10.4018/978-1-5225-3649-9.ch008

Bwalya, K. J. (2017). Next Wave of Tele-Medicine: Virtual Presence of Medical Personnel. In K. Moahi, K. Bwalya, & P. Sebina (Eds.), *Health Information Systems and the Advancement of Medical Practice in Developing Countries* (pp. 168–180). Hershey, PA: IGI Global. doi:10.4018/978-1-5225-2262-1.ch010

Carlton, E. L., Holsinger, J. W. Jr, & Anunobi, N. (2016). Physician Engagement with Health Information Technology: Implications for Practice and Professionalism. *International Journal of Computers in Clinical Practice*, *1*(2), 51–73. doi:10.4018/IJCCP.2016070103

Castillo-Page, L., Eliason, J., Conrad, S. S., & Nivet, M. A. (2016). Diversity in Undergraduate Medical Education: An Examination of Organizational Culture and Climate in Medical Schools. In C. Scott & J. Sims (Eds.), *Developing Workforce Diversity Programs, Curriculum, and Degrees in Higher Education* (pp. 304–326). Hershey, PA: IGI Global. doi:10.4018/978-1-5225-0209-8.ch016

Cebeci, H. I., & Hiziroglu, A. (2016). Review of Business Intelligence and Intelligent Systems in Healthcare Domain. In N. Celebi (Ed.), *Intelligent Techniques for Data Analysis in Diverse Settings* (pp. 192–206). Hershey, PA: IGI Global. doi:10.4018/978-1-5225-0075-9.ch009

Celik, G. (2018). Determining Headache Diseases With Genetic Algorithm. In U. Kose, G. Guraksin, & O. Deperlioglu (Eds.), *Nature-Inspired Intelligent Techniques for Solving Biomedical Engineering Problems* (pp. 249–262). Hershey, PA: IGI Global. doi:10.4018/978-1-5225-4769-3.ch012

Chakraborty, C., Gupta, B., & Ghosh, S. K. (2016). Mobile Telemedicine Systems for Remote Patient's Chronic Wound Monitoring. In A. Moumtzoglou (Ed.), *M-Health Innovations for Patient-Centered Care* (pp. 213–239). Hershey, PA: IGI Global. doi:10.4018/978-1-4666-9861-1.ch011

Chakraborty, S., Chatterjee, S., Ashour, A. S., Mali, K., & Dey, N. (2018). Intelligent Computing in Medical Imaging: A Study. In N. Dey (Ed.), *Advancements in Applied Metaheuristic Computing* (pp. 143–163). Hershey, PA: IGI Global. doi:10.4018/978-1-5225-4151-6.ch006

Chavez, A., & Kovarik, C. (2017). Open Source Technology for Medical Practice in Developing Countries. In K. Moahi, K. Bwalya, & P. Sebina (Eds.), *Health Information Systems and the Advancement of Medical Practice in Developing Countries* (pp. 33–59). Hershey, PA: IGI Global. doi:10.4018/978-1-5225-2262-1.ch003

Chen, E. T. (2016). Examining the Influence of Information Technology on Modern Health Care. In P. Manolitzas, E. Grigoroudis, N. Matsatsinis, & D. Yannacopoulos (Eds.), *Effective Methods for Modern Healthcare Service Quality and Evaluation* (pp. 110–136). Hershey, PA: IGI Global. doi:10.4018/978-1-4666-9961-8.ch006

Chin, S. (2016). Surviving Sandy: Recovering Collections after a Natural Disaster. In E. Decker & J. Townes (Eds.), *Handbook of Research on Disaster Management and Contingency Planning in Modern Libraries* (pp. 366–388). Hershey, PA: IGI Global. doi:10.4018/978-1-4666-8624-3.ch016

Chojnacki, M., & Wójcik, A. (2016). Security and the Role of New Technologies and Innovation in Medical Ethics. In A. Rosiek & K. Leksowski (Eds.), *Organizational Culture and Ethics in Modern Medicine* (pp. 52–77). Hershey, PA: IGI Global. doi:10.4018/978-1-4666-9658-7.ch003

Cılız, N., Yıldırım, H., & Temizel, Ş. (2016). Structure Development for Effective Medical Waste and Hazardous Waste Management System. In U. Akkucuk (Ed.), *Handbook of Research on Waste Management Techniques for Sustainability* (pp. 303–327). Hershey, PA: IGI Global. doi:10.4018/978-1-4666-9723-2.ch016

Ciufudean, C. (2018). Innovative Formalism for Biological Data Analysis. In M. Khosrow-Pour, D.B.A. (Ed.), Encyclopedia of Information Science and Technology, Fourth Edition (pp. 1814-1824). Hershey, PA: IGI Global. doi:10.4018/978-1-5225-2255-3.ch158

Ciufudean, C., & Ciufudean, O. (2016). Tele-Monitoring for Medical Diagnosis Availability. In M. Cruz-Cunha, I. Miranda, R. Martinho, & R. Rijo (Eds.), *Encyclopedia of E-Health and Telemedicine* (pp. 401–411). Hershey, PA: IGI Global. doi:10.4018/978-1-4666-9978-6.ch032

Colaguori, R., & Danesi, M. (2017). Medical Semiotics: A Revisitation and an Exhortation. *International Journal of Semiotics and Visual Rhetoric*, *1*(1), 11–18. doi:10.4018/IJSVR.2017010102

Cole, A. W., & Salek, T. A. (2017). Adopting a Parasocial Connection to Overcome Professional Kakoethos in Online Health Information. In M. Folk & S. Apostel (Eds.), *Establishing and Evaluating Digital Ethos and Online Credibility* (pp. 104–120). Hershey, PA: IGI Global. doi:10.4018/978-1-5225-1072-7.ch006

Contreras, E. C., & Puente, G. J. (2016). How to Identify Rheumatic Diseases by General Physicians. In T. Gasmelseid (Ed.), *Advancing Pharmaceutical Processes and Tools for Improved Health Outcomes* (pp. 136–166). Hershey, PA: IGI Global. doi:10.4018/978-1-5225-0248-7.ch006

D'Andrea, A., Ferri, F., & Grifoni, P. (2016). RFID Technologies in Healthcare Setting: Applications and Future Perspectives. *International Journal of Computers in Clinical Practice*, *1*(1), 15–27. doi:10.4018/IJCCP.2016010102

Damianakis, A., Kallonis, P., Loudos, G., Tsatsos, D., & Tsoukalis, A. (2016). Exploiting 3D Medical Equipment Simulations to Support Biomedical Engineering Academic Courses: Design Methodology and Implementation in a Small Scale National Project. In B. Khan (Ed.), *Revolutionizing Modern Education through Meaningful E-Learning Implementation* (pp. 277–295). Hershey, PA: IGI Global. doi:10.4018/978-1-5225-0466-5.ch015

Demiroz, E. (2016). Principles of Instructional Design for E-Learning and Online Learning Practices: Implications for Medical Education. In V. Wang (Ed.), *Handbook of Research on Advancing Health Education through Technology* (pp. 419–451). Hershey, PA: IGI Global. doi:10.4018/978-1-4666-9494-1.ch018

Deperlioglu, O. (2018). Intelligent Techniques Inspired by Nature and Used in Biomedical Engineering. In U. Kose, G. Guraksin, & O. Deperlioglu (Eds.), *Nature-Inspired Intelligent Techniques for Solving Biomedical Engineering Problems* (pp. 51–77). Hershey, PA: IGI Global. doi:10.4018/978-1-5225-4769-3.ch003

Dey, N., & Ashour, A. S. (2018). Meta-Heuristic Algorithms in Medical Image Segmentation: A Review. In N. Dey (Ed.), *Advancements in Applied Metaheuristic Computing* (pp. 185–203). Hershey, PA: IGI Global. doi:10.4018/978-1-5225-4151-6.ch008

Dey, N., Ashour, A. S., & Althoupety, A. S. (2017). Thermal Imaging in Medical Science. In V. Santhi (Ed.), *Recent Advances in Applied Thermal Imaging for Industrial Applications* (pp. 87–117). Hershey, PA: IGI Global. doi:10.4018/978-1-5225-2423-6.ch004

Di Virgilio, F., Camillo, A. A., & Camillo, I. C. (2017). The Impact of Social Network on Italian Users' Behavioural Intention for the Choice of a Medical Tourist Destination. *International Journal of Tourism and Hospitality Management in the Digital Age*, *1*(1), 36–49. doi:10.4018/IJTHMDA.2017010103

Dias, C. M., Ribeiro, A. G., & Furtado, S. F. (2016). An Overview about the Use of Healthcare Applications on Mobile Devices. In M. Cruz-Cunha, I. Miranda, R. Martinho, & R. Rijo (Eds.), *Encyclopedia of E-Health and Telemedicine* (pp. 285–298). Hershey, PA: IGI Global. doi:10.4018/978-1-4666-9978-6.ch024

Dogra, A. K., & Dogra, P. (2017). The Medical Tourism Industry in the BRIC Nations: An Indian Analysis. In M. Dhiman (Ed.), *Opportunities and Challenges for Tourism and Hospitality in the BRIC Nations* (pp. 320–336). Hershey, PA: IGI Global. doi:10.4018/978-1-5225-0708-6.ch020

Drowos, J. L., & Wood, S. K. (2017). Preparing Future Physicians to Adapt to the Changing Health Care System: Promoting Humanism through Curricular Design. In V. Bryan & J. Bird (Eds.), *Healthcare Community Synergism between Patients, Practitioners, and Researchers* (pp. 106–125). Hershey, PA: IGI Global. doi:10.4018/978-1-5225-0640-9.ch006

Dulam, K. (2017). Medical Patents and Impact on Availability and Affordability of Essential Medicines in India. In R. Aggarwal & R. Kaur (Eds.), *Patent Law and Intellectual Property in the Medical Field* (pp. 41–57). Hershey, PA: IGI Global. doi:10.4018/978-1-5225-2414-4.ch003

Dutta, P. (2017). Decision Making in Medical Diagnosis via Distance Measures on Interval Valued Fuzzy Sets. *International Journal of System Dynamics Applications, 6*(4), 63–83. doi:10.4018/IJSDA.2017100104

Edoh, T. O., Pawar, P. A., Brügge, B., & Teege, G. (2016). A Multidisciplinary Remote Healthcare Delivery System to Increase Health Care Access, Pathology Screening, and Treatment in Developing Countries: The Case of Benin. *International Journal of Healthcare Information Systems and Informatics, 11*(4), 1–31. doi:10.4018/IJHISI.2016100101

El Guemhioui, K., & Demurjian, S. A. (2017). Semantic Reconciliation of Electronic Health Records Using Semantic Web Technologies. *International Journal of Information Technology and Web Engineering, 12*(2), 26–48. doi:10.4018/IJITWE.2017040102

Ellouze, N., Rekhis, S., & Boudriga, N. (2016). Forensic Investigation of Digital Crimes in Healthcare Applications. In O. Isafiade & A. Bagula (Eds.), *Data Mining Trends and Applications in Criminal Science and Investigations* (pp. 169–210). Hershey, PA: IGI Global. doi:10.4018/978-1-5225-0463-4.ch007

Eneanya, A. N. (2016). Health Policy Implementation and Its Barriers: The Case Study of US Health System. In R. Gholipour & K. Rouzbehani (Eds.), *Social, Economic, and Political Perspectives on Public Health Policy-Making* (pp. 42–63). Hershey, PA: IGI Global. doi:10.4018/978-1-4666-9944-1.ch003

Entico, G. J. (2016). Knowledge Management and the Medical Health Librarians: A Perception Study. In J. Yap, M. Perez, M. Ayson, & G. Entico (Eds.), *Special Library Administration, Standardization and Technological Integration* (pp. 52–77). Hershey, PA: IGI Global. doi:10.4018/978-1-4666-9542-9.ch003

Ferradji, M. A., & Zidani, A. (2016). Collaborative Environment for Remote Clinical Reasoning Learning. *International Journal of E-Health and Medical Communications, 7*(4), 62–81. doi:10.4018/IJEHMC.2016100104

Fisher, J. (2018). Sociological Perspectives on Improving Medical Diagnosis Emphasizing CAD. In M. Khosrow-Pour, D.B.A. (Ed.), Encyclopedia of Information Science and Technology, Fourth Edition (pp. 1017-1024). Hershey, PA: IGI Global. doi:10.4018/978-1-5225-2255-3.ch088

Flores, C. D., Respício, A., Coelho, H., Bez, M. R., & Fonseca, J. M. (2016). Simulation for Medical Training. In M. Cruz-Cunha, I. Miranda, R. Martinho, & R. Rijo (Eds.), *Encyclopedia of E-Health and Telemedicine* (pp. 827–842). Hershey, PA: IGI Global. doi:10.4018/978-1-4666-9978-6.ch064

Frank, E. M. (2018). Healthcare Education: Integrating Simulation Technologies. In V. Bryan, A. Musgrove, & J. Powers (Eds.), *Handbook of Research on Human Development in the Digital Age* (pp. 163–182). Hershey, PA: IGI Global. doi:10.4018/978-1-5225-2838-8.ch008

Garner, G. (2018). Foundations for Yoga Practice in Rehabilitation. In S. Telles & N. Singh (Eds.), *Research-Based Perspectives on the Psychophysiology of Yoga* (pp. 263–307). Hershey, PA: IGI Global. doi:10.4018/978-1-5225-2788-6.ch015

Gasmelseid, T. M. (2016). Improving Pharmaceutical Care through the Use of Intelligent Pharmacoinformatics. In T. Gasmelseid (Ed.), *Advancing Pharmaceutical Processes and Tools for Improved Health Outcomes* (pp. 167–188). Hershey, PA: IGI Global. doi:10.4018/978-1-5225-0248-7.ch007

Gavurová, B., Kováč, V., & Šoltés, M. (2018). Medical Equipment and Economic Determinants of Its Structure and Regulation in the Slovak Republic. In M. Khosrow-Pour, D.B.A. (Ed.), Encyclopedia of Information Science and Technology, Fourth Edition (pp. 5841-5852). Hershey, PA: IGI Global. doi:10.4018/978-1-5225-2255-3.ch508

Ge, X., Wang, Q., Huang, K., Law, V., & Thomas, D. C. (2017). Designing Simulated Learning Environments and Facilitating Authentic Learning Experiences in Medical Education. In J. Stefaniak (Ed.), *Advancing Medical Education Through Strategic Instructional Design* (pp. 77–100). Hershey, PA: IGI Global. doi:10.4018/978-1-5225-2098-6.ch004

Gewald, H., & Gewald, C. (2018). Inhibitors of Physicians' Use of Mandatory Hospital Information Systems (HIS). *International Journal of Healthcare Information Systems and Informatics, 13*(1), 29–44. doi:10.4018/IJHISI.2018010103

Ghosh, D., & Dinda, S. (2017). Health Infrastructure and Economic Development in India. In R. Das (Ed.), *Social, Health, and Environmental Infrastructures for Economic Growth* (pp. 99–119). Hershey, PA: IGI Global. doi:10.4018/978-1-5225-2364-2.ch006

Ghosh, K., & Sen, K. C. (2017). The Potential of Crowdsourcing in the Health Care Industry. In N. Wickramasinghe (Ed.), *Handbook of Research on Healthcare Administration and Management* (pp. 418–427). Hershey, PA: IGI Global. doi:10.4018/978-1-5225-0920-2.ch024

Ghrab, S., & Saad, I. (2016). Identifying Crucial Know-How and Knowing-That for Medical Decision Support. *International Journal of Decision Support System Technology, 8*(4), 14–33. doi:10.4018/IJDSST.2016100102

Giokas, K., Tsirmpas, C., Anastasiou, A., Iliopoulou, D., Costarides, V., & Koutsouris, D. (2016). Contemporary Heart Failure Treatment Based on Improved Knowledge and Personalized Care of Comorbidities. In D. Fotiadis (Ed.), *Handbook of Research on Trends in the Diagnosis and Treatment of Chronic Conditions* (pp. 301–314). Hershey, PA: IGI Global. doi:10.4018/978-1-4666-8828-5.ch014

Gopalan, V., Chan, E., & Ho, D. T. (2018). Deliberate Self-Harm and Suicide Ideology in Medical Students. In C. Smith (Ed.), *Exploring the Pressures of Medical Education From a Mental Health and Wellness Perspective* (pp. 122–143). Hershey, PA: IGI Global. doi:10.4018/978-1-5225-2811-1.ch005

Goswami, S., Dey, U., Roy, P., Ashour, A., & Dey, N. (2017). Medical Video Processing: Concept and Applications. In N. Dey, A. Ashour, & P. Patra (Eds.), *Feature Detectors and Motion Detection in Video Processing* (pp. 1–17). Hershey, PA: IGI Global. doi:10.4018/978-1-5225-1025-3.ch001

Goswami, S., Mahanta, K., Goswami, S., Jigdung, T., & Devi, T. P. (2018). Ageing and Cancer: The Epigenetic Basis, Alternative Treatment, and Care. In B. Prasad & S. Akbar (Eds.), *Handbook of Research on Geriatric Health, Treatment, and Care* (pp. 206–235). Hershey, PA: IGI Global. doi:10.4018/978-1-5225-3480-8.ch012

Gouva, M. I. (2017). The Psychological Impact of Medical Error on Patients, Family Members, and Health Professionals. In M. Riga (Ed.), *Impact of Medical Errors and Malpractice on Health Economics, Quality, and Patient Safety* (pp. 171–196). Hershey, PA: IGI Global. doi:10.4018/978-1-5225-2337-6.ch007

Gürcü, M., & Tengilimoğlu, D. (2017). Health Tourism-Based Destination Marketing. In A. Bayraktar & C. Uslay (Eds.), *Strategic Place Branding Methodologies and Theory for Tourist Attraction* (pp. 308–331). Hershey, PA: IGI Global. doi:10.4018/978-1-5225-0579-2.ch015

Gürsel, G. (2016). Mobility in Healthcare: M-Health. In A. Panagopoulos (Ed.), *Handbook of Research on Next Generation Mobile Communication Systems* (pp. 485–511). Hershey, PA: IGI Global. doi:10.4018/978-1-4666-8732-5.ch019

Gürsel, G. (2017). For Better Healthcare Mining Health Data. In S. Bhattacharyya, S. De, I. Pan, & P. Dutta (Eds.), *Intelligent Multidimensional Data Clustering and Analysis* (pp. 135–158). Hershey, PA: IGI Global. doi:10.4018/978-1-5225-1776-4.ch006

Guzman-Lugo, G., Lopez-Martinez, M., Lopez-Ramirez, B., & Avila-Vazquez, D. (2016). City-Driven Approach to Determine Health Services Based on Current User Location and Collaborative Information. *International Journal of Knowledge Society Research, 7*(1), 53–62. doi:10.4018/IJKSR.2016010104

Gyaase, P. O., Darko-Lartey, R., William, H., & Borkloe, F. (2017). Towards an Integrated Electronic Medical Records System for Quality Healthcare in Ghana: An Exploratory Factor Analysis. *International Journal of Computers in Clinical Practice, 2*(2), 38–55. doi:10.4018/IJCCP.2017070103

Handayani, P. W., Sandhyaduhita, P. I., Hidayanto, A. N., Pinem, A. A., Fajrina, H. R., Junus, K. M., ... Ayuningtyas, D. (2016). Integrated Hospital Information System Architecture Design in Indonesia. In T. Iyamu & A. Tatnall (Eds.), *Maximizing Healthcare Delivery and Management through Technology Integration* (pp. 207–236). Hershey, PA: IGI Global. doi:10.4018/978-1-4666-9446-0.ch013

Hanel, P. (2017). Is China Catching Up?: Health-Related Applications of Biotechnology. In T. Bas & J. Zhao (Eds.), *Comparative Approaches to Biotechnology Development and Use in Developed and Emerging Nations* (pp. 465–520). Hershey, PA: IGI Global. doi:10.4018/978-1-5225-1040-6.ch016

Harmsen, C. A., & Royle, R. N. (2016). St. Stephen's Hospital Hervey Bay: Study of Developing a Digital Hospital. In J. Moon & M. Galea (Eds.), *Improving Health Management through Clinical Decision Support Systems* (pp. 127–153). Hershey, PA: IGI Global. doi:10.4018/978-1-4666-9432-3.ch006

Harp, D., Shim, R. S., Johnson, J., Harp, J. A., Wilcox, W. C., & Wilcox, J. K. (2016). Race and Gender Inequalities in Medicine and Biomedical Research. In U. Thomas & J. Drake (Eds.), *Critical Research on Sexism and Racism in STEM Fields* (pp. 115–134). Hershey, PA: IGI Global. doi:10.4018/978-1-5225-0174-9.ch006

Hartman, A., & Brown, S. (2017). Synergism through Therapeutic Visual Arts. In V. Bryan & J. Bird (Eds.), *Healthcare Community Synergism between Patients, Practitioners, and Researchers* (pp. 29–48). Hershey, PA: IGI Global. doi:10.4018/978-1-5225-0640-9.ch002

Hazra, J., Chowdhury, A. R., & Dutta, P. (2016). Cluster Based Medical Image Registration Using Optimized Neural Network. In S. Bhattacharyya, P. Banerjee, D. Majumdar, & P. Dutta (Eds.), *Handbook of Research on Advanced Hybrid Intelligent Techniques and Applications* (pp. 551–581). Hershey, PA: IGI Global. doi:10.4018/978-1-4666-9474-3.ch018

Hung, S., Huang, W., Yen, D. C., Chang, S., & Lu, C. (2016). Effect of Information Service Competence and Contextual Factors on the Effectiveness of Strategic Information Systems Planning in Hospitals. *Journal of Global Information Management, 24*(1), 14–36. doi:10.4018/JGIM.2016010102

Iltchev, P., Śliwczyński, A., Szynkiewicz, P., & Marczak, M. (2016). Mobile Health Applications Assisting Patients with Chronic Diseases: Examples from Asthma Care. In A. Moumtzoglou (Ed.), *M-Health Innovations for Patient-Centered Care* (pp. 170–196). Hershey, PA: IGI Global. doi:10.4018/978-1-4666-9861-1.ch009

Iqbal, S., Ahmad, S., & Willis, I. (2017). Influencing Factors for Adopting Technology Enhanced Learning in the Medical Schools of Punjab, Pakistan. *International Journal of Information and Communication Technology Education, 13*(3), 27–39. doi:10.4018/IJICTE.2017070103

Jagan, J., Dalkiliç, Y., & Samui, P. (2016). Utilization of SVM, LSSVM and GP for Predicting the Medical Waste Generation. In G. Hua (Ed.), *Smart Cities as a Solution for Reducing Urban Waste and Pollution* (pp. 224–251). Hershey, PA: IGI Global. doi:10.4018/978-1-5225-0302-6.ch008

Jagiello, K., Sosnowska, A., Mikolajczyk, A., & Puzyn, T. (2017). Nanomaterials in Medical Devices: Regulations' Review and Future Perspectives. *Journal of Nanotoxicology and Nanomedicine, 2*(2), 1–11. doi:10.4018/JNN.2017070101

Jena, T. K. (2018). Skill Training Process in Medicine Through Distance Mode. In U. Pandey & V. Indrakanti (Eds.), *Optimizing Open and Distance Learning in Higher Education Institutions* (pp. 228–243). Hershey, PA: IGI Global. doi:10.4018/978-1-5225-2624-7.ch010

Jesus, Â., & Gomes, M. J. (2016). Web 2.0 Tools in Biomedical and Pharmaceutical Education: Updated Review and Commentary. In T. Gasmelseid (Ed.), *Advancing Pharmaceutical Processes and Tools for Improved Health Outcomes* (pp. 52–78). Hershey, PA: IGI Global. doi:10.4018/978-1-5225-0248-7.ch003

Joseph, V., & Miller, J. M. (2018). Medical Students' Perceived Stigma in Seeking Care: A Cultural Perspective. In C. Smith (Ed.), *Exploring the Pressures of Medical Education From a Mental Health and Wellness Perspective* (pp. 44–67). Hershey, PA: IGI Global. doi:10.4018/978-1-5225-2811-1.ch002

Joyce, B. L., & Swanberg, S. M. (2017). Using Backward Design for Competency-Based Undergraduate Medical Education. In J. Stefaniak (Ed.), *Advancing Medical Education Through Strategic Instructional Design* (pp. 53–76). Hershey, PA: IGI Global. doi:10.4018/978-1-5225-2098-6.ch003

Kaljo, K., & Jacques, L. (2018). Flipping the Medical School Classroom. In M. Khosrow-Pour, D.B.A. (Ed.), Encyclopedia of Information Science and Technology, Fourth Edition (pp. 5800-5809). Hershey, PA: IGI Global. doi:10.4018/978-1-5225-2255-3.ch504

Karon, R. (2016). Utilisation of Health Information Systems for Service Delivery in the Namibian Environment. In T. Iyamu & A. Tatnall (Eds.), *Maximizing Healthcare Delivery and Management through Technology Integration* (pp. 169–183). Hershey, PA: IGI Global. doi:10.4018/978-1-4666-9446-0.ch011

Kasina, H., Bahubalendruni, M. V., & Botcha, R. (2017). Robots in Medicine: Past, Present and Future. *International Journal of Manufacturing, Materials, and Mechanical Engineering*, *7*(4), 44–64. doi:10.4018/IJMMME.2017100104

Katehakis, D. G. (2018). Electronic Medical Record Implementation Challenges for the National Health System in Greece. *International Journal of Reliable and Quality E-Healthcare*, *7*(1), 16–30. doi:10.4018/IJRQEH.2018010102

Katz, A., & Shtub, A. (2016). Design and Build a Wizard of Oz (WOZ) Telemedicine Simulator Platform. In M. Cruz-Cunha, I. Miranda, R. Martinho, & R. Rijo (Eds.), *Encyclopedia of E-Health and Telemedicine* (pp. 128–141). Hershey, PA: IGI Global. doi:10.4018/978-1-4666-9978-6.ch011

Kaur, P. D., & Sharma, P. (2017). Success Dimensions of ICTs in Healthcare. In B. Singh (Ed.), *Computational Tools and Techniques for Biomedical Signal Processing* (pp. 149–173). Hershey, PA: IGI Global. doi:10.4018/978-1-5225-0660-7.ch007

Kaushik, P. (2018). Comorbidity of Medical and Psychiatric Disorders in Geriatric Population: Treatment and Care. In B. Prasad & S. Akbar (Eds.), *Handbook of Research on Geriatric Health, Treatment, and Care* (pp. 448–474). Hershey, PA: IGI Global. doi:10.4018/978-1-5225-3480-8.ch025

Khachane, M. Y. (2017). Organ-Based Medical Image Classification Using Support Vector Machine. *International Journal of Synthetic Emotions*, *8*(1), 18–30. doi:10.4018/IJSE.2017010102

Kirci, P. (2018). Intelligent Techniques for Analysis of Big Data About Healthcare and Medical Records. In N. Shah & M. Mittal (Eds.), *Handbook of Research on Promoting Business Process Improvement Through Inventory Control Techniques* (pp. 559–582). Hershey, PA: IGI Global. doi:10.4018/978-1-5225-3232-3.ch029

Kldiashvili, E. (2016). Cloud Computing as the Useful Resource for Application of the Medical Information System for Quality Assurance Purposes. *International Journal of Computers in Clinical Practice*, *1*(2), 1–23. doi:10.4018/IJCCP.2016070101

Kldiashvili, E. (2018). Cloud Approach for the Medical Information System: MIS on Cloud. In M. Khosrow-Pour (Ed.), *Incorporating Nature-Inspired Paradigms in Computational Applications* (pp. 238–261). Hershey, PA: IGI Global. doi:10.4018/978-1-5225-5020-4.ch008

Kldiashvili, E., Burduli, A., Ghortlishvili, G., & Sheklashvili, I. (2016). Georgian Experience in Telecytology. In M. Cruz-Cunha, I. Miranda, R. Martinho, & R. Rijo (Eds.), *Encyclopedia of E-Health and Telemedicine* (pp. 62–71). Hershey, PA: IGI Global. doi:10.4018/978-1-4666-9978-6.ch006

Ko, H., Mesicek, L., Choi, J., Choi, J., & Hwang, S. (2018). A Study on Secure Contents Strategies for Applications With DRM on Cloud Computing. *International Journal of Cloud Applications and Computing*, *8*(1), 143–153. doi:10.4018/IJCAC.2018010107

Komendziński, T., Dreszer-Drogorób, J., Mikołajewska, E., Mikołajewski, D., & Bałaj, B. (2016). Interdisciplinary Education for Research and Everyday Clinical Practice: Lessons Learned from InteRDoCTor Project. In A. Rosiek & K. Leksowski (Eds.), *Organizational Culture and Ethics in Modern Medicine* (pp. 78–110). Hershey, PA: IGI Global. doi:10.4018/978-1-4666-9658-7.ch004

Komendziński, T., Mikołajewska, E., & Mikołajewski, D. (2018). Cross-Cultural Decision-Making in Healthcare: Theory and Practical Application in Real Clinical Conditions. In A. Rosiek-Kryszewska & K. Leksowski (Eds.), *Healthcare Administration for Patient Safety and Engagement* (pp. 276–298). Hershey, PA: IGI Global. doi:10.4018/978-1-5225-3946-9.ch015

Konecny, L. T. (2018). Medical School Wellness Initiatives. In C. Smith (Ed.), *Exploring the Pressures of Medical Education From a Mental Health and Wellness Perspective* (pp. 209–228). Hershey, PA: IGI Global. doi:10.4018/978-1-5225-2811-1.ch009

Konieczna, A., & Słomkowski, P. (2016). Confrontation of Human Rights in Daily Clinical Situations. In A. Rosiek & K. Leksowski (Eds.), *Organizational Culture and Ethics in Modern Medicine* (pp. 255–281). Hershey, PA: IGI Global. doi:10.4018/978-1-4666-9658-7.ch011

Kromrei, H., Solomonson, W. L., & Juzych, M. S. (2017). Teaching Residents How to Teach. In J. Stefaniak (Ed.), *Advancing Medical Education Through Strategic Instructional Design* (pp. 164–185). Hershey, PA: IGI Global. doi:10.4018/978-1-5225-2098-6.ch008

Kulkarni, S., Savyanavar, A., Kulkarni, P., Stranieri, A., & Ghorpade, V. (2018). Framework for Integration of Medical Image and Text-Based Report Retrieval to Support Radiological Diagnosis. In M. Kolekar & V. Kumar (Eds.), *Biomedical Signal and Image Processing in Patient Care* (pp. 86–122). Hershey, PA: IGI Global. doi:10.4018/978-1-5225-2829-6.ch006

Kumar, A., & Sarkar, B. K. (2018). Performance Analysis of Nature-Inspired Algorithms-Based Bayesian Prediction Models for Medical Data Sets. In U. Singh, A. Tiwari, & R. Singh (Eds.), *Soft-Computing-Based Nonlinear Control Systems Design* (pp. 134–155). Hershey, PA: IGI Global. doi:10.4018/978-1-5225-3531-7.ch007

Kurtz, R. S. (2016). Fortitude: A Study of African Americans in Surgery in New York City. In U. Thomas & J. Drake (Eds.), *Critical Research on Sexism and Racism in STEM Fields* (pp. 153–169). Hershey, PA: IGI Global. doi:10.4018/978-1-5225-0174-9.ch009

Labbadi, W., & Akaichi, J. (2017). Efficient Algorithm for Answering Fuzzy Medical Requests in Pervasive Healthcare Information Systems. *International Journal of Healthcare Information Systems and Informatics, 12*(2), 46–64. doi:10.4018/IJHISI.2017040103

Lagumdzija, A., & Swing, V. K. (2017). Health, Digitalization, and Individual Empowerment. In F. Topor (Ed.), *Handbook of Research on Individualism and Identity in the Globalized Digital Age* (pp. 380–402). Hershey, PA: IGI Global. doi:10.4018/978-1-5225-0522-8.ch017

Lamey, T. W., & Davidson-Shivers, G. V. (2017). Instructional Strategies and Sequencing. In J. Stefaniak (Ed.), *Advancing Medical Education Through Strategic Instructional Design* (pp. 30–52). Hershey, PA: IGI Global. doi:10.4018/978-1-5225-2098-6.ch002

Leon, G. (2017). The Role of Forensic Medicine in Medical Errors. In M. Riga (Ed.), *Impact of Medical Errors and Malpractice on Health Economics, Quality, and Patient Safety* (pp. 144–170). Hershey, PA: IGI Global. doi:10.4018/978-1-5225-2337-6.ch006

Lidia, B., Federica, G., & Maria, V. E. (2016). The Patient-Centered Medicine as the Theoretical Framework for Patient Engagement. In G. Graffigna (Ed.), *Promoting Patient Engagement and Participation for Effective Healthcare Reform* (pp. 25–39). Hershey, PA: IGI Global. doi:10.4018/978-1-4666-9992-2.ch002

Love, L., & McDowelle, D. (2018). Developing a Comprehensive Wellness Program for Medical Students. In C. Smith (Ed.), *Exploring the Pressures of Medical Education From a Mental Health and Wellness Perspective* (pp. 190–208). Hershey, PA: IGI Global. doi:10.4018/978-1-5225-2811-1.ch008

Lovell, K. L. (2017). Development and Evaluation of Neuroscience Computer-Based Modules for Medical Students: Instructional Design Principles and Effectiveness. In J. Stefaniak (Ed.), *Advancing Medical Education Through Strategic Instructional Design* (pp. 262–276). Hershey, PA: IGI Global. doi:10.4018/978-1-5225-2098-6.ch013

Lubin, R., & Hamlin, M. D. (2018). Medical Student Burnout: A Social Cognitive Learning Perspective on Medical Student Mental Health and Wellness. In C. Smith (Ed.), *Exploring the Pressures of Medical Education From a Mental Health and Wellness Perspective* (pp. 92–121). Hershey, PA: IGI Global. doi:10.4018/978-1-5225-2811-1.ch004

Luk, C. Y. (2018). Moving Towards Universal Health Coverage: Challenges for the Present and Future in China. In B. Fong, A. Ng, & P. Yuen (Eds.), *Sustainable Health and Long-Term Care Solutions for an Aging Population* (pp. 19–45). Hershey, PA: IGI Global. doi:10.4018/978-1-5225-2633-9.ch002

Mahat, M., & Pettigrew, A. (2017). The Regulatory Environment of Non-Profit Higher Education and Research Institutions and Its Implications for Managerial Strategy: The Case of Medical Education and Research. In L. West & A. Worthington (Eds.), *Handbook of Research on Emerging Business Models and Managerial Strategies in the Nonprofit Sector* (pp. 336–351). Hershey, PA: IGI Global. doi:10.4018/978-1-5225-2537-0.ch017

Maitra, I. K., & Bandhyopadhyaay, S. K. (2017). Adaptive Edge Detection Method towards Features Extraction from Diverse Medical Imaging Technologies. In S. Bhattacharyya, S. De, I. Pan, & P. Dutta (Eds.), *Intelligent Multidimensional Data Clustering and Analysis* (pp. 159–192). Hershey, PA: IGI Global. doi:10.4018/978-1-5225-1776-4.ch007

Mangu, V. P. (2017). Mobile Health Care: A Technology View. In C. Bhatt & S. Peddoju (Eds.), *Cloud Computing Systems and Applications in Healthcare* (pp. 1–18). Hershey, PA: IGI Global. doi:10.4018/978-1-5225-1002-4.ch001

Manirabona, A., Fourati, L. C., & Boudjit, S. (2017). Investigation on Healthcare Monitoring Systems: Innovative Services and Applications. *International Journal of E-Health and Medical Communications, 8*(1), 1–18. doi:10.4018/IJEHMC.2017010101

Mannai, M. M., & Karâa, W. B. (2016). Biomedical Image Processing Overview. In W. Karâa & N. Dey (Eds.), *Biomedical Image Analysis and Mining Techniques for Improved Health Outcomes* (pp. 1–12). Hershey, PA: IGI Global. doi:10.4018/978-1-4666-8811-7.ch001

Manzoor, A. (2016). RFID in Health Care-Building Smart Hospitals for Quality Healthcare. *International Journal of User-Driven Healthcare*, *6*(2), 21–45. doi:10.4018/IJUDH.2016070102

Marwan, M., Kartit, A., & Ouahmane, H. (2018). A Framework to Secure Medical Image Storage in Cloud Computing Environment. *Journal of Electronic Commerce in Organizations*, *16*(1), 1–16. doi:10.4018/JECO.2018010101

Masoud, M. P., Nejad, M. K., Darebaghi, H., Chavoshi, M., & Farahani, M. (2018). The Decision Support System and Conventional Method of Telephone Triage by Nurses in Emergency Medical Services: A Comparative Investigation. *International Journal of E-Business Research*, *14*(1), 77–88. doi:10.4018/IJEBR.2018010105

McDonald, W. G., Martin, M., & Salzberg, L. D. (2018). From Medical Student to Medical Resident: Graduate Medical Education and Mental Health in the United States. In C. Smith (Ed.), *Exploring the Pressures of Medical Education From a Mental Health and Wellness Perspective* (pp. 145–169). Hershey, PA: IGI Global. doi:10.4018/978-1-5225-2811-1.ch006

Medhekar, A. (2017). The Role of Social Media for Knowledge Dissemination in Medical Tourism: A Case of India. In R. Chugh (Ed.), *Harnessing Social Media as a Knowledge Management Tool* (pp. 25–54). Hershey, PA: IGI Global. doi:10.4018/978-1-5225-0495-5.ch002

Medhekar, A., & Haq, F. (2018). Urbanization and New Jobs Creation in Healthcare Services in India: Challenges and Opportunities. In U. Benna & I. Benna (Eds.), *Urbanization and Its Impact on Socio-Economic Growth in Developing Regions* (pp. 198–218). Hershey, PA: IGI Global. doi:10.4018/978-1-5225-2659-9.ch010

Mehta, G., Dutta, M. K., & Kim, P. S. (2016). An Efficient and Lossless Cryptosystem for Security in Tele-Ophthalmology Applications Using Chaotic Theory. *International Journal of E-Health and Medical Communications*, *7*(4), 28–47. doi:10.4018/IJEHMC.2016100102

Mehta, P. (2017). Framework of Indian Healthcare System and its Challenges: An Insight. In V. Bryan & J. Bird (Eds.), *Healthcare Community Synergism between Patients, Practitioners, and Researchers* (pp. 247–271). Hershey, PA: IGI Global. doi:10.4018/978-1-5225-0640-9.ch011

Metelmann, B., & Metelmann, C. (2016). M-Health in Prehospital Emergency Medicine: Experiences from the EU funded Project LiveCity. In A. Moumtzoglou (Ed.), *M-Health Innovations for Patient-Centered Care* (pp. 197–212). Hershey, PA: IGI Global. doi:10.4018/978-1-4666-9861-1.ch010

Mi, M. (2017). Informal Learning in Medical Education. In J. Stefaniak (Ed.), *Advancing Medical Education Through Strategic Instructional Design* (pp. 225–244). Hershey, PA: IGI Global. doi:10.4018/978-1-5225-2098-6.ch011

Miglioretti, M., Mariani, F., & Vecchio, L. (2016). Could Patient Engagement Promote a Health System Free From Malpractice Litigation Risk? In G. Graffigna (Ed.), *Promoting Patient Engagement and Participation for Effective Healthcare Reform* (pp. 240–264). Hershey, PA: IGI Global. doi:10.4018/978-1-4666-9992-2.ch012

Misra, S. C., & Bisui, S. (2016). Feasibility of Large Scale Implementation of Personalized Medicine in the Current Scenario. *International Journal of E-Health and Medical Communications*, *7*(2), 30–49. doi:10.4018/IJEHMC.2016040103

Misra, S. C., Bisui, S., & Fantazy, K. (2016). Identifying Critical Changes in Adoption of Personalized Medicine (PM) in Healthcare Management. *International Journal of E-Health and Medical Communications*, *7*(3), 1–15. doi:10.4018/IJEHMC.2016070101

Mohammadian, M., Hatzinakos, D., Spachos, P., & Jentzsh, R. (2016). An Intelligent and Secure Framework for Wireless Information Technology in Healthcare for User and Data Classification in Hospitals. In V. Wang (Ed.), *Handbook of Research on Advancing Health Education through Technology* (pp. 452–479). Hershey, PA: IGI Global. doi:10.4018/978-1-4666-9494-1.ch019

Mokeddem, S., & Atmani, B. (2016). Assessment of Clinical Decision Support Systems for Predicting Coronary Heart Disease. *International Journal of Operations Research and Information Systems*, *7*(3), 57–73. doi:10.4018/IJORIS.2016070104

Mokrzycka, A., & Kowalska-Bobko, I. (2016). Public Health Legislation and Patient's Rights: Health2020 Strategy, European Perspective. In A. Rosiek & K. Leksowski (Eds.), *Organizational Culture and Ethics in Modern Medicine* (pp. 298–322). Hershey, PA: IGI Global. doi:10.4018/978-1-4666-9658-7.ch013

Moon, J. D., & Galea, M. P. (2016). Overview of Clinical Decision Support Systems in Healthcare. In J. Moon & M. Galea (Eds.), *Improving Health Management through Clinical Decision Support Systems* (pp. 1–27). Hershey, PA: IGI Global. doi:10.4018/978-1-4666-9432-3.ch001

Mosadeghrad, A. M., & Woldemichael, A. (2017). Application of Quality Management in Promoting Patient Safety and Preventing Medical Errors. In M. Riga (Ed.), *Impact of Medical Errors and Malpractice on Health Economics, Quality, and Patient Safety* (pp. 91–112). Hershey, PA: IGI Global. doi:10.4018/978-1-5225-2337-6.ch004

Moumtzoglou, A. (2017). Digital Medicine: The Quality Standpoint. In A. Moumtzoglou (Ed.), *Design, Development, and Integration of Reliable Electronic Healthcare Platforms* (pp. 179–195). Hershey, PA: IGI Global. doi:10.4018/978-1-5225-1724-5.ch011

Moumtzoglou, A., & Pouliakis, A. (2018). Population Health Management and the Science of Individuality. *International Journal of Reliable and Quality E-Healthcare*, *7*(2), 1–26. doi:10.4018/IJRQEH.2018040101

Mpofu, C. (2016). International Medical Experiences Outbound New Zealand: An Economic and Medical Workforce Strategy. In D. Velliaris & D. Coleman-George (Eds.), *Handbook of Research on Study Abroad Programs and Outbound Mobility* (pp. 446–469). Hershey, PA: IGI Global. doi:10.4018/978-1-5225-0169-5.ch018

Mukhtar, W. F., & Abuelyaman, E. S. (2017). Opportunities and Challenges of Big Data in Healthcare. In N. Wickramasinghe (Ed.), *Handbook of Research on Healthcare Administration and Management* (pp. 47–58). Hershey, PA: IGI Global. doi:10.4018/978-1-5225-0920-2.ch004

Munugala, S., Brar, G. K., Syed, A., Mohammad, A., & Halgamuge, M. N. (2018). The Much Needed Security and Data Reforms of Cloud Computing in Medical Data Storage. In M. Lytras & P. Papadopoulou (Eds.), *Applying Big Data Analytics in Bioinformatics and Medicine* (pp. 99–113). Hershey, PA: IGI Global. doi:10.4018/978-1-5225-2607-0.ch005

Narasimhamurthy, A. (2016). An Overview of Machine Learning in Medical Image Analysis: Trends in Health Informatics. In N. Dey & A. Ashour (Eds.), *Classification and Clustering in Biomedical Signal Processing* (pp. 23–45). Hershey, PA: IGI Global. doi:10.4018/978-1-5225-0140-4.ch002

Ngara, R. (2017). Multiple Voices, Multiple Paths: Towards Dialogue between Western and Indigenous Medical Knowledge Systems. In P. Ngulube (Ed.), *Handbook of Research on Theoretical Perspectives on Indigenous Knowledge Systems in Developing Countries* (pp. 332–358). Hershey, PA: IGI Global. doi:10.4018/978-1-5225-0833-5.ch015

O'Connor, Y., & Heavin, C. (2018). Defining and Characterising the Landscape of eHealth. In M. Khosrow-Pour, D.B.A. (Ed.), Encyclopedia of Information Science and Technology, Fourth Edition (pp. 5864-5875). Hershey, PA: IGI Global. doi:10.4018/978-1-5225-2255-3.ch510

Ochonogor, W. C., & Okite-Amughoro, F. A. (2018). Building an Effective Digital Library in a University Teaching Hospital (UTH) in Nigeria. In A. Tella & T. Kwanya (Eds.), *Handbook of Research on Managing Intellectual Property in Digital Libraries* (pp. 184–204). Hershey, PA: IGI Global. doi:10.4018/978-1-5225-3093-0.ch010

Olaniran, B. A. (2016). ICTs, E-health, and Multidisciplinary Healthcare Teams: Promises and Challenges. *International Journal of Privacy and Health Information Management*, *4*(2), 62–75. doi:10.4018/IJPHIM.2016070105

Olaniran, B. A. (2016). ICT Use and Multidisciplinary Healthcare Teams in the Age of e-Health. *International Journal of Reliable and Quality E-Healthcare*, *5*(1), 18–31. doi:10.4018/IJRQEH.2016010102

Olivares, S. L., Cruz, A. G., Cabrera, M. V., Regalado, A. I., & García, J. E. (2017). An Assessment Study of Quality Model for Medical Schools in Mexico. In S. Mukerji & P. Tripathi (Eds.), *Handbook of Research on Administration, Policy, and Leadership in Higher Education* (pp. 404–439). Hershey, PA: IGI Global. doi:10.4018/978-1-5225-0672-0.ch016

Omidoyin, E. O., Opeke, R. O., & Osagbemi, G. K. (2016). Utilization Pattern and Privacy Issues in the use of Health Records for Research Practice by Doctors: Selected Nigerian Teaching Hospitals as Case Study. *International Journal of Privacy and Health Information Management*, *4*(1), 1–11. doi:10.4018/IJPHIM.2016010101

Omoruyi, E. A., & Omidele, F. (2018). Resident Physician and Medical Academic Faculty Burnout: A Review of Current Literature. In C. Smith (Ed.), *Exploring the Pressures of Medical Education From a Mental Health and Wellness Perspective* (pp. 171–189). Hershey, PA: IGI Global. doi:10.4018/978-1-5225-2811-1.ch007

Osop, H., & Sahama, T. (2016). Data-Driven and Practice-Based Evidence: Design and Development of Efficient and Effective Clinical Decision Support System. In J. Moon & M. Galea (Eds.), *Improving Health Management through Clinical Decision Support Systems* (pp. 295–328). Hershey, PA: IGI Global. doi:10.4018/978-1-4666-9432-3.ch014

Ossowski, R., & Izdebski, P. (2016). Ethical Aspects of Talking to a Patient. In A. Rosiek & K. Leksowski (Eds.), *Organizational Culture and Ethics in Modern Medicine* (pp. 203–235). Hershey, PA: IGI Global. doi:10.4018/978-1-4666-9658-7.ch009

Pandian, P. S. (2016). An Overview of Telemedicine Technologies for Healthcare Applications. *International Journal of Biomedical and Clinical Engineering*, *5*(2), 29–52. doi:10.4018/IJBCE.2016070103

Papadopoulou, P., Lytras, M., & Marouli, C. (2018). Bioinformatics as Applied to Medicine: Challenges Faced Moving from Big Data to Smart Data to Wise Data. In M. Lytras & P. Papadopoulou (Eds.), *Applying Big Data Analytics in Bioinformatics and Medicine* (pp. 1–25). Hershey, PA: IGI Global. doi:10.4018/978-1-5225-2607-0.ch001

Paraskou, A., & George, B. P. (2018). An Overview of Reproductive Tourism. In *Legal and Economic Considerations Surrounding Reproductive Tourism: Emerging Research and Opportunities* (pp. 1–17). Hershey, PA: IGI Global. doi:10.4018/978-1-5225-2694-0.ch001

Park, S., & Moon, J. (2016). Strategic Approach towards Clinical Information Security. In J. Moon & M. Galea (Eds.), *Improving Health Management through Clinical Decision Support Systems* (pp. 329–359). Hershey, PA: IGI Global. doi:10.4018/978-1-4666-9432-3.ch015

Pereira, D., Castro, A., Gomes, P., Areias, J. C., Reis, Z. S., Coimbra, M. T., & Cruz-Correia, R. (2016). Digital Auscultation: Challenges and Perspectives. In M. Cruz-Cunha, I. Miranda, R. Martinho, & R. Rijo (Eds.), *Encyclopedia of E-Health and Telemedicine* (pp. 910–927). Hershey, PA: IGI Global. doi:10.4018/978-1-4666-9978-6.ch070

Peters, R. A., & Cruz, M. (2016). The States as Generators of Incremental Change in American Health Care Policy: 1935 to 1965. In R. Gholipour & K. Rouzbehani (Eds.), *Social, Economic, and Political Perspectives on Public Health Policy-Making* (pp. 86–114). Hershey, PA: IGI Global. doi:10.4018/978-1-4666-9944-1.ch005

Phuritsabam, B., & Devi, A. B. (2017). Information Seeking Behavior of Medical Scientists at Jawaharlal Nehru Institute of Medical Science: A Study. In S. Ram (Ed.), *Library and Information Services for Bioinformatics Education and Research* (pp. 177–187). Hershey, PA: IGI Global. doi:10.4018/978-1-5225-1871-6.ch010

Pieczka, B. (2018). Management of Risk and Adverse Events in Medical Entities. In A. Rosiek-Kryszewska & K. Leksowski (Eds.), *Healthcare Administration for Patient Safety and Engagement* (pp. 31–46). Hershey, PA: IGI Global. doi:10.4018/978-1-5225-3946-9.ch003

Poduval, J. (2016). Curriculum Development. In *Optimizing Medicine Residency Training Programs* (pp. 45–102). Hershey, PA: IGI Global. doi:10.4018/978-1-4666-9527-6.ch003

Poduval, J. (2016). Ethics and Professionalism. In *Optimizing Medicine Residency Training Programs* (pp. 103–133). Hershey, PA: IGI Global. doi:10.4018/978-1-4666-9527-6.ch004

Poduval, J. (2016). Management Skills and Leadership. In *Optimizing Medicine Residency Training Programs* (pp. 182–205). Hershey, PA: IGI Global. doi:10.4018/978-1-4666-9527-6.ch008

Poduval, J. (2016). Medicine Residency Training. In *Optimizing Medicine Residency Training Programs* (pp. 1–27). Hershey, PA: IGI Global. doi:10.4018/978-1-4666-9527-6.ch001

Poduval, J. (2016). Personal Issues. In *Optimizing Medicine Residency Training Programs* (pp. 206–221). Hershey, PA: IGI Global. doi:10.4018/978-1-4666-9527-6.ch009

Poduval, J. (2017). Medical Errors: Impact on Health Care Quality. In M. Riga (Ed.), *Impact of Medical Errors and Malpractice on Health Economics, Quality, and Patient Safety* (pp. 33–60). Hershey, PA: IGI Global. doi:10.4018/978-1-5225-2337-6.ch002

Politis, D., Stagiopoulos, P., Aidona, S., Kyriafinis, G., & Constantinidis, I. (2018). Autonomous Learning and Skill Accreditation: A Paradigm for Medical Studies. In A. Kumar (Ed.), *Optimizing Student Engagement in Online Learning Environments* (pp. 266–296). Hershey, PA: IGI Global. doi:10.4018/978-1-5225-3634-5.ch012

Pomares-Quimbaya, A., Gonzalez, R. A., Quintero, S., Muñoz, O. M., Bohórquez, W. R., García, O. M., & Londoño, D. (2016). A Review of Existing Applications and Techniques for Narrative Text Analysis in Electronic Medical Records. In M. Cruz-Cunha, I. Miranda, R. Martinho, & R. Rijo (Eds.), *Encyclopedia of E-Health and Telemedicine* (pp. 796–811). Hershey, PA: IGI Global. doi:10.4018/978-1-4666-9978-6.ch062

Pomares-Quimbaya, A., González, R. A., Sierra, A., Daza, J. C., Muñoz, O., García, A., ... Bohórquez, W. R. (2017). ICT for Enabling the Quality Evaluation of Health Care Services: A Case Study in a General Hospital. In A. Moumtzoglou (Ed.), *Design, Development, and Integration of Reliable Electronic Healthcare Platforms* (pp. 196–210). Hershey, PA: IGI Global. doi:10.4018/978-1-5225-1724-5.ch012

Pouliakis, A., Margari, N., Karakitsou, E., Archondakis, S., & Karakitsos, P. (2018). Emerging Technologies Serving Cytopathology: Big Data, the Cloud, and Mobile Computing. In I. El Naqa (Ed.), *Emerging Developments and Practices in Oncology* (pp. 114–152). Hershey, PA: IGI Global. doi:10.4018/978-1-5225-3085-5.ch005

Queirós, A., Silva, A. G., Ferreira, A., Caravau, H., Cerqueira, M., & Rocha, N. P. (2016). Assessing Mobile Applications Considered Medical Devices. In M. Cruz-Cunha, I. Miranda, R. Martinho, & R. Rijo (Eds.), *Encyclopedia of E-Health and Telemedicine* (pp. 111–127). Hershey, PA: IGI Global. doi:10.4018/978-1-4666-9978-6.ch010

Raffaeli, L., Spinsante, S., & Gambi, E. (2016). Integrated Smart TV-Based Personal e-Health System. *International Journal of E-Health and Medical Communications*, *7*(1), 48–64. doi:10.4018/IJEHMC.2016010103

Rai, A., Kothari, R., & Singh, D. P. (2017). Assessment of Available Technologies for Hospital Waste Management: A Need for Society. In R. Singh, A. Singh, & V. Srivastava (Eds.), *Environmental Issues Surrounding Human Overpopulation* (pp. 172–188). Hershey, PA: IGI Global. doi:10.4018/978-1-5225-1683-5.ch010

Ramamoorthy, S., & Sivasubramaniam, R. (2018). Image Processing Including Medical Liver Imaging: Medical Image Processing from Big Data Perspective, Ultrasound Liver Images, Challenges. In M. Lytras & P. Papadopoulou (Eds.), *Applying Big Data Analytics in Bioinformatics and Medicine* (pp. 380–392). Hershey, PA: IGI Global. doi:10.4018/978-1-5225-2607-0.ch016

Rathor, G. P., & Gupta, S. K. (2017). Improving Multimodality Image Fusion through Integrate AFL and Wavelet Transform. In V. Tiwari, B. Tiwari, R. Thakur, & S. Gupta (Eds.), *Pattern and Data Analysis in Healthcare Settings* (pp. 143–157). Hershey, PA: IGI Global. doi:10.4018/978-1-5225-0536-5.ch008

Rawat, D. B., & Bhattacharya, S. (2016). Wireless Body Area Network for Healthcare Applications. In N. Meghanathan (Ed.), *Advanced Methods for Complex Network Analysis* (pp. 343–358). Hershey, PA: IGI Global. doi:10.4018/978-1-4666-9964-9.ch014

Rea, P. M. (2016). Advances in Anatomical and Medical Visualisation. In M. Pinheiro & D. Simões (Eds.), *Handbook of Research on Engaging Digital Natives in Higher Education Settings* (pp. 244–264). Hershey, PA: IGI Global. doi:10.4018/978-1-5225-0039-1.ch011

Rexhepi, H., & Persson, A. (2017). Challenges to Implementing IT Support for Evidence Based Practice Among Nurses and Assistant Nurses: A Qualitative Study. *Journal of Electronic Commerce in Organizations, 15*(2), 61–76. doi:10.4018/JECO.2017040105

Reychav, I., & Azuri, J. (2016). Including Elderly Patients in Decision Making via Electronic Health Literacy. In M. Cruz-Cunha, I. Miranda, R. Martinho, & R. Rijo (Eds.), *Encyclopedia of E-Health and Telemedicine* (pp. 241–249). Hershey, PA: IGI Global. doi:10.4018/978-1-4666-9978-6.ch020

Richards, D., & Caldwell, P. H. (2016). Gamification to Improve Adherence to Clinical Treatment Advice: Improving Adherence to Clinical Treatment. In D. Novák, B. Tulu, & H. Brendryen (Eds.), *Handbook of Research on Holistic Perspectives in Gamification for Clinical Practice* (pp. 47–77). Hershey, PA: IGI Global. doi:10.4018/978-1-4666-9522-1.ch004

Rissman, B. (2016). Medical Conditions Associated with NLD. In B. Rissman (Ed.), *Medical and Educational Perspectives on Nonverbal Learning Disability in Children and Young Adults* (pp. 27–66). Hershey, PA: IGI Global. doi:10.4018/978-1-4666-9539-9.ch002

Rosiek, A. (2018). The Assessment of Actions of the Environment and the Impact of Preventive Medicine for Public Health in Poland. In A. Rosiek-Kryszewska & K. Leksowski (Eds.), *Healthcare Administration for Patient Safety and Engagement* (pp. 106–119). Hershey, PA: IGI Global. doi:10.4018/978-1-5225-3946-9.ch006

Rosiek, A., Leksowski, K., Goch, A., Rosiek-Kryszewska, A., & Leksowski, Ł. (2016). Medical Treatment and Difficult Ethical Decisions in Interdisciplinary Hospital Teams. In A. Rosiek & K. Leksowski (Eds.), *Organizational Culture and Ethics in Modern Medicine* (pp. 121–153). Hershey, PA: IGI Global. doi:10.4018/978-1-4666-9658-7.ch006

Rosiek, A., & Rosiek-Kryszewska, A. (2018). Managed Healthcare: Doctor Life Satisfaction and Its Impact on the Process of Communicating With the Patient. In A. Rosiek-Kryszewska & K. Leksowski (Eds.), *Healthcare Administration for Patient Safety and Engagement* (pp. 244–261). Hershey, PA: IGI Global. doi:10.4018/978-1-5225-3946-9.ch013

Rosiek-Kryszewska, A., Leksowski, Ł., Rosiek, A., Leksowski, K., & Goch, A. (2016). Clinical Communication in the Aspect of Development of New Technologies and E-Health in the Doctor-Patient Relationship. In A. Rosiek & K. Leksowski (Eds.), *Organizational Culture and Ethics in Modern Medicine* (pp. 18–51). Hershey, PA: IGI Global. doi:10.4018/978-1-4666-9658-7.ch002

Rosiek-Kryszewska, A., & Rosiek, A. (2018). The Involvement of the Patient and his Perspective Evaluation of the Quality of Healthcare. In A. Rosiek-Kryszewska & K. Leksowski (Eds.), *Healthcare Administration for Patient Safety and Engagement* (pp. 121–144). Hershey, PA: IGI Global. doi:10.4018/978-1-5225-3946-9.ch007

Rosiek-Kryszewska, A., & Rosiek, A. (2018). The Impact of Management and Leadership Roles in Building Competitive Healthcare Units. In A. Rosiek-Kryszewska & K. Leksowski (Eds.), *Healthcare Administration for Patient Safety and Engagement* (pp. 13–30). Hershey, PA: IGI Global. doi:10.4018/978-1-5225-3946-9.ch002

Roşu, S. M., Păvăloiu, I. B., Dragoi, G., Apostol, C. G., & Munteanu, D. (2016). Telemedicine Based on LMDS in the Urban/Metropolitan Area: A Romanian Case Study. In M. Cruz-Cunha, I. Miranda, R. Martinho, & R. Rijo (Eds.), *Encyclopedia of E-Health and Telemedicine* (pp. 96–109). Hershey, PA: IGI Global. doi:10.4018/978-1-4666-9978-6.ch009

Rouzbehani, K. (2017). Health Policy Implementation: Moving Beyond Its Barriers in United States. In N. Wickramasinghe (Ed.), *Handbook of Research on Healthcare Administration and Management* (pp. 541–552). Hershey, PA: IGI Global. doi:10.4018/978-1-5225-0920-2.ch032

Ruiz, I. M., Cohen, D. S., & Marco, Á. M. (2016). ISO/IEEE11073 Family of Standards: Trends and Applications on E-Health Monitoring. In M. Cruz-Cunha, I. Miranda, R. Martinho, & R. Rijo (Eds.), *Encyclopedia of E-Health and Telemedicine* (pp. 646–660). Hershey, PA: IGI Global. doi:10.4018/978-1-4666-9978-6.ch050

Sam, S. (2017). Mobile Phones and Expanding Human Capabilities in Plural Health Systems. In K. Moahi, K. Bwalya, & P. Sebina (Eds.), *Health Information Systems and the Advancement of Medical Practice in Developing Countries* (pp. 93–114). Hershey, PA: IGI Global. doi:10.4018/978-1-5225-2262-1.ch006

Sankaranarayanan, S., & Ganesan, S. (2016). Applications of Intelligent Agents in Health Sector-A Review. *International Journal of E-Health and Medical Communications*, *7*(1), 1–30. doi:10.4018/IJEHMC.2016010101

Santos-Trigo, M., Suaste, E., & Figuerola, P. (2018). Technology Design and Routes for Tool Appropriation in Medical Practices. In M. Khosrow-Pour, D.B.A. (Ed.), Encyclopedia of Information Science and Technology, Fourth Edition (pp. 3794-3804). Hershey, PA: IGI Global. doi:10.4018/978-1-5225-2255-3.ch329

Sarivougioukas, J., Vagelatos, A., Parsopoulos, K. E., & Lagaris, I. E. (2018). Home UbiHealth. In M. Khosrow-Pour, D.B.A. (Ed.), Encyclopedia of Information Science and Technology, Fourth Edition (pp. 7765-7774). Hershey, PA: IGI Global. doi:10.4018/978-1-5225-2255-3.ch675

Sarkar, B. K. (2017). Big Data and Healthcare Data: A Survey. *International Journal of Knowledge-Based Organizations*, *7*(4), 50–77. doi:10.4018/IJKBO.2017100104

Saxena, K., & Banodha, U. (2017). An Essence of the SOA on Healthcare. In R. Bhadoria, N. Chaudhari, G. Tomar, & S. Singh (Eds.), *Exploring Enterprise Service Bus in the Service-Oriented Architecture Paradigm* (pp. 283–304). Hershey, PA: IGI Global. doi:10.4018/978-1-5225-2157-0.ch018

Schmeida, M., & McNeal, R. (2016). Consulting Online Healthcare Information: E-Caregivers as Knowledgeable Decision Makers. *International Journal of Computers in Clinical Practice*, *1*(1), 42–52. doi:10.4018/IJCCP.2016010104

Sen, K., & Ghosh, K. (2018). Incorporating Global Medical Knowledge to Solve Healthcare Problems: A Framework for a Crowdsourcing System. *International Journal of Healthcare Information Systems and Informatics*, *13*(1), 1–14. doi:10.4018/IJHISI.2018010101

Shakdher, A., & Pandey, K. (2017). REDAlert+: Medical/Fire Emergency and Warning System using Android Devices. *International Journal of E-Health and Medical Communications*, *8*(1), 37–51. doi:10.4018/IJEHMC.2017010103

Shekarian, E., Abdul-Rashid, S. H., & Olugu, E. U. (2017). An Integrated Fuzzy VIKOR Method for Performance Management in Healthcare. In M. Tavana, K. Szabat, & K. Puranam (Eds.), *Organizational Productivity and Performance Measurements Using Predictive Modeling and Analytics* (pp. 40–61). Hershey, PA: IGI Global. doi:10.4018/978-1-5225-0654-6.ch003

Shi, J., Erdem, E., & Liu, H. (2016). Expanding Role of Telephone Systems in Healthcare: Developments and Opportunities. In A. Dwivedi (Ed.), *Reshaping Medical Practice and Care with Health Information Systems* (pp. 87–131). Hershey, PA: IGI Global. doi:10.4018/978-1-4666-9870-3.ch004

Shijina, V., & John, S. J. (2017). Multiple Relations and its Application in Medical Diagnosis. *International Journal of Fuzzy System Applications*, *6*(4), 47–62. doi:10.4018/IJFSA.2017100104

Shipley, N., & Chakraborty, J. (2018). Big Data and mHealth: Increasing the Usability of Healthcare Through the Customization of Pinterest – Literary Perspective. In J. Machado, A. Abelha, M. Santos, & F. Portela (Eds.), *Next-Generation Mobile and Pervasive Healthcare Solutions* (pp. 46–66). Hershey, PA: IGI Global. doi:10.4018/978-1-5225-2851-7.ch004

Singh, A., & Dutta, M. K. (2017). A Reversible Data Hiding Scheme for Efficient Management of Tele-Ophthalmological Data. *International Journal of E-Health and Medical Communications*, *8*(3), 38–54. doi:10.4018/IJEHMC.2017070103

Sivaji, A., Radjo, H. K., Amin, M., & Abu Hashim, M. A. (2016). Design of a Hospital Interactive Wayfinding System: Designing for Malaysian Users. In N. Mohamed, T. Mantoro, M. Ayu, & M. Mahmud (Eds.), *Critical Socio-Technical Issues Surrounding Mobile Computing* (pp. 88–123). Hershey, PA: IGI Global. doi:10.4018/978-1-4666-9438-5.ch005

Skourti, P. K., & Pavlakis, A. (2017). The Second Victim Phenomenon: The Way Out. In M. Riga (Ed.), *Impact of Medical Errors and Malpractice on Health Economics, Quality, and Patient Safety* (pp. 197–222). Hershey, PA: IGI Global. doi:10.4018/978-1-5225-2337-6.ch008

Smith, C. R. (2018). Medical Students' Quest Towards the Long White Coat: Impact on Mental Health and Well-Being. In C. Smith (Ed.), *Exploring the Pressures of Medical Education From a Mental Health and Wellness Perspective* (pp. 1–42). Hershey, PA: IGI Global. doi:10.4018/978-1-5225-2811-1.ch001

Smith, S. I., & Dandignac, M. (2018). Perfectionism: Addressing Lofty Expectations in Medical School. In C. Smith (Ed.), *Exploring the Pressures of Medical Education From a Mental Health and Wellness Perspective* (pp. 68–91). Hershey, PA: IGI Global. doi:10.4018/978-1-5225-2811-1.ch003

Sobrinho, Á. A., Dias da Silva, L., Perkusich, A., Cunha, P., Pinheiro, M. E., & Melo de Medeiros, L. (2016). Towards Medical Systems to Aid the Detection and Treatment of Chronic Diseases. In D. Fotiadis (Ed.), *Handbook of Research on Trends in the Diagnosis and Treatment of Chronic Conditions* (pp. 50–69). Hershey, PA: IGI Global. doi:10.4018/978-1-4666-8828-5.ch003

Soczywko, J., & Rutkowska, D. (2018). The Patient/Provider Relationship in Emergency Medicine: Organization, Communication, and Understanding. In A. Rosiek-Kryszewska & K. Leksowski (Eds.), *Healthcare Administration for Patient Safety and Engagement* (pp. 74–105). Hershey, PA: IGI Global. doi:10.4018/978-1-5225-3946-9.ch005

Sołtysik-Piorunkiewicz, A., Furmankiewicz, M., & Ziuziański, P. (2016). Web Healthcare Applications in Poland: Trends, Standards, Barriers and Possibilities of Implementation and Usage of E-Health Systems. In I. Deliyannis, P. Kostagiolas, & C. Banou (Eds.), *Experimental Multimedia Systems for Interactivity and Strategic Innovation* (pp. 258–283). Hershey, PA: IGI Global. doi:10.4018/978-1-4666-8659-5.ch013

Soni, P. (2018). Implications of HIPAA and Subsequent Regulations on Information Technology. In M. Gupta, R. Sharman, J. Walp, & P. Mulgund (Eds.), *Information Technology Risk Management and Compliance in Modern Organizations* (pp. 71–98). Hershey, PA: IGI Global. doi:10.4018/978-1-5225-2604-9.ch004

Spinelli, R., & Benevolo, C. (2016). From Healthcare Services to E-Health Applications: A Delivery System-Based Taxonomy. In A. Dwivedi (Ed.), *Reshaping Medical Practice and Care with Health Information Systems* (pp. 205–245). Hershey, PA: IGI Global. doi:10.4018/978-1-4666-9870-3.ch007

Srivastava, A., & Aggarwal, A. K. (2018). Medical Image Fusion in Spatial and Transform Domain: A Comparative Analysis. In M. Anwar, A. Khosla, & R. Kapoor (Eds.), *Handbook of Research on Advanced Concepts in Real-Time Image and Video Processing* (pp. 281–300). Hershey, PA: IGI Global. doi:10.4018/978-1-5225-2848-7.ch011

Srivastava, S. K., & Roy, S. N. (2018). Recommendation System: A Potential Tool for Achieving Pervasive Health Care. In J. Machado, A. Abelha, M. Santos, & F. Portela (Eds.), *Next-Generation Mobile and Pervasive Healthcare Solutions* (pp. 111–127). Hershey, PA: IGI Global. doi:10.4018/978-1-5225-2851-7.ch008

Stancu, A. (2016). Correlations and Patterns of Food and Health Consumer Expenditure. In A. Jean-Vasile (Ed.), *Food Science, Production, and Engineering in Contemporary Economies* (pp. 44–101). Hershey, PA: IGI Global. doi:10.4018/978-1-5225-0341-5.ch003

Stanimirovic, D. (2017). Digitalization of Death Certification Model: Transformation Issues and Implementation Concerns. In S. Saeed, Y. Bamarouf, T. Ramayah, & S. Iqbal (Eds.), *Design Solutions for User-Centric Information Systems* (pp. 22–43). Hershey, PA: IGI Global. doi:10.4018/978-1-5225-1944-7.ch002

Stavros, A., Vavoulidis, E., & Nasioutziki, M. (2016). The Use of Mobile Health Applications for Quality Control and Accreditational Purposes in a Cytopathology Laboratory. In A. Moumtzoglou (Ed.), *M-Health Innovations for Patient-Centered Care* (pp. 262–283). Hershey, PA: IGI Global. doi:10.4018/978-1-4666-9861-1.ch013

Sukkird, V., & Shirahada, K. (2018). E-Health Service Model for Asian Developing Countries: A Case of Emergency Medical Service for Elderly People in Thailand. In M. Khosrow-Pour (Ed.), *Optimizing Current Practices in E-Services and Mobile Applications* (pp. 214–232). Hershey, PA: IGI Global. doi:10.4018/978-1-5225-5026-6.ch011

Sygit, B., & Wąsik, D. (2016). Patients' Rights and Medical Personnel Duties in the Field of Hospital Care. In A. Rosiek & K. Leksowski (Eds.), *Organizational Culture and Ethics in Modern Medicine* (pp. 282–297). Hershey, PA: IGI Global. doi:10.4018/978-1-4666-9658-7.ch012

Sygit, B., & Wąsik, D. (2016). The Idea of Human Rights in Conditions of Hospital Treatment. In A. Rosiek & K. Leksowski (Eds.), *Organizational Culture and Ethics in Modern Medicine* (pp. 236–254). Hershey, PA: IGI Global. doi:10.4018/978-1-4666-9658-7.ch010

Talbot, T. B. (2017). Making Lifelike Medical Games in the Age of Virtual Reality: An Update on "Playing Games with Biology" from 2013. In B. Dubbels (Ed.), *Transforming Gaming and Computer Simulation Technologies across Industries* (pp. 103–119). Hershey, PA: IGI Global. doi:10.4018/978-1-5225-1817-4.ch006

Tamposis, I., Pouliakis, A., Fezoulidis, I., & Karakitsos, P. (2016). Mobile Platforms Supporting Health Professionals: Need, Technical Requirements, and Applications. In A. Moumtzoglou (Ed.), *M-Health Innovations for Patient-Centered Care* (pp. 91–114). Hershey, PA: IGI Global. doi:10.4018/978-1-4666-9861-1.ch005

Tiago, M. T., Tiago, F., Amaral, F. E., & Silva, S. (2016). Healthy 3.0: Healthcare Digital Dimensions. In A. Dwivedi (Ed.), *Reshaping Medical Practice and Care with Health Information Systems* (pp. 287–322). Hershey, PA: IGI Global. doi:10.4018/978-1-4666-9870-3.ch010

Tripathy, B. (2016). Application of Rough Set Based Models in Medical Diagnosis. In S. Dash & B. Subudhi (Eds.), *Handbook of Research on Computational Intelligence Applications in Bioinformatics* (pp. 144–168). Hershey, PA: IGI Global. doi:10.4018/978-1-5225-0427-6.ch008

Turcu, C. E., & Turcu, C. O. (2017). Social Internet of Things in Healthcare: From Things to Social Things in Internet of Things. In C. Reis & M. Maximiano (Eds.), *Internet of Things and Advanced Application in Healthcare* (pp. 266–295). Hershey, PA: IGI Global. doi:10.4018/978-1-5225-1820-4.ch010

Unwin, D. W., Sanzogni, L., & Sandhu, K. (2017). Developing and Measuring the Business Case for Health Information Technology. In K. Moahi, K. Bwalya, & P. Sebina (Eds.), *Health Information Systems and the Advancement of Medical Practice in Developing Countries* (pp. 262–290). Hershey, PA: IGI Global. doi:10.4018/978-1-5225-2262-1.ch015

Urooj, S., & Singh, S. P. (2016). Wavelet Transform-Based Soft Computational Techniques and Applications in Medical Imaging. In P. Saxena, D. Singh, & M. Pant (Eds.), *Problem Solving and Uncertainty Modeling through Optimization and Soft Computing Applications* (pp. 339–363). Hershey, PA: IGI Global. doi:10.4018/978-1-4666-9885-7.ch016

Vasant, P. (2018). A General Medical Diagnosis System Formed by Artificial Neural Networks and Swarm Intelligence Techniques. In U. Kose, G. Guraksin, & O. Deperlioglu (Eds.), *Nature-Inspired Intelligent Techniques for Solving Biomedical Engineering Problems* (pp. 130–145). Hershey, PA: IGI Global. doi:10.4018/978-1-5225-4769-3.ch006

Waegemann, C. P. (2016). mHealth: History, Analysis, and Implementation. In A. Moumtzoglou (Ed.), M-Health Innovations for Patient-Centered Care (pp. 1-19). Hershey, PA: IGI Global. doi:10.4018/978-1-4666-9861-1.ch001

Watfa, M. K., Majeed, H., & Salahuddin, T. (2016). Computer Based E-Healthcare Clinical Systems: A Comprehensive Survey. *International Journal of Privacy and Health Information Management*, *4*(1), 50–69. doi:10.4018/IJPHIM.2016010104

Wietholter, J. P., Coetzee, R., Nardella, B., Kincaid, S. E., & Slain, D. (2016). International Healthcare Experiences: Caring While Learning and Learning While Caring. In D. Velliaris & D. Coleman-George (Eds.), *Handbook of Research on Study Abroad Programs and Outbound Mobility* (pp. 470–496). Hershey, PA: IGI Global. doi:10.4018/978-1-5225-0169-5.ch019

Witzke, K., & Specht, O. (2017). M-Health Telemedicine and Telepresence in Oral and Maxillofacial Surgery: An Innovative Prehospital Healthcare Concept in Structurally Weak Areas. *International Journal of Reliable and Quality E-Healthcare*, *6*(4), 37–48. doi:10.4018/IJRQEH.2017100105

Wójcik, A., & Chojnacki, M. (2016). Behavior and Ethical Problems in the Functioning of the Operating Theater (Case Study). In A. Rosiek & K. Leksowski (Eds.), *Organizational Culture and Ethics in Modern Medicine* (pp. 154–179). Hershey, PA: IGI Global. doi:10.4018/978-1-4666-9658-7.ch007

Wolk, K., & Marasek, K. P. (2016). Translation of Medical Texts using Neural Networks. *International Journal of Reliable and Quality E-Healthcare*, *5*(4), 51–66. doi:10.4018/IJRQEH.2016100104

Wong, A. K., & Lo, M. F. (2018). Using Pervasive Computing for Sustainable Healthcare in an Aging Population. In B. Fong, A. Ng, & P. Yuen (Eds.), *Sustainable Health and Long-Term Care Solutions for an Aging Population* (pp. 187–202). Hershey, PA: IGI Global. doi:10.4018/978-1-5225-2633-9.ch010

Wu, W., Martin, B. C., & Ni, C. (2017). A Systematic Review of Competency-Based Education Effort in the Health Professions: Seeking Order Out of Chaos. In K. Rasmussen, P. Northrup, & R. Colson (Eds.), *Handbook of Research on Competency-Based Education in University Settings* (pp. 352–378). Hershey, PA: IGI Global. doi:10.4018/978-1-5225-0932-5.ch018

Yadav, N., Aliasgari, M., & Poellabauer, C. (2016). Mobile Healthcare in an Increasingly Connected Developing World. *International Journal of Privacy and Health Information Management*, *4*(2), 76–97. doi:10.4018/IJPHIM.2016070106

Yadav, S., Ekbal, A., Saha, S., Pathak, P. S., & Bhattacharyya, P. (2017). Patient Data De-Identification: A Conditional Random-Field-Based Supervised Approach. In S. Saha, A. Mandal, A. Narasimhamurthy, S. V, & S. Sangam (Eds.), Handbook of Research on Applied Cybernetics and Systems Science (pp. 234-253). Hershey, PA: IGI Global. doi:10.4018/978-1-5225-2498-4.ch011

Yu, B., Wijesekera, D., & Costa, P. C. (2017). Informed Consent in Healthcare: A Study Case of Genetic Services. In A. Moumtzoglou (Ed.), *Design, Development, and Integration of Reliable Electronic Healthcare Platforms* (pp. 211–242). Hershey, PA: IGI Global. doi:10.4018/978-1-5225-1724-5.ch013

Yu, B., Wijesekera, D., & Costa, P. C. (2017). Informed Consent in Electronic Medical Record Systems. In I. Management Association (Ed.), Healthcare Ethics and Training: Concepts, Methodologies, Tools, and Applications (pp. 1029-1049). Hershey, PA: IGI Global. doi:10.4018/978-1-5225-2237-9.ch049

Yu, M., Li, J., & Wang, W. (2017). Creative Life Experience among Students in Medical Education. In C. Zhou (Ed.), *Handbook of Research on Creative Problem-Solving Skill Development in Higher Education* (pp. 158–184). Hershey, PA: IGI Global. doi:10.4018/978-1-5225-0643-0.ch008

Zarour, K. (2017). Towards a Telehomecare in Algeria: Case of Diabetes Measurement and Remote Monitoring. *International Journal of E-Health and Medical Communications*, *8*(4), 61–80. doi:10.4018/IJEHMC.2017100104

Zavyalova, Y. V., Korzun, D. G., Meigal, A. Y., & Borodin, A. V. (2017). Towards the Development of Smart Spaces-Based Socio-Cyber-Medicine Systems. *International Journal of Embedded and Real-Time Communication Systems*, *8*(1), 45–63. doi:10.4018/IJERTCS.2017010104

Zeinali, A. A. (2018). Word Formation Study in Developing Naming Guidelines in the Translation of English Medical Terms Into Persian. In M. Khosrow-Pour, D.B.A. (Ed.), Encyclopedia of Information Science and Technology, Fourth Edition (pp. 5136-5147). Hershey, PA: IGI Global. doi:10.4018/978-1-5225-2255-3.ch446

Ziminski, T. B., Demurjian, S. A., Sanzi, E., & Agresta, T. (2016). Toward Integrating Healthcare Data and Systems: A Study of Architectural Alternatives. In T. Iyamu & A. Tatnall (Eds.), *Maximizing Healthcare Delivery and Management through Technology Integration* (pp. 270–304). Hershey, PA: IGI Global. doi:10.4018/978-1-4666-9446-0.ch016

Ziminski, T. B., Demurjian, S. A., Sanzi, E., Baihan, M., & Agresta, T. (2016). An Architectural Solution for Health Information Exchange. *International Journal of User-Driven Healthcare*, *6*(1), 65–103. doi:10.4018/IJUDH.2016010104

Zineldin, M., & Vasicheva, V. (2018). Reducing Medical Errors and Increasing Patient Safety: TRM and 5 Q's Approaches for Better Quality of Life. In *Technological Tools for Value-Based Sustainable Relationships in Health: Emerging Research and Opportunities* (pp. 87–115). Hershey, PA: IGI Global. doi:10.4018/978-1-5225-4091-5.ch005

About the Author

Jennifer Lynne Bird is the Director of the Writing and Reading Center (WRC) and teaches literature and writing classes at Oxbridge Academy in West Palm Beach, Florida. She previously taught current and future teachers at Florida Atlantic University. She received her Bachelor of Science in Education in Secondary English Education, Master of Education in Secondary English Education, and Doctor of Philosophy degrees from Miami University in Oxford, Ohio and her health coach certification from Duke University Integrative Medicine in Durham, North Carolina. She is a National Board Certified Health and Wellness Coach. Her research in writing and healing led to the publication of her book Innovative Collaborative Practice and Reflection in Patient Education (2015).

Index

S

U

W

CPSIA information can be obtained
at www.ICGtesting.com
Printed in the USA
BVHW012125100921
616055BV00045B/27

9 781799 89051